The Psychotherapists' Guide To Managed Care in the 21st Century

The Psychotherapists' Guide to Managed Care in the 21st Century

Surviving Big Brother and Providing Quality Mental Health Services

Sondra Tuckfelt, Ph.D.,
Jeri Fink, D.S.W., and
Muriel Prince Warren, D.S.W.

JASON ARONSON INC.
Northvale, New Jersey
London

Director of Editorial Production: Robert D. Hack

This book was set in 11 pt. Bodoni by Alpha Graphics of Pittsfield, NH and printed and bound by Book-mart Press, Inc. of North Bergen, NJ.

10 9 8 7 6 5 4 3 2 1

Library of Congress Cataloging-in-Publication Data

Tuckfelt, Sondra.
The psychotherapists' guide to managed care in the 21st century : surviving big brother and providing quality mental health services / Sondra Tuckfelt, Jeri Fink & Muriel Prince Warren.
p. cm.
Includes bibliographical references and index.
ISBN 0-7657-0002-6 (alk. paper)
1. Managed mental health care–United States. I. Fink, Jeri. II. Warren, Muriel. III. Title.
RA790.6.T83 1997
362.2'0973–DC21 96-40915

Printed in the United States of America on acid-free paper. For information and catalog write to Jason Aronson Inc., 230 Livingston Street, Northvale, New Jersey 07647-1731. Or visit our website: http://www.aronson.com

From the age of uniformity, from the age of solitude, from the age of Big Brother, from the age of doublethink–greetings!

–George Orwell, *1984*

CONTENTS

ACKNOWLEDGMENTS

We could not have written this book without the vision, trust, and encouragement of our publisher, Michael B. Moskowitz.

We thank Jason Aronson, for lifting our spirits from the inception through the completion of this book. We also thank Bob Hack, Director of Editorial Production, who responded to our problems with intelligence, patience, and guidance; and Norma Pomerantz, Director of Author Relations, who shared with us the benefits of her expertise and hopefulness.

We would also like to add individual acknowledgments. Sondra Tuckfelt thanks Shelley Malin for her tireless administrative skills and good cheer. Mark Tuckfelt provided ideas, labor, and focus, and gave the loving support that made progress with this work possible. The parts of this book written by Sondra with Mark's help are dedicated to their families, friends and children, who never lost faith.

Jeri Fink lovingly thanks her husband, Richard, and sons, David and Russell, for their support, encouragement and inimitable sense of humor for Big Brother. A special thanks goes to all the social workers in the virtual community at the NFSCSW website who shared their time, insights, experiences, and e-mail.

Muriel Warren is extremely grateful to her husband Howard Matus for his editorial acumen, sensibility, supersonic typing, and wry way of being in the world. She also thanks her children and children's children for their loving support and their ability to cope with sibling rivalry toward "Big Brother."

To Health!

ABOUT THE AUTHORS

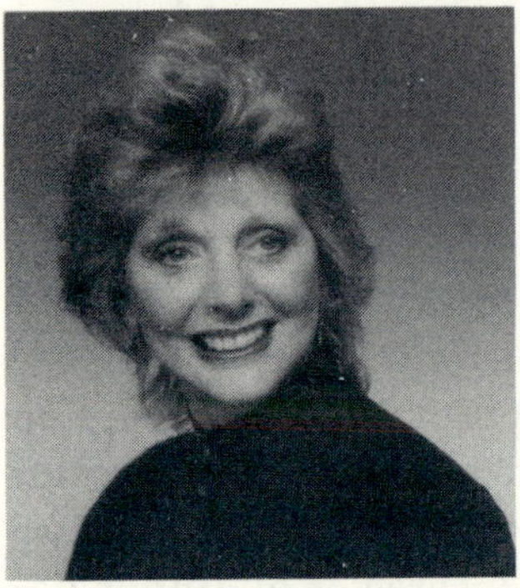

Sondra Tuckfelt is a clinical psychologist engaged in the private practice of psychotherapy with adults and adolescents in Warwick, New York. She has worked with child, family, and prison populations and has consulted to the Orange County, New York, Departments of Health and Social Services in addition to teaching in the New York City Public School and City College systems. Dr. Tuckfelt holds degrees in English and Education from Columbia University, a Ph.D. in Clinical Psychology from Long Island University, and a certificate in psychoanalysis from The Psychoanalytic Center for Communicative Education.

Jeri Fink, D.S.W., is a psychotherapist, author, and adjunct professor of sociology. As a clinician, she treats individuals, couples, families, and groups in private practice in Merrick, New York. Also a specialist in online mental health, Dr. Fink's work has appeared in over 60 publications. She has designed one of the first Internet courses for professionals on human behavior in cyberspace and is the author of *Psychotechnology: The Online Couch* (in press). Dr. Fink can be reached at her website, http://www.psychotechnology.com.

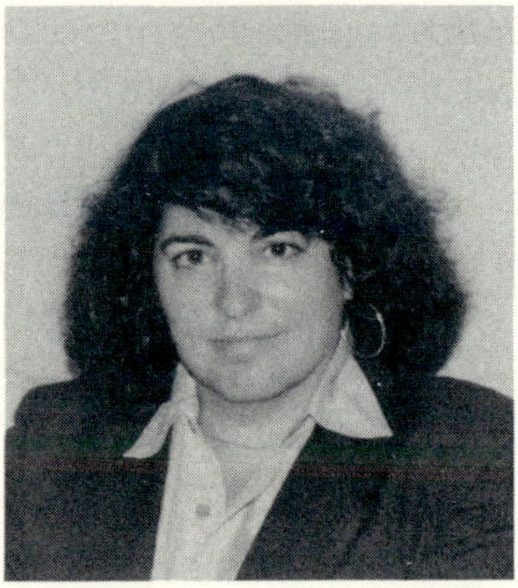

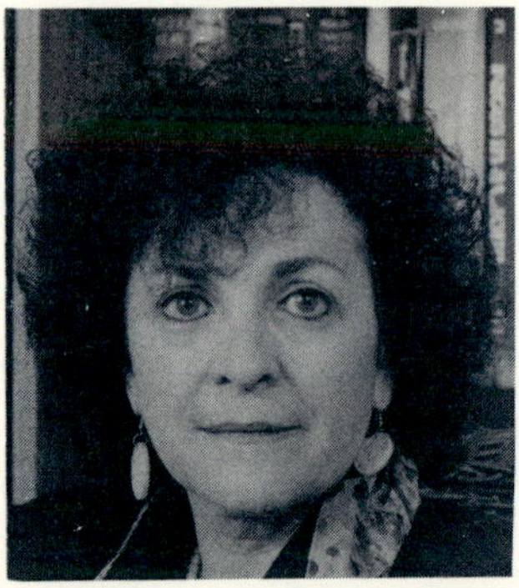

Muriel Warren, D.S.W., executive director of The Psychoanalytic Center for Communicative Education, is a psychoanalyst, writer, and educator. Past president of the International Society for Psychoanalysis, from which she has won three awards, Dr. Warren maintains private practices in Manhattan and Rockland County, New York. She is the author of *Sons: A Mother's Manual* as well as numerous articles on empathy and narcissistic personality disorders.

PROLOGUE

Psychotherapy is changing. It was once a profession practiced by highly trained, caring individuals. It is becoming an industry operated by business administrators.

This book describes the changes brought by managed mental health care and tells how to adapt to them, whether by choosing to work within managed care, outside of managed care, or in a combination of the two. It addresses the essential issue faced by psychotherapists today: how to maintain professional integrity while protecting income in the world of managed care.

This book is not an indictment of the managed health care system. Managed care will continue to evolve under the pressures of national and state legislation, of litigation, and of concerns about responsibility, confidentiality, and accountability. Many of the problems that clinicians face relate to the business approach to psychotherapy practiced by managed care organizations (MCOs). The delivery of mental health services is being orchestrated by people who specialize in business management, economics, and administration. Their goal is to make money by reducing costs while offering the most commercially attractive product possible. Financial, legal, technological, and governmental mechanisms, all relatively invisible to practitioner and patient, affect the ways in which MCOs choose to implement cost control and quality assurance. This business approach to health care may be a shock to professionals whose goal has been to earn a living by healing people in an ethical and responsible manner. Many psychotherapists have experienced difficulty making the ideological leap to a business perspective. Conversely, many managed care administrators have difficulty understanding the ideology of traditionally autonomous, professional clinicians in private practices.

Knowing that the differences in perspective between managed care administrators and psychotherapists were causing problems for both sides, we began to write a guide for helping psychotherapists work with MCOs. Two of us who planned this project have been working with MCOs for several years and were able to work out professional and ethical problems at a time when the MCOs were eager to have us. The third person brought more recent experiences with evaluating and attempting to join various managed care systems.

As we developed our lists of suggestions, directions, cautions, and resources, we found that MCOs were growing and changing at a rate that made it very difficult to document their policies before the organizations or its policies changed again. MCOs changed internal structures and procedures as they grew, and they changed in response to external occurrences such as acquisitions and mergers as well.

In order to try to keep our suggestions relevant in a changing managed care environment, we examined the principles on which managed care is based. We found that frequently the principles of managed care systems are in conflict with the traditional principles of mental health professionals. We also found that many professionals, although not all, wanted to find ways to resolve the conflicts between their values and goals and those of the MCOs.

As psychotherapists, our professional experience leads us to explore options and generate choices when we are faced with obstacles to the further development of our relationships. We therefore could not resist the need to look for solutions to the conflicts uncovered by the advent of managed care. Ultimately, we looked at a range of solutions from modest, short-range modifications in private practices to ambitious plans to restructure the mental health care delivery system in this country.

Thus, we now present a book that roughly follows the parts of a psychotherapy session. Part I provides information about problems with managed care that is intended to help psychotherapists make choices consistent with their own needs and commitments. Part II contains suggestions for participating in managed care systems. This part is the distillation of our original guide, intended for psychotherapists who decide that they want to become providers for MCOs, or for psychotherapists who just are curious about the steps involved in participation. The suggestions are based on our own experiences, on interviews with managed care representatives, and on reading many of the books and seminar papers that are already on the office shelves of our colleagues. What makes our advice somewhat different is that we are extremely cautious at this point and try to point out, specifically, the places where we believe caution is necessary. Part III is a collection of ideas for practical actions and possible solutions to extend the choices proposed in Part I and the suggestions in Part II. Our original purpose was the description of solutions that could be used to work with managed care, or to work outside of managed care, or in a combination of professional practice choices.

The intent of the authors is to present the conflicts between MCOs and psychotherapists in as fair and useful a manner as possible. For this book we interviewed managed care providers, independent professionals, administrators, investment analysts, attorneys, technological experts, political activists, people in business, people in government, and patients throughout the country. We changed the names of all patients, as well as the names of psychotherapists whose patients otherwise might be identified. We included resources we thought might be useful or interesting, as well as ones that we had actually used in our practices. Because we could not adequately research all included materials, we cannot endorse specific resources, individuals, organizations, or schools.

I

Meet Big Brother

1

Where Did It All Come From?

This is business, not ethics.
–Robert Daly, Ph.D., former ethicist at Beth Israel Medical Center, referring to managed health care.

In the late 1960s, President Nixon needed a health care plan to offer to the American public as an alternative to plans proposed by his opponents. Paul Ellwood, Jr., a practicing pediatric neurologist and a member of the think tank of the American Rehabilitation Institute, proposed a system of care that would provide incentives to promote health rather than treat illness. Ellwood coined the term "health maintenance organization" (HMO) and provided Nixon with a plan that had competing HMOs at its center. Ellwood's plan became the basis for the Health Maintenance Organization Act, signed by Nixon in 1973–a bill that promoted HMOs, but under conditions so restrictive that only a few organizations became successful.

In the early 1990s, President Clinton needed a health care plan to offer the American public as an alternative to the increasingly expensive plans current at the time. Paul Ellwood, Jr., now chief executive of the think tank *Interstudy* in Minnesota and the Jackson Hole group in Wyoming, again proposed a system of care that would provide incentives to promote health rather than treat illness. Ellwood's group proposed the term "managed competition" and provided Clinton with a plan that had competing managed care organizations (MCOs) at its center. The system proposed by Ellwood and his colleagues became the basis for the Clinton administration's health care proposals.

During the two years that Congress debated the Clinton plan before rejecting the proposals for change, pre-existing private industries took over the health care systems. These large and powerful companies argued against the Clinton plan claiming that it would cause rationing of health care, overwhelming paperwork, and limitations of choices among health care professionals. By the time Congress rejected the proposals for change, large profit seeking industries had established MCOs that practiced the cost cutting methods they said they opposed—only now they were able to establish themselves while there were gaps in the regulation of health care policy and financing. At present, the legislative system is producing laws to curtail the most egregious practices of MCOs, such as refusing to accept responsibility for the consequences of their decisions and prohibiting providers from discussing managed care limitations with their patients.

With modifications of the current system underway, what is the best plan for professionals in the mental health field? Many professionals believe that working from within the managed care industry provides the best chance to contribute to changes beneficial to mental health services. Others argue for the establishment of a completely different system, such as national health care. As expected in a field of people with diverse orientations, psychotherapists vary not only in their choices but also in the reasons for their choices.

Many psychotherapists have chosen to work with managed care organizations because they believe that the current managed care health care system offers a preferable alternative to the mental health delivery system of the past. Thomas D. Kalous (1996), for example, a Colorado psychologist, urges fellow members of the American Psychological Association (APA) to participate in the development of affordable mental health care. Kalous states that contrary to prevalent beliefs about managed care, many MCOs ". . . are interested in quality. But, they define quality as the most effective treatment provided in the most cost-efficient way. As scientists, psychologists can help managed-care companies sort out what works best for whom in the most cost-conscious manner" (p. 3).

Ronald Fox (1994), past president of the APA, takes a position that is more cautious about the interests of MCOs as they currently function. Fox apparently appreciates at least some of the cost containment principles advanced by the managed care industry. Fox himself is integrating managed care techniques and direct employer services into his own Chapel Hill, North Carolina, practice. According to an article in *Psychotherapy Finances* (1994), Fox said that he would use a managed care system but not under the MCO-promoted premise that extensive utilization review is cost effective, a model that Fox says has made managed care firms wealthy while hurting providers.

Fox's point about the wealth of the managed care industry is important because the major argument in support of MCOs is that the managed care industry saves money. The argument that MCOs are demonstrating decreased health care costs is supported if decreased costs refer to the savings incurred through denied health care and denied or decreased fees for health care providers. Virtually all MCOs report reduced expenses for health care, but it is doubtful that any of these savings come from reduced administrative costs, reduced consequences of inappropriate care, or correction of misappropriation of funds intended for people in need of health care. It is also difficult to determine how much of the savings in health care actually appears as savings for the employers, government agencies, and individuals who pay the money that MCOs manage.

Psychotherapists are likely to find issues other than the finances of MCOs more directly relevant to their practices. The denial of benefits to the needy and subsequent increases in human suffering, the degradation of the professional psychotherapeutic process by limiting it to methods deemed most appropriate by MCO employees, and damage to patients through the loss of confidentiality are among the potential ill effects of managed care procedures that need to be evaluated and limited in order to reduce the potential for serious damage to human beings. Because these issues are complicated and difficult to observe and to quantify, they will be discussed separately in this book. Financial issues, on the other hand, represent the more obvious and quantifiable aspects of MCOs and consequently are presented before the more subtle, professionally important issues. As everyone knows, the notorious gangster Al Capone was not convicted for the egregious crimes he allegedly committed, but for income tax evasion. With major criminal activities, as with most other complicated organized activities, it is easier to demonstrate abuses of financial arrangements than abuses of human beings.

While the MCOs may be cutting costs in ways that are not in violation of current laws, the methods that they are using are frequently controversial. Further, the ways that the money cut from health care is then appropriated does appear to be at odds with the intentions of the payers or the consumers. For example, information presented in *U.S. News & World Report* (Geier 1996) supports the suspicion that managed care is exceedingly profitable for organizations other than those for whom the profits were intended. The report states that "the mob is in it. New Jersey officials reported busting a Mafia ring for allegedly siphoning money from a health care management company that serves one million patients in five states" (p. 14).

MANAGED CARE PROFITS

The profits reported by one MCO provide some insight into the benefits of heavy utilization review and decreased fees for treatment. The New York

State Psychological Association *Newsgram* (Glazer 1994a) printed the following summary of the earnings of U.S. Healthcare, a fast-growing MCO headed by one-time taxicab driver Leonard Abramson.

> While the labor department reported that third quarter medical prices climbed just 4.2%, U.S. Healthcare says their earnings have advanced 63% for the same quarter. They attribute this growth to managed-care's effectiveness in controlling the use of medical services. According to the New York Post, this allows them to pay Leonard Abramson, their C.E.O., $10 million a year, with another $800,000 in salaries and bonuses to his family members. It has also allowed the company to lend $10 million to a business started by one of Abramson's daughters. [p. 4]

Leslie Eaton (1996) reported in *The New York Times* the sale by Leonard Abramson of U.S. Healthcare, his enormously successful MCO, to Aetna Life and Casualty Company for $8.8 billion. Abramson stands to receive about $500 million in cash, plus over $3 million in common shares of Aetna which make him the company's largest individual shareholder.

On June 14, 1996, *The New York Times* printed an article entitled "U.S. Healthcare Chief Will Get $1 Billion," stating that Abramson will get about $970 million in cash and stock, plus a $25 million corporate jet. This article also stated that Mr. Abramson will act as a consultant to Aetna, after the merger under a five-year agreement that will pay him $10 million. Further, Joseph T. Sebastianelli, co-president of U.S. Healthcare, will get $5.6 million in cash and restricted stock to join Aetna, and Michael J. Cardillo, co-president and marketing officer, will receive over $6 million in cash and stock to join Aetna. The combined company will cover 23 million people, or one in every 12 Americans, and will be the fourth-largest company nationwide operating health maintenance organizations (HMOs). U.S. Healthcare had acquired MetraHealth the previous year, a company that in turn was the product of the merger of Metropolitan Life Insurance and Travelers Life Insurance. The sale of U.S. Healthcare to Aetna is the biggest deal in the wave of consolidations as health care companies seek to become big enough to get the upper hand in negotiating prices with their suppliers.

What does the merger mean for people enrolled with Aetna? For psychotherapists and other clinicians? For health care organizations seeking to compete with managed care? The consequences of this particular merger are representative of the far-reaching consequences of the numerous mergers that are taking place in the health care industry. According to *New York Times* news analyst Kirk Johnson (1996), people covered by the traditional health insurance plans provided by Aetna will be faced with pressure to join one of the merged company's managed care programs. Subscribers will also find that U.S. Healthcare provides a particularly restrictive health care plan that limits access to specialists and other kinds of treatment.

U.S. Healthcare insists on capitation policies and closely monitors services provided by clinicians and hospitals. The combined company, as the fourth-largest institute in the country operating health maintenance organizations, has a huge advantage in negotiating with health care providers and hospitals for lower fees and for controlling the access of patients to health care services. For psychotherapists who have resisted working with companies such as U.S. Healthcare, there are now fewer choices for working with insurance companies.

As for hospitals that have been trying to establish independent health care networks, they will find it even more difficult to compete with a company with as vast resources as the one resulting from the U.S. Healthcare–Aetna merger. Kenneth E. Raske, the president of the Greater New York Hospital Association, said that any hospital system would be in an enormously difficult situation attempting to confront the combined company, which he describes as a large and aggressive managed care company merged with an extremely well-financed insurance company (Johnson 1996).

The case of the U.S. Healthcare–Aetna merger demonstrates exorbitant profit making, but other examples of questionable MCO profits are plentiful. In this respect, it is worth noting that the U.S. Healthcare–Aetna merger produced the second-largest managed care system in New York City, second only to the Health Insurance Plan of Greater New York (HIP). Just one day before the announcement of the U.S. Healthcare–Aetna merger, *The New York Times* (Special Report 1996) presented a special report that found that HIP, the state's largest and oldest health maintenance organization, routinely fails to pay millions of dollars of its members' medical bills each year. The report revealed that the health care organization has for years delayed paying for treatment that it authorized outside its regular network of doctors, leaving members to either cover bills themselves or fight collection agencies representing medical practitioners who are seeking payment for their services.

The managed care industry has, in fact, saved money. Some of these savings may have benefited the patients and their employers, but a remarkable amount of the savings has gone into the pockets of managed care administrators and stockholders. The profitability of the various types of MCOs has made them popular as investments on Wall Street, according to financial analyst Joe Niedzielski (1996) writing for the National Underwriter Life and Financial Services. Frequent newspaper reports document successful managed care acquisitions, mergers, and managed care empires in the making (Freudenheim 1996a,b).

The financial success of the managed care industry and of its executives illustrates a classic problem in American entrepreneurial economics. Ideally, when a new product or service is conceived, it is then tested in the marketplace, and if it is accepted by its potential consumers, it is widely sold. This process benefits all participants in the system. Consumers have a product that helps them or pleases them, and the originators, manufacturers, and distributors make money. Obviously, a great deal of money can be made with a product that many people want. Although some people may then express outrage at the income of a sports or entertainment star or of a software or manufacturing CEO, at the same time most of the people know that those successes are earned because individual consumers made their choices from among an array of similar heroes, products, or services that they are competent to evaluate. Thus, the public buys the products endorsed by their heroes, and they do not mind that their purchases contribute to the fortunes of the heroes, because they are still making choices among products they know, such as sneakers, hamburgers, or computer games.

In the ideal entrepreneurial model, the transformation of a taxi driver into a multimillionaire by providing a desirable product or service would be a classic and praiseworthy accomplishment. In the case of MCOs, however, the method by which they market their product and make their profit removes them from the realm of the ideal entrepreneur and illustrates a particular problem in the entrepreneurial system. Although problems arise in the entrepreneurial markets in many ways, the most important problems arise when the consumers either do not have enough information with which to judge the product or when they have limited choices among similar products. Health care consumers have always had the first problem and, with the ascendance of managed care, they now have the second as well. Choosing a good doctor has never been easy and patients have had to rely on such factors as word of mouth, the doctor's bedside manner, and the courtesy of the office staff as surrogates for evidence of clinical skill. Usually, however, there were many doctors among which to choose, and patients were free to choose another if they felt they were not getting the quality for which they were paying. At present, many people are choosing health insurance companies, including MCOs, from limited lists. The average consumer does not have the training necessary to evaluate these providers and/or their standards, yet he or she usually must make a choice long before services are needed and therefore long before the plan's benefits are experienced and can be evaluated directly. These perturbations of the entrepreneurial system have allowed MCOs and their executives to profit not by developing a better health care product but merely by developing a cheaper one.

The claim by MCOs that there is a need to monitor health care is probably justified. It is true that health care costs have been increasing at higher rates than most other costs, but the frequently cited explanation—that health care professionals have been charging high fees and patients have been requiring many treatment appointments and laboratory tests—refers to only part of the problem. There are many reasons for the increased cost of health care, such as advanced technology for detecting and treating disorders; new treatment possibilities for people who would not have been alive many years ago, including extremely premature infants and a large number of needy, elderly people; concepts of health that include entitlement to all conventional and experimental treatments; lack of sufficient willingness to look at issues of rationing of resources; high administrative costs, including unnecessary duplications; waste, fraud, and other deceptive practices; high fees for questionable services; legal flaws that permit expensive litigation and consequent high malpractice insurance costs that are frequently passed on in higher medical fees; and greed.

Health care costs have increased rapidly, first with the availability of new resources, and second with the demand to use these resources to provide the best treatment possible with little regard to the financial consequences. The situation became ripe for MCOs to enter with their methods of health care controls. Of the many areas in the health care delivery system that were in need of evaluation and possible control, however, the MCOs began with the most superficially obvious ones, and they began without evaluation of long-range effects. They cut costs in the areas that are most dramatic and short-term effective: the areas of access to care and payment to professional health care providers. MCOs implemented their business methods quickly and the results appeared quickly. MCOs rapidly demonstrated savings in health care. Indeed, greed on the part of patients who wanted all the health care that is available and greed on the part of unethical health care providers have been curtailed. Yet, as the public is now discovering, most of the financial greed simply has moved over to the MCOs.

FEES, CLAIMS, AND FRUSTRATION

Although managed care systems have reduced the amount of money paid for the services of health care providers, many psychotherapists do not consider the reduced fees to be the critical issue in their participation in MCOs. For one thing, if an MCO actually does provide the services for psychotherapists that many MCOs claim to provide, such as appropriate referrals and simple billing procedures with timely payments, then the fees paid to MCO providers would be at least comparable to fees non-MCO health care professionals routinely accept if allowance is made for the 5 to 20 percent write-offs that non-MCO therapists commonly accept for adjustments and bad debt. In addition, private practice billing procedures can be quite cumbersome, requiring, for example, billing of two separate insurance companies for one patient. Some psychotherapists are therefore willing to accept the discounted fees for services offered by MCOs in exchange for a steady patient flow and a simple and reliable method for getting paid. The problem arises when therapists agree to the discounted fee and then find themselves accepting a new kind of bad debt write-off: denied claims.

MCOs deny provider claims for payment for many reasons. A common reason for denial is simply, either on the part of the MCO or the part of the provider, sending the form to the wrong address. In that case, when an inquiry is sent, the MCO may respond that the claim was never received. Sometimes, the MCO will refuse to consider a claim that is made after 30 days, even if an earlier claim was sent to an incorrect division or branch of the MCO.

There are a myriad of reasons for sending a claim to an incorrect address. A provider, or even a billing service, may inadvertently send a claim to an address previously listed but now changed because of provider merger or relocation. Claims are sometimes sent to an incorrect office such as the one where records rather than claims are assigned. The confusion about where to send a claim is sometimes the result of the necessity of sending claims to a completely different company from the company that provides initial and ongoing certification. For example, some patients who present with initial forms for Value Behavioral Health (VBH), an MCO with offices in New York, Texas, and other states, need to have their visits precertified by VBH but their visits are paid by submitting claims either to VBH or to another organization, such as MetraHealth in the New York area. Another example is found with U.S. Healthcare, which has its precertifications issued by a company called MBC, a company that replaced Achievement and Guidance Centers of America (AGCA). Blue Cross of Western Pennsylvania depends on Green Spring of Western Pennsylvania for some of the precertification process. Independent Health, listed in *Newsweek* (Spragins et al. 1996) as one of the best HMOs in the country, sent providers a newsletter with an article entitled "Where to Send Your Independent Health Documents." The article lists six types of documents that providers may need to send to Independent Health in order to present a claim for payment. Along with the document types are five addresses for electronic billing and five for paper billing. Independent Health acknowledged the complications involved in applying for payment by developing a chart to use as a reference when sending documents. Following a request to clip the chart, Independent Health asked providers, "Please be sure to attach a copy of either the corresponding voucher or a detailed note documenting the patient's name, ID number, DOS and claim number when submitting operative reports, EOBs and EOMBs" (p. 11). Despite the apparently sincere effort of Independent Health to provide these instructions as a service, the process has become too complicated to present in simple terms. Even billing specialists are having trouble following the guidelines.

Sometimes a provider submits a claim form with a minor omission or error, such as omitting a zip code, or missing a day in the date of birth of a subscriber's child or other family member. Despite the fact that the MCOs have this information on file, they may send the claim back denied for lack of completion. Sometimes the error is the result of idiosyncratic policies on the part of the MCO. For example, there are instances where an MCO requires a particular procedure code even when the required code is different from the code used by Medicare, most insurance companies, and the majority of MCOs. The particular code may, in fact, be a less accurate code. Psychotherapists, who usually use the procedure code 90844 (individual psychotherapy for approximately 45 to 50 minutes) for provided services, as listed in *Current Procedural Terminology* (CPT) (1996), would be denied payment by MCOs that require that psychotherapists treat patients for at least 45 minutes but require that they use the code 90841 (individual psychotherapy: no length of time given). Another example of idiosyncratic policies is the inconsistency of MCOs in requiring special codes for psychologists and social workers during some periods of time and not at others. For example, psychologists have been required to use the letters AH after procedure codes at some periods of time and not at others for Medicare payment. Whatever the reason for the error, the correction of the error is likely to require that the provider spend time-consuming efforts attempting to collect the fees that they have earned. In some cases, psychotherapists need to spend more time in collecting fees for a particular patient than the time spent in treating the patient.

An additional caution about precertification is in order here. Precertification of a claim does not mean that that claim will be paid, even when the provider fulfills all of the requirements of his or her contract. Let us look, for example, at procedures used by one of the companies mentioned previously, Value Behavioral Health, Inc. (VBH). VBH has contractual responsibility to precertify the medical necessity of all mental health and substance abuse covered services provided by mental health clinicians to New York State employees insured with the Empire Plan Mental Health and Substance Abuse Program. VBH, in common with most precertification businesses, notifies providers that the precertification review process is a review of requests to provide treatment for patients. Precertification is based on a review of only the medical necessity of treatment (see Part II for an explanation of medical necessity). VBH states that precertification is not a guarantee that benefits will be paid; that all provider requirements must be met before benefits are payable; that the patient must be eligible for coverage at time of service; and that a completed claim form must be submitted within the time specified to MetraHealth Service Corporation, the administrator for MetLife for processing some aspects of claims. While the process is complicated, it does not sound as unfair in this presentation as it can become. VBH and other MCOs omit a further reason for failure to provide benefits even when a claim has been precertified. A psychotherapist can be dropped from a provider list for many reasons, including a change of the company that does the precertification. This means that although a psychotherapist may be treating several people for conditions that have been precertified as medically necessary, if the company changes procedures and drops the psychotherapist, the psychotherapist remains ethically and even legally responsible for continuing to care for these patients, but the MCO no longer accepts any responsibility for payment of treatment. When VBH terminated several providers, the New York State Psychological Association contacted representatives of VBH to try to learn the basis for dropping mental health practitioners from provider lists. When questioned, VBH representatives responded that they had been advised by counsel not to discuss reasons for eliminating any provider from their lists (Glazer 1994).

Another frustrating aspect of payment for health care providers is the system of intentional delay of payment followed by MCOs. Bill Alpert, writing in *Barrons* (1996) reports investigations of the payment policies of

Wellcare Management Group, an MCO based in Kingston, New York. Although Wellcare is one of the smaller publicly traded MCOs, it dominates medical care in the Hudson Valley region of New York state. According to Alpert, Wellcare has been a favorite of Wall Street, with high profits and prestigious accounts that have included IBM and the Archdiocese of New York. In the *Barrons* article, Alpert documents complaints that Wellcare became a chronically late payer after it went on the public exchange. Examination of Wellcare documents and the records of a state insurance department examination suggest that Wellcare's delay of payment tactics resulted in the appearance of inflated profits. While it is apparently not illegal to withhold payment of fees to health care providers, the question of an attempt by Wellcare to appear even more profitable than was actually the case is currently being investigated. Wellcare's problems are particularly disturbing because Edward A. Ulmann, Wellcare's charismatic chief executive, has convinced many people that MCOs are efficient, effective, and in fact, more responsive and helpful to the public than any other type of health delivery system. In 1994, Ulmann lectured to the United States Senate on how MCOs like Wellcare could bring efficiency to government health programs such as Medicare and Medicaid. At present Wellcare, despite its stated intentions and goals, appears to be in trouble. MCOs in trouble frequently are purchased by large business entities such as insurance companies that include managed care divisions. Although Wellcare might meet the fate of being bought out by another company, it is unlikely that its major executives will lose money.

While practical issues concerning fees and claims can be annoying, some more fundamental problems with MCOs are being neglected. Many of these practical problems can be solved as increased attention is given to errors and injustices in the system. The fundamental problems that are more important to psychotherapists center on professional and ethical commitments. These will be more difficult to solve.

CONSCIENCE AND CONFLICTS

Psychotherapists are concerned with the industrialization of mental health services, that is, with the change from a service to a business. The American Psychological Association (APA) has taken the position that "those managed care entities which focus primarily on cost containment may be unresponsive to the psychological needs and confidentiality of patients and the professional judgment and autonomy of psychologists" and that the APA is committed to continuing its efforts to "strongly promote and defend the imperativeness of quality care in an ethical fashion to all consumers of psychological services" (DeLeon 1995, p. 671). The ethical and professional conflicts between therapists and MCOs are sometimes so subtle that even psychotherapists themselves sometimes may not be immediately aware of the impact of MCO procedures on their ability to practice. The following case narrative is told from the position of a psychotherapist who has been working with people referred by an MCO.

CASE NARRATIVE: CONFLICTS OF A MENTAL HEALTH PROVIDER

For a psychotherapist, the initial encounter with a prospective patient usually starts with a telephone message left by a person requesting an appointment. Dr. Howard Furst, a psychotherapist and mental health care provider for a major MCO, listened carefully to his messages. In addition to the name and telephone number of the caller, Dr. Furst wrote in his telephone log any special communications, such as a stated or implied sense of urgency that might require an immediate return call and readiness for emergency services. Because of his MCO commitment, Dr. Furst also listened for information that identified the caller as a person referred by the MCO.

Dr. Furst took pride in his ability to detect clues in telephone messages that were helpful in establishing a therapeutic relationship. He was always alert for information in a message that produced professional and ethical conflict in him. He is now apprehensive when he hears a caller communicating both that the situation is urgent and that there is insurance coverage with an MCO. Dr. Furst knows that the MCO may not agree with his assessment of an urgent situation. Neither Dr. Furst nor any other mental health specialist in this MCO system will be paid for sessions unless those sessions are precertified, and the precertification process can take days or even weeks.

Thus, it was with relief that Dr. Furst listened to the message from an MCO subscriber whose call he was expecting. The caller gave his name as Dan Gross and asked for an appointment to discuss a problem he had at the place where he worked. Dr. Furst had been alerted to expect Dan Gross's phone call by an MCO case manager with whom he had developed a cordial relationship. The particular MCO where Dr. Furst was listed as a behavioral health care provider has a policy of calling psychotherapists to be sure that they have time in their schedules for a client before giving the therapist's name to the client. The MCO telephone call to him was a courtesy that Dr. Furst appreciated.

Dan Gross had left both his work and home numbers. Dr. Furst looked at his watch and then dialed the home number. "Hello, this is Dr. Howard Furst. I am returning a call from Mr. Dan Gross."

"Yes, thanks for calling right back. It's about my job," said the 24-year-old transit department employee. "I have a problem because I don't want to take this promotion I was offered. I work downtown and the company wants me to work uptown. I got mugged last year going uptown to cover another guy's work. My supervisor wants to keep me here, too, but he says the company has a policy about refusing promotions. He says you need a letter from a doctor telling them your reasons. I guess the administration people don't understand why someone would turn down a promotion." His voice trailed off a little and he continued, in a humorous tone, "But I can see that. They all got promoted to where they are." Mr. Gross's chuckle was audible and Dr. Furst laughed in response.

Dr. Furst thought that it was a good sign that Mr. Gross had a sense of humor. He looked forward to meeting the young welder who was turning down a promotion. The case manager had told Dr. Furst that this young man had a preliminary diagnosis of adjustment reaction with anxiety. Probably an appropriate diagnosis, Dr. Furst thought, in view of Mr. Gross's declining a promotion. This could be a rather easy task for a trained psychotherapist. It would bring some satisfaction to Dr. Furst to be able to meet Mr. Gross's request within the three sessions that had been precertified.

Dan Gross, in person, did not present so easy a case. He was a small, slight man, not what one might expect to see in a welder. Gross trembled when he spoke about being mugged. "I was broken up bad; I wasn't conscious for days. When I left the hospital, I thought I would never be able to go back into those tunnels. But after a month I missed going to work. I like to weld." He forced a laugh and then said, "Maybe it's because I like the fire. I used to set fires when I was a kid. Nothing too bad. I didn't set fires outside or anything like that. Once or twice it was in a wastepaper basket in the bathroom. What I liked best was rolling a piece of cardboard into a tight roll and watching the fire burn down toward my fingers. I would see how long I could hold on before dropping the paper into the bathroom sink . . . sometimes it was close. Sometimes my mother or father smelled the burning paper and pounded on the door. They seemed scared. I was scared, too, but I couldn't stop for a long time. Then I forgot about it. I got interested in cars and parties and girls."

A few questions revealed that until the mugging last year, this young man had managed to keep thoughts about his fire-setting episodes out of his awareness. During the time of recovery from his injuries, the memories came back. Mr. Gross suffered nightmares about setting fires that went out of control. He had a girlfriend who had stood by him through the hospitalization and recovery, but he felt that he was now at risk of losing her because he was reluctant to go out socially after he returned home from work. He was afraid of crowded movie theaters, enclosed malls, elevators and escalators, and traveling more than a few miles in any direction from his home.

Dr. Furst sighed to himself. There were several problems to address. The situation included an apparently cooperative person, a challenging problem, and, as yet, an unpredictable course. It was important to acknowledge signs of potential danger. He would have to explore with Mr. Gross to find out how serious this situation was and how much Mr. Gross was able to do about his needs and fears. As for me, thought Dr. Furst, I am in for a struggle to get more sessions than the three that were approved. I will once again have to face my own conflicts about giving information to the MCO and about other issues of confidentiality and about the need to consult with people who do not know Dan Gross or understand the complications involved in helping him. I will not get paid for at least some of the sessions, and I will not be able to discuss fees with this patient although the issue of fees might become therapeutically important.

If Dr. Furst together with Mr. Gross decided that it was important to continue psychotherapy, then Dr. Furst would have to work on a treatment plan with the MCO's case manager. After each few sessions, the case manager would have to ask the reasons for continuing psychotherapy, the progress in terms of the stated goals, the ways in which progress was being measured, why alternate methods were not being used, and whole sets of other questions that made Dr. Furst feel helpless to secure what he thought was best for his patient. He searched for the terms that were acceptable to the MCO to describe the suffering of this young man.

In his mind, Dr. Furst next saw his treatment plan placed on the desk of the case manager, who would study the steps in his plan to compare them to the guidelines set by the MCO for each acceptable diagnosis. He saw the agents of the MCO coming to check his charts because there was a question about sufficient documentation to support the number of sessions requested. Dr. Furst felt like Big Brother was watching him.

COST, QUALITY, AND CONFLICT

George Orwell (1949) gave the name "Big Brother" to an entity that was capable of continuously monitoring an individual's every action, from brushing one's teeth to having sex. The goal was complete control of behavior and full compliance with government regulations. There was no escape from observation. People were rendered helpless because the government behind Big Brother had assumed control over their lives.

Today, psychotherapists often view managed care as a mental health Big Brother appearing on an invisible screen in their offices and collecting information about the psychotherapist and the patient. To many, it seems as if a new partner has materialized to enforce a set of rules and regulations that complicate the delivery of mental health services. Managed care's rules and regulations often result in two kinds of conflicts for the psychotherapist. The first generally involves the psychotherapist's desire to act on behalf of the patient and the desire to fulfill contractual terms for reimbursement. This type of conflict has always been a problem for therapists—does one continue treatment for a needy patient who cannot pay for treatment? Under managed care, the problem has become much more complicated. In a traditional independent practice, the therapist addresses these problems directly with the patient, using clinical skills to evaluate the patient's needs and to balance those needs with his or her own professional ethics, needs, and feelings. For a therapist under contract with an MCO, the same problem must be resolved with a case manager. A case manager's understanding of the problem can sometimes be influenced by the therapist's clinical skills and ethical principles, but the work of the case manager is conceptually different from that of the professional psychotherapist. The case manager's work is not based on ethical principles but rather on contractual and legal obligations that are far less protective of the patient than are the therapist's ethical obligations. Managed care is not a professional practice organization established to promote the well-being of patients and the ethical behavior of practitioners; it is essentially a business—an economic entity that operates on fundamental entrepreneurial principles.

In addition to conflicts that psychotherapists feel between themselves and MCO regulations, therapists working with MCOs have to confront problems within themselves. Some examples of internal conflicts are reflected in the following questions: Is the duration of therapy approved by the MCO adequate to address the problems of a particular patient? Am I doing the right thing by not discussing the MCO limitations with the patient? Will the MCO consider it fraudulent if I fail to collect or waive the co-payment for a needy patient?

The new industry of psychotherapy, as part of the health care system, has been restructured as a business with a product to sell. As with other products in successful businesses, the psychotherapy product must be competitive in price and quality. Managed health care industry leaders have centered their competitive efforts in psychotherapy on marketing and price. In order to reduce prices, these health care leaders attempt to reduce costs. They aim to reduce costs by reducing inefficiency in administration, reducing fees paid for individual services, and eliminating services considered by them to be unnecessary. Unfortunately, the MCOs themselves have been the judges of what services are necessary. Moreover, the MCOs do not take responsibility for the consequences of denying services. The representatives of the MCOs claim that they are making business, not medical, decisions even when their decisions result in injurious or fatal medical outcomes. Robert Daly (1996), director of the Behavioral Health Division for the Building Services Union, observes that as a health care system gets closer and closer to profit margins, it reaches a critical point where the only way to cut costs is to reduce benefits.

MCOs limit the number of allowed psychotherapy sessions in subtle ways. For example, a psychotherapist and a patient may believe that the patient is entitled to 20 psychotherapy sessions a year based on their reading of the health care contract. Yet, when the psychotherapist requests more than the number of sessions originally certified, the MCO representative may inform the psychotherapist that the "20 covered sessions" stipulated in the contract refers to a maximum number. Although the patient's contract does state that there are 20 sessions available for psychotherapy, the contract does not provide the information that neither the psychotherapist nor the patient decides how many sessions are actually allowed. The case manager follows directives to decide if the psychotherapist has reported a sufficient defense of psychotherapeutic interventions to warrant additional sessions. For the psychotherapist, each additional set of treatment reports brings with it concerns about exposure and consequent feelings of anger and helplessness.

There are other cost-cutting techniques that do not, at first, appear to be what they are. Recently a large and successful MCO notified psychotherapists that their fees would be increased at the beginning of the new year. Following the list of increased fees, there was a statement to the effect that the increases would come not from the MCO but from patients in the form of a higher co-payment. A little arithmetic showed that this MCO was planning actually to pay less to their providers in the coming year than they had been paying during the current year. Another rather questionable tactic involves simply withholding payments for many months. The money in the bank earns interest for the MCOs at the expense of the providers (Alpert 1996).

There is also the issue of having two methods to count psychotherapy sessions, with the choice of method dependent on the financial interest of the MCO. Dr. Sage's situation illustrates the problem.

> Dr. Sage had just recently become a provider for a major MCO. The MCO referred a patient to him for a consultation with one precertified session. During that session, Dr. Sage found that the patient was responding to a critical situation with overwhelming anxiety. Dr. Sage made an appointment with the patient to continue the evaluation and treatment. He followed the session with a call to the MCO as directed in his contract and negotiated with the case manager for three more sessions to take place during the three weeks after that initial session.
>
> A problem occurred for Dr. Sage when the patient called that evening, a time when case managers generally are not available. The patient urgently requested a session. Based on his clinical judgment, Dr. Sage saw the patient and, following that session, was satisfied that the patient felt sufficiently supported to endure his situation until the next scheduled session. Dr. Sage treated the patient for a total of four sessions and billed for these four sessions. Dr. Sage was paid several months later for three sessions. A careful reading of the explanation of benefits (EOB) that accompanied the payment revealed that someone at the MCO thought the second session was not precertified. After several phone calls and a letter of grievance, Dr. Sage found that the second session indeed was not certified because it had taken place shortly after the first session rather than a week after the first session as he and the case man-

ager had originally planned. Dr. Sage considered several options and then graciously gave up the attempt to get paid for his work.

Now, here is the worst part of the manipulations experienced by Dr. Sage in the area of counting sessions. The same patient called Dr. Sage several months later to request help in coping with another critical situation. Dr. Sage dutifully called the MCO requesting precertification for three sessions, the maximum number he had learned would be precertified without having to submit a time-consuming outpatient treatment report (OTR). The case manager responded that there were only two sessions that could be approved for this patient without an OTR. "Hold it. Something is wrong with your numbers," Dr. Sage told the case manager. "Although I did have four sessions with this patient, your company paid for only three, saying that they had not precertified the second session. Therefore, of those six session to which the patient is entitled, you can still precertify three, which is the number I am requesting."

"No," said the case manager, "we subtract all the sessions for which you billed. We count *billed* sessions, not *paid* sessions. Members are allowed six sessions before the OTR is required. This patient has had four sessions according to our records, leaving two more before the OTR."

"Let's return to counting sessions, please. If this patient uses all the sessions allowed in his contract, he will have had 20 hours of treatment but the MCO will have paid for 19. Is that right?"

"Yes, I guess it is. Unless the provider fails to get precertification or fails to submit statements on time, or uses codes not specified in the contract, or does something else like that—then this organization is obliged to refuse payment for those sessions only. But the sessions still count towards the total number allowed."

"I am having trouble believing that you have two systems for counting sessions, one for payment and one for the number of allowed sessions. Is that legal?"

"I believe it is. Can I do something else for you?"

In addition to limiting access to benefits, MCOs reduce costs for the benefits they do provide. One method for reducing costs involves reducing the fees paid to therapists for each unit of service. MCOs decrease psychotherapists' fees in several ways. One way is quite direct: some MCOs simply offer lower rates in subsequent contracts than they offered in the original contract.

The American Managed Behavior Healthcare Association (AMBHA) (1996) reported dramatic growth of MCO membership rates, which the association attributed to the success of management techniques. Between 1993 and 1994 membership grew by 58 percent. The following year it grew by 35 percent. The estimated growth for 1996 was 11 percent. This adds up to over 74 million Americans covered by the 19 AMBHA companies. According to Neal M. Lonky's (1995) report on *Mental Health Net*, the value of publicly traded, for-profit health plans was over $35 billion at that time.

MCOs have rewarded their top managers handsomely for the financial success of their businesses. An analysis of the compensation for the chief executive officers of ten leading MCOs was compiled from health plan proxy statements (1995). The analysis shows salaries plus bonuses and stock options for 1993 averaging $4.4 million for each executive. At the head of the list at that time was Daniel D. Crowley, Chief Executive Officer of Foundation Health, with a salary and bonus of $3.6 million, plus $15 million in stock options.

Managed health care today is a profitable industry owned by corporations and their stockholders. Portfolio managers are advertising the health care industry as a lucrative investment for both individuals and funds. Major investment groups are buying and selling health care industry stock every day. A recent advertisement by a prominent New York investment firm offered customers a way to give their investment portfolio a healthy boost (Gruntal & Co. 1996). The firm recommends taking advantage of the bright financial future of the health care and medical services industries and their exciting "potential in capital appreciation." Because MCOs are thriving, psychotherapists are facing the prospect of becoming businesspeople in order to survive. For many, this means struggling with one's identity and ideals. "I never used to worry about referrals," Sherry Milton, Ph.D., a clinical psychologist from Atlanta, sighs. "Now I constantly speak to people, making contacts and selling myself, so I can be sure the phone will ring." Dr. Milton's story has become familiar.

LANGUAGE AS A BUSINESS TECHNIQUE

The term *psychotherapist* usually refers to those professionals who provide treatment of mental disorders. Traditionally, psychotherapists are psychiatrists, psychologists, social workers, and psychiatric nurses who are educated and trained to treat mental problems and who receive a license from their states allowing them to practice their profession. In the literature of managed care, psychotherapists are included in a category called mental health care providers or, more recently, behavioral health care providers. The difference between a professional person and a provider reflects the emphasis on the part of the MCOs to include, in the category of mental health care providers, many different types of professions and occupations. With the divisions erased, it is easy to erase individuality and respect for specialized skills. A mental health clinician goes from being a professional person to being a bureaucrat, from being a trained person with a code of ethics to being an employee whose code is meeting the requirements of the employer.

The act of changing what someone is called or changing the title of what someone does is a technique deliberately used in business management. A change in a title often is accompanied by a change in attitude, making it easy to use a change in title as a means of reward, of penalty, and of other tokens of control.

Changes in the names of positions or of departments within a organization can also serve to obscure the activities or the aims of that position or department. In this light, it is noteworthy that at the same time in the late 1940s that the United States Department of War became the Department of Defense, George Orwell completed the novel *1984*, in which he describes the creation of language to control the thoughts of the people.

In his novel, Orwell (1949) introduces the language systems of *newspeak* and *doublethink*. Orwell invented newspeak to demonstrate the control of thought through the control of language. Just as psychologists propose that vocabulary is an essential instrument in advanced mental processes, Orwell proposed that the limitation of vocabulary limits thought. Vocabulary and intelligence are connected because, in general, people think with words. Consequently, the more words a person knows, the more ideas that person may be expected to generate. In order to limit thinking, newspeak eliminated all undesirable words. The words that remained were stripped of secondary meanings. The example that Orwell gives is the word *free*. The word existed in the sense that a dog could be declared free of fleas or a forest free of deer, but no one could be described as free to make choices. In essence, newspeak was designed to diminish the range of thought by "cutting the choice of words down to a minimum" (p. 247).

Karen Shore, President of the National Coalition for Mental Health Professionals and Consumers, also observes that the industrialization of health care has changed the language so that psychotherapists sign contracts that refer to "covered lives," rather than people, and to "providers" rather than to specialists in medicine, psychiatry, psychology, social work, or nursing.

Shore (1995a) comments, "If Communist Russia or China had devised managed care, we would have criticized it as another manifestation of authoritarian control over worker-clinicians, over citizens, and over education professionals. But when we do it, we call it 'good business'" (p. 4).

Doublethink refers to the process of holding two contradictory thoughts in one's mind at the same time. In the Afterword to *1984*, Erich Fromm (1961) gives as an example of doublethink the observation that the people of this country spend a considerable part of the national income on the development of thermonuclear weapons while closing their minds to the possibility that bombs could detonate and destroy half of the population. Additional examples of doublethink can be found in the language of MCOs. Ivan Miller (1994), psychotherapist and co-founder of the Boulder Psychotherapist's Guild, points out two examples of MCO expressions that are misleading because they convey contradictory meanings: *quality assurance* and *focused therapy*. Quality assurance programs are usually aimed at reducing costs, not at improving quality of care. At the same time, these programs are aimed at assuring a type of quality, and that type is the *minimum* quality that the MCOs can possibly offer while still maintaining (assuring) that they have a salable product. Focused therapy uses the concept of *being focused* because that concept is associated with positive qualities, such as the ability to concentrate, to be centered, to be given attention, to bring intensity to a situation In reality, MCOs have policies that focus on their agenda for psychotherapy, and MCO representatives do not attend to any other issue no matter how important it might be to psychotherapists or their patients.

In a recent article in the *American Journal of Psychotherapy*, Abram Chipman (1995) discusses the crises in identity and values for psychotherapists. Chipman explains the relationship between changes in semantics and changes in attitude in the health care industry. He observes that the health care industry has become less concerned with ameliorating disease and with solving the problems of patients, and more concerned with the process of purchasing a commodity. Further, Chipman suggests that the shift in the focus of concern promotes increasing emotional distance between therapists and patients.

PAST HISTORY

The current changes in health care delivery can be traced back to World War II. The initial changes began as a response to wage and price controls. During the war, workers were scarce, and employers could not compete for them by offering increased wages because wage controls were in effect. Thus, to attract workers, employers looked for new ways other than increased wages. They found the unregulated benefit of employer-paid medical care insurance. Health care benefits increased the compensation received by workers and also provided the advantage of being tax exempt for both employer and employee (Friedman 1994).

Health care benefits gave insured workers access to health care, generally with only a 10–20 percent co-payment. This access produced what health care investment analysts call a "blank-check market." Karen Shore (1995a) also points out the lack of financial incentives to control misuse of health care benefits. Shore notes that the small co-payment was not enough to cause patients to be cost-and-utilization conscious.

In 1965 another large group was added to those who paid for health care through a third party. Medicare and Medicaid provided essentially unlimited medical services with little or no co-payment and little or no incentive for patients or practitioners to limit services.

The absence of cost incentives combined with the marked presence in this country of a sense of entitlement left little reason for Americans to be concerned about their increasing health care demands. Most people seemed to believe that they and their parents, grandparents, even great-grandparents deserved the best treatment money could buy for as long as they could be kept alive. Because health care expenses did not come directly out of the pockets of patients, there was little respect for the balancing of money spent against treatment obtained.

The entrepreneurs of the marketplace rushed to meet accelerating health care demands in many ways, building hospitals and facilities, and increasing the availability of expensive, sophisticated technology that was not imaginable twenty years earlier. People never saw what they were spending and they appeared to have no control over themselves or their health expenses. Employers eventually took the growing benefit costs of health care out of various other expense areas in the corporation, primarily employee wages. Employees rarely were aware that increasing costs and demands for health care affected their income. Health care costs increased at a greater rate than the costs, for example, of education and defense. The statistics in Robert G. Frank's (1993) proposal for health care reform are: the cost of health care grew from approximately 6 percent of the gross national product (GNP) in 1965 to 13.2 percent in 1992. In comparison, spending on education in 1992 was approximately 7.2 percent of the GNP while defense was below 6 percent. Health care was estimated to cost 40 percent more in the United States than any other developed nation in the world and still did not insure adequate health care for everyone.

The time was right for public examination of the appropriate use of medical care. The separation of individuals from the payment process had contributed unreasonable expectations for health care. Healthy people wanted low premiums; sick people wanted unlimited benefits. There seemed to be little awareness in the general population that these goals were incompatible. Elected officials did not promote public debate, perhaps because of the political consequences. There were no proposals to limit benefits because people in elected positions feared alienating voters, especially the elderly. The officials did not dare to propose paying premiums through payroll deductions or taxes because increases in payments through any means would likely anger other voters, especially younger, working people. The business people involved in managed care systems rushed into this political situation appearing to offer both reduced premiums and increased benefits. As costs continued to spiral, indemnity insurance plans became too expensive for businesses and employees. Given the extreme expenses of health care at that time, Shore (1995a) noted that it was inevitable that the pendulum had to swing to the other extreme, to managed care with large-scale, dramatic cost containment. The time was right for the entrance of MCOs. MCOs used techniques for control of health care that came straight from *1984*. The monitoring tactics of the MCOs especially evoked in practitioners the feeling that Big Brother was watching.

Suddenly, psychotherapists who saw themselves as autonomous and skilled in the treatment room were faced with an uncomfortable ideology. Patients or clients became consumers, psychotherapists became providers, and the goal of treatment had to match the requirements of managed care.

MCOs attempted to reduce health care expenditures and to make profits by making decisions for everyone, especially for patients, doctors, and hospitals. MCOs also attacked the entire health care system as it existed by cutting payments for treatment, for tests, and for the utilization of services and equipment. MCOs continued to sell their plans to employers searching for ways to cut health care benefit costs. They expanded into various regions of the country, establishing themselves especially in California, Minnesota, and Massachusetts. Their programs spread quickly. Employers, eager to save money, bought the new contracts. Patients, unhappy with high deductibles and co-payments, confusing paperwork, high cost of prescription medications, and increasing complaints about the high cost of their health care, enrolled in the new systems. Many people believed that managed care would save money through reduced administrative costs and investigations of waste and fraud.

In mental health the idea of affordable treatment for a greater number of people was compelling. The new managed care system promised access to psychotherapy for many people who otherwise would never have sought help for emotional problems. MCOs applied the same model to both physical and mental health. In order to cut the costs of psychotherapy, MCOs imposed requirements on psychotherapy that permitted limited treatment for most people.

It is ironic that MCOs have targeted mental health as an area in which to curtail services. Psychotherapeutic treatment reduces the expense of *total* medical care for many conditions, most obviously in the areas of alcohol and chemical dependency where, with the control of addiction, medical costs may decline dramatically (Bonstedt 1992).

In considering the relative expense of psychotherapy, it is important to study the impact of mental health issues on primary care. According to Behavioral HealthCare CEO Errol Nadler (1995), approximately 75 percent of visits to primary care physicians (PCPs) involve psychological concern or distress, and, in addition, 80 percent of patients who actually need mental health services will seek instead medical care. Nadler reported studies that found that overtime at work and excess levels of stress can lead to reduced productivity, greater absenteeism, accidents, and illness. The report further stated that treatment for the consequences of excess stress is expensive and takes employees away from work. Stress prevention programs have been shown to decrease visits to medical and mental health professionals by 35–50 percent. It appears that attention to mental health problems leads to improvement of economic outcomes.

Mental health services have never shared the same blank-check marketplace as medical care. One reason for the more modest use of mental health care services might be that insurance companies generally required a larger co-payment for mental health services, often as high as 50 percent. The higher co-payment may have lead the consumers of mental health services to be more conscious of costs and utilization of services. In fact, mental health care accounted for only 3 to 4 percent of all health care expenses (Miller 1994). However, as Kiesler (1992) notes, mental health care policy has followed the growth and development of medical health care policy; and now as the failings and problems of the American health care system become the target of reform, mental health services are swept into the changes of the general health care system.

LIMITATIONS ON PSYCHOTHERAPY

Two problems created by the new relationship between psychotherapists and MCOs are especially critical. These problems are the limitation of therapy sessions and the limitation of confidentiality, both very complicated issues. While there are places where limiting sessions can be effective, each situation requires careful evaluation of the patient's needs. As a result of the MCO insistence on short-term therapy, two major categories of people are ignored or underserved in the system. The first group includes patients who need in-depth, long-term psychotherapy for significant personality change. Their problems can impair their basic ability to function, let alone their productivity, self-fulfillment, and happiness. MCOs force these patients to choose between limited sessions and assumption of financial responsibility. The second group of people who are shortchanged by MCO insistence on brief therapy are people with severe and chronic psychological problems. Long-term treatment is considered too expensive. MCOs frequently insist on psychotropic medication or self-help groups as ways to replace individual therapy.

The second problem in the new relationship is the limitation of confidentiality. Traditionally, the psychotherapy dyad involves two parties: the therapist and the person called the patient or client. In most cases their relationship is viewed as private, and confidentiality is seen as essential for successful psychotherapy. In fact it has been said that confidentiality is as essential for psychotherapy as sterility is for surgery. Third parties in treatment are sometimes not avoidable, such as in those situations where the psychotherapist needs to share the case with a clinical supervisor or uses the case experience in a training institute. In these cases, everyone is in agreement that the patient's identity and the details of his or her life are disguised or concealed, and, if information is inadvertently revealed, all professionals respect the information as private. In the clinic or agency setting, the patient is generally more aware of the fact that his or her case may be reported to a staff or committee, but as much is done as possible to protect privacy. The breaches of confidentiality that do occur frequently result in patients' fantasies about breaches. If such fantasies occur, the psychotherapist can interpret the symbolic meaning for the patient and, together, the psychotherapist and patient can work through the issues as part of therapy. The addition of a managed-care business partner alters the essential nature of the therapeutic relationship. The manager is not concerned with the material of traditional psychotherapy, such as structural change, ego strength, insufficient sense of self, quality of object relations, style of coping, and other clinical issues, but instead the manager is concerned with the issues of the business of managed care. MCO case managers become overseers in the offices of psychotherapists. The case manager intrudes into psychotherapy, and interferes with psychotherapy to the extent that the benefits are limited.

FUTURE HISTORY

Managed care as a new economic product may be a rising star in the investment industry, but managed care will change greatly in response to market forces, public scrutiny, and government regulation. Competitive forces will push MCOs to further reduce their costs. One method of reducing costs is to use less expensive providers. In mental health, the most expensive providers, psychiatrists, are increasingly delegated to psychopharmacology. Referrals to psychiatrists for medication makes sense if the psychiatrist has interest and expertise in psychopharmacology. Psychiatrists who specialize in medication, known as psychopharmacologists, work with primary care physicians and psychotherapists to treat patients. Problems occur when pressure is applied to primary care physicians to administer psychotropic medications instead of psychotherapy. In many situations, a psychological evaluation is needed, perhaps an extended one. Who shall provide this evaluation to determine the most appropriate treatment? The answer from MCOs, frequently, is to use the least expensive provider, not the most appropriate one. In psychotherapy, psychologists are usually paid slightly higher than social workers. Consequently, managed care has encouraged using social workers.

According to Behavioral HealthCare CEO Errol Nadler (1995), demand management may be the wave of the future (see Chapter 3). Demand management supports preventative treatment to avoid more expensive interventions. One type of preventative treatment is called a wellness program. Wellness programs are educational workshops that deal with behaviors such as smoking, stress management, drug and alcohol abuse, and related issues. Because MCOs pay less to case managers than they pay to psychotherapists, MCOs are likely to train case managers to conduct community wellness groups.

Another method of reducing expenses is capitation. In a typical capitation arrangement, a provider or group of providers is paid a fixed amount of money to assume the health care responsibility for a designated population (e.g., a corporation's employees or residents of a geographic area). The providers have full responsibility and authority for the treatment of the population. If the cost of that treatment for all covered lives exceeds the fixed amount paid, the providers take the loss. If it is less than the paid amount, the providers profit. This gives some incentive to the provider to control treatment costs, but it is also bound to create conflicts of interest for the provider.

A market force outside of MCOs may influence the delivery of health care services. At present there are groups of physicians that are joining with hospitals to create physician–hospital organizations (PHOs) to contract directly with large employers for the care of their employees or with the state or county for the care of Medicare and Medicaid patients. PHOs do not need to earn a profit for outside investors and can therefore provide services for lower premium payments. Because PHOs operate, in some respects, as managed care systems, they do not resolve all of the professional conflicts faced by health care providers, but the PHOs do provide more opportunities for the providers to change the problems that occur.

Mergers will also alter the health care market. A trend to consolidate managed care companies has become obvious. "The mergers of MCOs appear to be managed care empires in the making" (Freudenheim 1996a, p. D1). These health conglomerates may become so powerful that they will be able to regulate fee schedules with medical suppliers and attract more employers with low-cost plans.

Societal influences will also affect health care delivery and managed care in the future. Public sentiment and needs will affect judicial and legislative actions. As more people are exposed to the practices of managed care, they are becoming disillusioned with the services they receive. The disillusionment is likely to result in pressure on employers and other payers of health care to either find better solutions or return to at least some aspects of more traditional indemnity plans for health care.

Capitation is an increasingly widespread development in managed care. It is more common in the medical field than in the mental health field because capitation plans are usually offered to primary care physicians. Mental health professionals, however, are affected by capitation because primary care providers are not as likely to refer patients for psychotherapy when MCOs encourage the primary care providers to follow psychotherapy guidelines themselves. Robert Daly (1996) points out that the concept of capitation may ultimately backfire on MCOs. Large hospitals or practitioner systems can bypass MCOs and contract directly with payers to provide specific health care services. Arrangements of this type that are already in existence are now working out ways to coordinate their services with the services of other health care providers.

Daly predicts that profit-driven MCOs ultimately will be forced to face the courts. He suggests that lawsuits resulting from radical cost-containment measures, denial of benefits, negligence, and malpractice will use up profits and compel managed care to change. Bryant L. Welch (1996b) writes that "the most effective and comprehensive shield to protect quality care may well be the very same sword which many health providers have come to dread, to wit, the malpractice case" (p. 15). Welch suggests that the need to use malpractice suits against corporate health providers is far greater than the need to use it against the traditional target, individual practitioners. It is difficult to regulate corporate MCOs, which, unlike practitioners, do not have to face professional and state boards. Ironically, the current progress toward limiting malpractice awards in certain cases may put MCOs in an advantageous position. If MCOs can anticipate minimal malpractice penalties, they will be more likely to take greater risks in causing harm by denying or limiting access to health care benefits.

Other forms of public pressure are certain to affect managed care's methods. Numerous articles from professional journals to supermarket tabloids have pointed out the dangers of the managed care approach to limiting cost by limiting treatment. When *Redbook* magazine, with Oprah Winfrey on the cover, carries an article called "Some HMOs Are Bad News" (McCall 1996) and *Glamour* presents a tragedy called "Death by HMO" (Dolnick 1996), there can be no doubt that public awareness is growing and that public pressure will lead to legislative controls on MCOs. A major control of MCO activities occurred with the passing of the Health Insurance Portability and Accountability Act, a federal bill signed by President Clinton on August 21, 1996. William Yurkowski (1996), executive director of Independent Health, states that this law "is one of the most comprehensive federal health policy accomplishments. It provides increased protection for workers and their families by eliminating preexisting condition exclusions when people with health care coverage change jobs or health plans" (p. 25).

Universal health care was an important issue in the 1992 presidential election. The failure of the administration and the Congress to move toward a solution did not erase the issue from the public forum. Public pressure may demand scrutiny of a variety of health care delivery systems in this country and around the world. The results of experimental systems such as the rationing program in the state of Oregon will influence the development of future health care systems.

Although MCOs will change in response to new laws and regulations, some form of managed health care system is probably here to stay. The need to reconcile cost containment with the provision of quality services will become more difficult as new useful services—almost always more expensive than the older ones—become available. Adapting to the current system while it is changing presents problems for all health care practitioners. The demands on mental health practitioners will be more severe than the demands on physicians, for example, because the problems of definition of illness and of confidentiality in the mental health field are more difficult to resolve than the problems of definition in the treatment of anatomic, physiological illness.

Mental health practitioners will need to evaluate their concepts of themselves and their practices in light of the changing health care system. There are many ways to try to accommodate to the current managed care situation and many ways to resist or actively fight. The following six suggestions will be discussed further in Parts II and III of this book. They are mentioned here as options for consideration as further discussions about living in an MCO era are presented. They are, of course, noninclusive. A psychotherapist can:

1. become a managed care clinician and accept referrals through the system;
2. devote part of her or his practice to managed care and part to traditional fee-for-service patients or part to performing other clinical services, such as testing and evaluation or consulting to hospital or school programs;
3. maintain an independent practice, entirely outside the scope of managed care;
4. practice as part of a group, agency, or institution on a salaried basis;
5. practice as part of a nonmanaged care network, guild, or cooperative;
6. find new ways to use psychotherapy skills or learn new skills based on his or her interests and the needs of his or her community. Study of hypnosis or psychopharmacology, for example, may satisfy old dreams and provide new professional work.

It will be a formidable challenge for psychotherapists to find satisfying ways to practice their profession in these days of constantly shifting systems and frequent challenges to professional identity. As Abram Chipman (1995) writes in the *American Journal of Psychotherapy*, "The generalized effect of managed care . . . is to radically alter the behaviors and internalized paradigms of those who struggle to adapt to the realities of contemporary 'providership'" (p. 565).

CONCLUSION

Traditionally, mental health clinicians provided health care services for patients in as professional and ethical manner as possible and, generally, they derived satisfaction from the practice of their profession. In most cases, the patients or their families paid for their health care services directly. Under this traditional fee-for-service health care system, there were financial incentives to provide treatment. There has been recent concern with overuse of medical services, such as excessive and redundant testing or automatic heroic efforts to prolong life. Unfortunately, excesses in the medical field lead to restrictions that affect psychotherapists, often unjustifiably.

On the other hand, there is also concern that MCO incentives to reduce health care expenditures may result in undertreatment. This would occur through restricted access to primary care and failure to recommend sufficient diagnostic tests, specialty care, hospitalization, and rehabilitation efforts, and from failure to appropriately recommend treatment by out-of-plan providers.

Psychotherapists suffer additional conflicts because many MCOs constrain the providers from making negative remarks about the MCO plan and keep them from encouraging patients to advocate for their own care and for timely payments. Providers frequently feel intimidated in pleading too extensively for their patients because they know that their contracts may not be renewed if they request more sessions for their patients than the MCO case worker certifies, or if they generate more health care expenditures on behalf of their patients than some MCO-calculated average for mental health treatment.

Psychotherapists experience conflicts with regard to their control of the treatment that they assess as best for their patients. The health care allowed for patients and the fees paid to providers are controlled by MCOs with business ethics and goals that are sometimes at odds with the ethics and goals of professional health care providers. There is no doubt that MCOs are responding to market forces that demand health care services at reduced costs. "Not surprisingly, the organizations that deliver for these payors are the primary beneficiaries of change," says Amanda Bowman (1994), specialist in communication strategies for managed care.

While many psychotherapists support MCO policies as the best attempt at treatment outcomes in terms of cost efficiency, many other psychotherapists, whether participating in MCO networks or practicing outside of MCOs, are experiencing problems with MCOs, including identity conflicts and reduced freedoms. Financial issues seem especially relevant because the profits MCOs report are spectacular, while incomes of health care providers and benefits to patients are generally at reduced levels. By denying payment and other techniques, MCOs reduce the psychotherapy services received by patients both in frequency of sessions and duration of treatment. Psychotherapists may need to consider several approaches to protecting their visions of themselves and their practices.

2

The Impact of Managed Care

We are under attack by a rapacious, dishonest, disruptive, greed-driven insurance-managed care big business combine that is in the process of decimating all health care in America, but most egregiously, the care of the mentally ill.

–Harold Eist, President-elect of the American Psychiatric Association [quoted in Saeman 1996a, p. 1]

Dr. Paul Ling, a clinical psychologist in Quincy, Massachusetts, said he had to tell a case reviewer for a managed care company "the most gory of details" about a patient who had been raped repeatedly by a family member when she was a child. "Variations on this theme occur all the time," Dr. Ling said.

–quoted by Gina Kolata, "When Patients' Records Are Commodities for Sale" [New York Times, *November 15, 1995, p. A1*]

"I feel like killing myself," Shannon Rose said.

Dr. Beverly Davis watched her patient silently. She had been treating the 32-year-old woman for a year. In that time Mrs. Rose had revealed the horrors of her childhood: repeatedly raped by her father, seemingly unattended by her cocaine-addicted mother, and enmeshed in constant battles with an older sister for the clothes and costume jewelry that she claimed as her only belongings.

"I feel like I was put on this earth to be abused." The content of Mrs. Rose's statement was dramatic but her tone and her facial expression were flat.

Predictably, Shannon Rose had married a man who continued to abuse her, throwing her so hard against the walls of their apartment that her head left imprints in the plaster. At the beginning of treatment, Mrs. Rose insisted that she had no skills to do anything. She said that she did not know anything except how to be hurt.

It took a long time for Mrs. Rose to trust Dr. Davis. For this traumatized woman, the year had been spent learning that she could have a relationship where she was not abused. This knowledge enabled her to realize that she could have some control over her life. She was even talking about getting a part-time job. The prognosis was good until Dr. Davis and Mrs. Rose received the information about the new managed care coverage.

"They're taking it all away from me," Mrs. Rose said when she was talking about the fact that her husband's employer had signed a contract with a new MCO. "They're taking it all away from me and I can't do anything about it." Mrs. Rose was too afraid of confrontation to advocate for herself with the MCO representative. Dr. Davis was able to become a provider for this particular MCO because it has a policy of accepting those psychotherapists who are already treating a number of people who subscribe to the MCO.

Dr. Davis argued with the MCO case manager, saying that Mrs. Rose had accomplished so much in that year and that continued treatment would help her to move toward a productive life.

"I can certify three sessions," the case manager said, "and then we will need an outpatient treatment report (OTR) before any more sessions can be certified." Dr. Davis explained that, in her opinion, the time involved in filing the OTR and waiting for approval represented a violation that would interfere with treatment. Dr. Davis tried to describe the anxiety that her patient experienced worrying about the continuation of sessions. Noting that frequent and extensive reports would interfere with Mrs. Rose's ability to benefit from treatment, Dr. Davis requested certification for at least 10 sessions. The case manager sounded upset by Dr. Davis's arguments but he continued to insist that the regulations permitted precertification for no more than three sessions.

Traditional psychotherapy creates an essential two-person relationship that is the instrument for change. The entrance of managed care into psychotherapy created three additional active relationships in treatment. The resulting four relationships are as follows:

1) Psychotherapist–Patient–MCO
2) Psychotherapist–Patient
3) Psychotherapist–MCO
4) Patient–MCO

The outcome of psychotherapy depends on interactions in each of these relationships. In traditional therapy, the patient–therapist relationship was enhanced by the skill of the therapist. It was vulnerable to limitations in the nature and circumstances of the patient's problems and to the limitations of psychotherapy itself.

In the new managed care structure, the problems of the original relationship still exist, but in addition, each new relationship adds its own vulnerabilities. Although every clinical problem in which there is a third-party payer involves all three parties, it is useful to look at each set separately.

THE PSYCHOTHERAPIST–PATIENT–MCO RELATIONSHIP

Simon Redd, a clinical social worker, worked with an employee assistance program (EAP) that provided up to six sessions of counseling. Fortunately, some of the problems of the EAP patients involved crisis situations that actually could be addressed in six sessions of solution focused therapy. In addition, many of the people with whom this particular EAP worked carried insurance that could be used if the EAP coverage was not sufficient. Thus, if a patient showed serious problems, Simon Redd would contact the insurer and advocate for longer therapy or inpatient treatment.

Bruce was a cocaine addict. His wife had thrown him out of the house. His boss had thrown him off the job. Bruce had spent his last dollars on a line of coke six hours before he showed up at Simon Redd's office.

"I believe we can get you help," Mr. Redd said softly.

"I don't know if I can hold on," Bruce said.

Simon Redd immediately called the managed care company. "I have an emergency," he explained. "The patient is a cocaine addict. He is experiencing withdrawal symptoms and psychological decompensation. He needs hospitalization. Please authorize inpatient treatment immediately." The case manager asked many questions and left Mr. Redd with the impression that she would provide authorization within a few hours.

Bruce showed up the next day.

"I'm losing it," he said. "What did the insurance company say?"

"They haven't called yet. I'll call them right now with you here." The voice mail of the case manager said that she was temporarily away from her desk. Mr. Redd left his name and telephone number and said that it was an urgent situation. Turning to his patient, who looked as though he had not slept at all, Mr. Redd asked Bruce if he could talk about what was going on for him. Bruce was able to stay for the whole session although he had to jump up several times and he kept looking at the door as though he were about to bolt out of the room.

Mr. Redd called the MCO again. By the end of the day, he had put in four telephone calls. Each time, the case manager told him that she would get back to him with the information.

The next day Bruce arrived without his jacket. His face was streaked with dirt and sweat.

"I don't know what to do," he cried, his voice full of rage and fear.

"You need to go into the hospital now," Mr. Redd said. "Insurance approval or not."

"No." Bruce shook his head. "There's no money. They won't take me."

He ran out of the office.

Mr. Redd called the managed care company after every patient he saw that day. At one point, the case manager told him that the computers were down. At another, the case manager apologized for the delay, explaining that there had been a change in procedures for hospitalization.

"If you do not hear from the authorization department by the end of the day, please call me."

At 4:30, her voice message informed him that she was not at her desk. At 5:00, she had left.

On the fourth day, Bruce didn't show up at Mr. Redd's office. The MCO representative who covered hospital authorization for this case returned Simon Redd's call.

"Hospitalization is approved," the authorization manager said. "Please ask him to wait at home until he is called with an authorization number."

Bruce called later that day distraught and incoherent. He said he was on his way to the city. Both therapist and patient knew that meant he was going to meet the people with whom he got high on cocaine. Mr. Redd pleaded with him to go home to get the authorization number and promised to meet him at the hospital. Bruce went home, but there were no messages on his answering machine. He found the licensed pistol that he kept in a locked box in the bedroom. He started driving to meet his friends, but for some reason, he took a detour back to work. He started walking toward his office. When his boss called a greeting out to him, Bruce turned and fired at his boss, killing him instantly.

There was talk of a major lawsuit against the managed care company. Investigation, however, revealed that Bruce's urine had been tested soon after he arrived at jail. Because it had been four days since his last line of cocaine, the urine came back clean. That meant there was no evidence of drug abuse. The insurance company was not liable.

The story of Simon Redd's attempt to get help for his patient illustrates the frustration that many psychotherapists are experiencing as they try to provide psychotherapy for their patients. MCOs interfere with the psychotherapist–patient relationship by violating confidentiality, by overriding the psychotherapist's clinical judgment, and by intrusions into the therapeutic interventions that comprise the relationship between the psychotherapist and the patient.

THE PSYCHOTHERAPIST–PATIENT RELATIONSHIP

Karen Shore (1996c) maintains that each individual considering psychotherapy is entitled to three essential rights: (1) the right of choice, (2) the right to make decisions, and (3) the right to privacy. MCOs have taken over all three of these patients' rights in psychotherapy. The right of choice is denied when patients must use only network providers, short-term therapy, and a system of utilization determined by established protocols and implemented by case managers, or gatekeepers.

"The case reviewers," writes John Iglehart (1996) "using clinical protocols to guide them, assign patients to the least expensive appropriate treatment" (p. 133). Consequently, the right to participate in decisions is also relinquished. A case manager or gatekeeper might insist on medication, termination of sessions, referral to self-help groups, or community services. Neither the patient nor clinician has any choice. The psychotherapist can appeal the denial, which often entails a long process that sometimes leads to peer review and sometimes to another denial. At each step of the process, the patient's right to privacy is jeopardized.

Studies have shown that when patients lose the rights to choice, decision, and privacy, psychotherapy is compromised. Denkers and Clifford (1994) reported that 57 percent of 173 psychologists participating in a study indicated that managed care denials had damaged their patients' progress. In the same year, the *Consumer Reports* (Seligman 1996) study of 4000 readers who sought professional help found that respondents who had insurance plans that limited length, frequency, and type of therapist reported poorer outcomes than patients whose treatment was not restricted in these ways. In an earlier Lou Harris Poll (1991), nearly 80 percent of the subjects regarded privacy as a fundamental right, while 70 percent believed that they had lost control over personal information (EPIC 1996a).

Most patients have not had the experience to fully understand the significance of Big Brother in the treatment room. They assume that managed care will take care of the money and stay out of the therapy. Patients are often reluctant to recognize that Big Brother's surveillance is not benign. Many patients appear satisfied with having the psychotherapist submit the claims and receive the fees without their input, thus eliminating themselves from the loop. They do not understand that they have given up control of their therapy. They surrender choices of therapist, type of therapy, control of payment arrangements, and privacy. "I explain the realities of managed care to patients all the time without regard to MCO restrictions on what I am supposed to conceal," says a clinical social worker, "but they don't really understand the significance of what I am saying. Sure, they are afraid of the financial cost of treatment, but it's more than that. You can't expect patients to know about the principles of psychotherapy and you can't expect the industries to care. Yet MCO therapists have to negotiate with the industry on behalf of the patient. They can't do it alone. That's why I keep trying to get patients to advocate for themselves. If patients take care of their insurance issues, maybe we can get back to the fundamental psychotherapist–patient relationship."

There has been increasing concern in this country with issues of privacy and confidentiality for the general public (e.g. Alderman and Kennedy 1995) and with confidentiality in the psychotherapist–patient relationship, in particular (e.g., Bollas and Sundelson 1995). Bollas and Sundelson discuss several critical ways in which confidentiality is betrayed in psychotherapy. With regard to insurance companies, they take the position that psychoanalysis for certain, and many other forms of psychotherapy as well, cannot be effective when practiced in conjunction with MCO regulations. They state that psychoanalysts and their patients under managed care cannot form the inner psychic space that is essential to the creation of psychoanalysis, and further, "Without that space, the form of treatment that has carefully evolved for over 100 years cannot exist" (p. 99).

In a special report on the loss of confidence in psychotherapy, Tamar Lewin (1996) reports the case of Arnold Holzman, a Connecticut psychologist. According to Lewin, Dr. Holzman thought he was making progress with an upper-level manager who came to psychotherapy only after his wife threatened to leave him if he did not gain control of his angry outbursts. The patient developed sufficient trust in Dr. Holzman to talk about the sources of his anger and depression. Dr. Holzman worried about what would happen to that trust when he told the patient that the MCO paying for the treatment was coming to inspect the therapist's files.

Dr. Holzman's concern was justified. Following the inspection of Dr. Holzman's files by the MCO, the patient became more concerned about what he was saying and whether the psychotherapist would have to write it down. The patient stopped coming to therapy a few visits later. Dr. Holzman is convinced that his patient left treatment because he knew that his privacy could be compromised.

Lewin points out that confidentiality has been considered one of the fundamentals of treatment, a prerequisite for giving patients the freedom to explore their innermost feelings and fantasies. "Indeed, many therapists say confidentiality is to therapy what a sterile field is to surgery—a basic requirement of good practice" (p. 1).

Dr. Hera had been a school psychologist who had gone on to complete a clinical internship and to successfully pass state tests for licensing in psychology. He continued his studies to include special training in the techniques of crisis intervention and also in the treatment of adolescents. With his background and license, Dr. Hera had a successful private practice. When managed care expanded into his region, Dr. Hera enrolled with several different organizations, and the struggle to keep up with their demands began. One day, an adolescent patient with suicidal ideation was referred to him. The patient's family was covered by one of Dr. Hera's MCOs, and precertification was required before therapy could begin. Hera made numerous calls for precertification but was met with busy signals, long waits, and the intricacies of computerized voice mail. Assessing that the patient was in crisis, he scheduled the first session without precertification. Over the next several weeks he called repeatedly and left voice mail messages on the MCO's provider relations line. Despite the lack of response, Hera continued to see the patient. After five weeks he finally made contact with the MCO. The patient authorization was denied. Dr. Hera never got paid.

"It wasn't just the money," said Hera, "it was the way they treated the whole situation. It didn't matter that the patient was suicidal. It did not matter that the patient and I had developed a caring relationship. It did not matter that ethics required me to continue seeing him. It didn't matter that their telephone lines were jammed and no one returned messages. All that mattered was the precertification. And I never got it."

Dr. Hera was in the enviable position of having options. Working part time now at a private secondary school, he is writing a book about treating adolescent patients in crisis situations, but he worries that psychotherapists in managed care practices may not be able to follow even minimal guidelines for appropriate treatment.

Dr. Hera left his private practice to work in other ways within the field. Not all psychotherapists are willing or able to make the same choice. There are other choices. For example, Edward Shapiro, Ph.D. (1996) developed a program at Austin Riggs that encourages patients to advocate on their own with insurance carriers. Despite the obvious therapeutic value of Shapiro's procedures, not all psychotherapists have found success with the same method.

Certainly, in some situations, the patient can argue his or her case directly with the MCO. If that does not work, the patient can terminate therapy and live with the problem or arrange for private sessions on a fee for service basis. However, many MCOs do not allow providers to see patients privately. In many cases the patient does not have the resources for private therapy, leaving both patient and therapist at risk. Can a psychotherapist ethically deny a patient treatment because he or she has run out of sessions? Should a psychotherapist work for little or no fee because an MCO decides to reduce expenses even further? Is there any compromise between the position of the MCOs, on the one hand, and the psychotherapist–patient dyad on the other?

When psychotherapists cannot find ways to practice with integrity and satisfaction, they look for ways to regain control of their profession. When patients feel that their integrity is being violated, they cannot benefit from psychotherapy. The Coalition of Mental Health Professionals and Consumers, Inc. in Commack, New York, keeps records of complaints about psychotherapists and patient experiences with MCOs. There are many examples of people who left psychotherapy rather than allow the continuation of divulging deeply personal information to MCOs.

THE PSYCHOTHERAPIST–MCO RELATIONSHIP

Dr. Devon listened carefully when the new patient called for an appointment.

"I'm covered by Life Healthcare of Rhode Island," she explained.

Devon got off the telephone with her new client. She knew that Life covered her for psychotherapy but was unaware of the specifics. Devon called Life Healthcare.

"Thank you for calling Life," a recorded voice said. "All our representatives are busy. We appreciate your call. Please hold for the next available representative."

A half hour later a live voice came on the wire. "Can I help you?"

Devon explained the case and was told she had the wrong number to register patients. She was given another number. She dialed the second number and was told that the client had a $200 individual deductible, $350 family deductible, and they would pay 80 percent for the first 30 visits and 60 percent for the next 30 visits up to a $3500 annual maximum. Patient registration was not required. Devon quickly wrote down the numbers and hung up.

It was then that she realized that she did not know whether the deductibles were only for mental health or could be applied for all health care. A repeat call brought her through two voice menus and a 20-minute wait. The new live voice told Devon that she could not possibly have received that information because mental health had to be registered at their office on Long Island, New York. Devon wrote down the new number and, feeling quite annoyed, thanked the representative.

After several attempts, Devon finally got through to a live voice at the Long Island office.

"I'm sorry," the Long Island representative said sweetly, "but we are not directly responsible for registering mental health patients. You have to contact Comprehensive Health Benefits."

Once again, Devon scratched out a telephone number and replaced it with a new one.

Comprehensive Health Benefits also had a lengthy voice menu system. Every time she made a menu selection she was greeted by telephone music. Devon did not have time to enjoy the music.

A live voice finally responded, informing Devon that she was called "Mary." No last name was offered.

"Of course I can register your client," Mary said, "I just need a little information."

Devon read the demographics.

When she was finished there was a long pause.

"I'm sorry," Mary said. "There is a problem with the computers. I can only authorize two sessions right now. You will have to call back in two weeks for additional sessions."

Devon glanced at her watch. The entire process had taken 1½ hours. "Thank you Mary," she said. And slammed the telephone into its receiver.

But it wasn't over.

When the new client showed up for her first session, she was apologetic. She had made a terrible mistake. Life was her secondary insurance company. Her primary insurance company was Employee Benefit Plan.

Devon had to start all over again.

Many psychotherapists believe that it is their duty to interpret to their patients the meanings of having Big Brother as an economic partner in treatment. This can be a very delicate process, particularly if an MCO prohibits or discourages disclosing information to patients. Patients frequently find it difficult to understand how an earned benefit can work against the beneficiary. In most cases, the alternative—paying out of pocket—is not an available option. "When managed care focuses on money and in turn, the therapist focuses on dealing with the MCO, patient treatment becomes secondary," adds Daly (1996).

How can mental health care professionals accept a situation in which the psychotherapist–patient relationship is secondary to the psychotherapist–MCO relationship? Obviously, they cannot both remain committed to their profession and accept being unable to practice with integrity. For most psychotherapists, there are only two paths to follow. Psychotherapists can work to change MCO regulations or they can practice outside of the managed care industry.

There are training seminars and established groups to support a psychotherapist's choice. For example, *Professional Health Plan Publications* (Polonsky 1996a) offers a guide to working in a practice free of managed care. The Coalition of Mental Health Professionals and Consumers offers guidance in ways to advocate for change and in procedures for practice outside of managed care.

Managed care may affect practitioners by limiting their access to patients. Managed care panels are closed to two types of practitioners: those who have been terminated and those who have not been accepted initially. Termination can come at any time, without any warning, in many situations for reasons that may never be known to the practitioner. Termination can be the ultimate MCO punishment. MCOs can also reject applicants without providing explanation. A case in point is the situation reported in many communities of well-established clinicians who refused to join managed care when it first came to town. These clinicians usually had a good reason to be reluctant. Why become part of a system that regulated treatment and reduced fees? Most did not foresee the inevitability of MCO penetration.

Among those who were reluctant to join MCOs were the highly trained psychoanalysts who believed that third-party payments interfered with treatment. Although these practitioners traditionally have been reluctant to be involved with insurance issues, at present they may be feeling pressure to become part of an MCO system in order to accommodate patients in treatments other than psychoanalysis. However, it appears that many MCOs reject providers if they indicate a psychoanalytic degree or training.

Recent predictions about the end of solo practices has had an impact on many psychotherapists. Accordingly, the managed care provider is often very careful to maintain participation. Usually they are "so scared of being dropped from panels they carefully adhere to both the spirit and the letter of their managed care agreements," observes Hillowe (1996).

While there seems to be agreement that MCOs intrude on treatment and create difficulties for patients, there has not been very much discussion about the effects of managed care on the psychotherapist. Henry Saeman (1996b), editor *of The National Psychologist*, reports a study in which 75 percent of the respondents, all psychologists, answered that their experiences with managed care were unfavorable. There was also a general dejection reported by the psychotherapists who also reported being disheartened by the current health care environment. When asked to describe their greatest concerns about the future of professional psychology, the psychotherapists reported that they were concerned with survival, the demise of private practice, and the "loss of enthusiasm for doing a very fascinating job" (p. 1).

The contracts that psychotherapists must sign are sometimes at odds with both their own professional ethics and assumptions made by patients. Chad Breckenridge (1995) expressed concern about these contracts in his "President's Report" to the National Federation of Societies for Clinical Social Workers. "Increasingly . . . the membership is being asked to sign on to contract language and then practice in ways that place the member in violation of the code of ethics of a variety of professions they belong to and/or state boards" (p. 3).

D. G. Phillips (1995), Co-Chair of the Committee on Professional Standards at the National Federation of Societies for Clinical Social Work, suggests that psychotherapists suffer inner conflicts that interfere with psychotherapy when they enter into a managed care arrangement in which they receive financial benefits for providing a level of care below what is optimum for a patient. Conflicts of conscience definitely occur when psychotherapists are told to provide short-term treatment when they believe that long-term psychotherapy would better serve a patient's needs. This issue has become so controversial that numerous bills in state and federal legislatures have been proposed to establish "anti-gag" rules in managed health care (see Chapter 5). Many of these proposals would prohibit MCOs from limiting a provider's right to discuss a condition or course of treatment with the patient. The provider would be guaranteed the right to initiate or participate in an appeal when treatment has been denied. In addition, if a psychotherapist believes that long-term treatment is necessary, he or she would be able to address this option with the patient and appeal a case manager's denial without fearing that there might be unfavorable consequences as a result of advocating for the patient.

MCOs are continuously presenting ways to shorten psychotherapy. Based on the belief that medication is a cost-effective treatment, MCO policies instruct case managers to encourage the use of drugs in psychotherapy. In an article concerning MCO pressure to use medication in psychotherapy, E. J. Pollack (1995) quotes Dr. Gottlieb, a Chicago psychiatrist: "Pressure from managed care firms to choose drugs over therapy ranges from subtle to explicit" (p. A1). Gottlieb also states that he is encouraged by MCOs to find some symptom that responds to medication. Gottlieb reports that he and his colleagues often are given only one session to evaluate a patient for medication. Follow-ups are limited to periodic 10- to 20-minute "med-checks" to review dosages. Most MCOs discourage psychiatrists from doing any assessments other than the proscribed procedures for assessing medication.

According to Pollack (1995), the economics are clear. Drugs are cheaper than psychotherapy. A managed care plan can save up to 30 percent in treatment costs by using psychiatric consultations and medications in place of psychotherapy. Managed care administrators argue that medications are better for patients because, among other things, drug therapy relieves pain faster that psychotherapy.

Many MCOs, suggests Pollack, contain costs by establishing a hierarchy of preferred treatments for mental illness. For example, they begin with using the older, less expensive tricyclic antidepressants such as imipramine, desipramine, and amitriptyline, which cost about six cents a pill wholesale. Patients are expected to endure the side affects which may include weight gain, dry mouth, and irregular heartbeat. For most patients, the newer antidepressants—selective serotonin reuptake inhibitors such as Prozac, Paxil, and Zoloft—are as good or better than the tricyclics. There are fewer side effects and it is more difficult to take a fatal overdose. But often cost considerations prevail. The average wholesale price of Prozac is $2.24 per pill resulting in a typical retail price of $77.40 for a 30-day supply of Prozac

(20mg daily) for a patient who lives in Long Island, New York. The same patient would be charged $3.95 for a 30-day supply of imipramine (75mg daily). Which drug will MCOs endorse?

Most psychotherapists maintain that medication is indicated when the condition warrants its use, not when it is a cost containment effort by managed care. Bollas and Sundelson (1995) say that "No drug, in and of itself, consistently resolves human pain and conflict. The health care industry, however, looks for the quick fix: a worker ready to go back on the job and no longer a burden to company funds" (p. 64).

The business regulations and corporate structures of MCOs create further complications with regard to medications. Many health insurance plans (Winslow 1996) provide formularies to doctors who prescribe drugs for their patients. The goal of a formulary, which is simply a list of approved medications, is to limit the use of expensive medicines, encouraging the cheaper, generic versions. One way to compile formularies is the cost containment hierarchy previously mentioned. However, there are cases where the MCO is owned by a pharmaceutical company. Pharmaceutical companies make money by selling their more expensive brand name drugs. These interlocking financial relationships can directly affect the formulary. Robert Daly (1996b) observes that when drug companies own MCOs, they preferentially list their own drugs on the formulary.

The Wall Street Journal (Winslow 1996) reported a study of cost containment practices with 13,000 patients in five HMOs. Ironically, the results indicated that patients who had the most restricted access to prescription drugs also had the highest overall health care costs. Patients in an MCO with an unrestricted formulary incurred the lowest costs in this study.

MCO procedures with regard to medication are even more alarming when one considers how professionals are being encouraged to use psychotropic drugs with children. Psychotherapy with children usually involves a more complex effort that addresses individual and family problems. This is costly. It is far less expensive to prescribe Ritalin or Prozac and let the schools deal with the problem. Providers under contract to managed care experience the conflict produced by the pressure to rely on prescription drugs to treat a range of problems.

Although mild depression may be the presenting problem, underlying problems may exist, creating potential dangers for the patient, the family, and the community. When the problem is not amenable to brief therapy, the therapist faces a battle with a managed care case manager over additional sessions. Who are the case managers? Many of them lack sufficient past experience or formal education, and lack current training or support in understanding the ramifications of the decisions they are expected to provide. Although MCOs now expect case managers to participate in a formal credentialing system, the case managers are not expected to question the principles that are taught.

If the patient in therapy has not improved and further certification is denied, what happens next? The psychotherapist can appeal the denial of benefits. Appelbaum (1993) suggests that providers may have an obligation to advocate for their patients. In a case where a patient was suing a state Medicaid plan for damages resulting from denial of care, the California Judge who heard the case wrote that "The physician who complies without protest with the limitations imposed by a third-party payer, when his medical judgment dictates otherwise, cannot avoid his ultimate responsibility for the patient's care" (Appelbaum 1993, p. 253). The obligation to advocate for patients opens up a Pandora's Box. Who is ultimately responsible for denial of benefits and the consequent risk of malpractice litigation? If providers must pursue appeals, how far must they go? How much unpaid time should be spent on the appeal? How does a provider select which cases to appeal and which to ignore? Is a provider obligated to appeal when there is little or no chance of success? And how does a provider balance the obligation to advocate for the patient with the reality of retaliation from the MCO?

DR. HIMMELSTEIN'S STORY

What happens when a provider protests too loudly?

Dr. Himmelstein's story was told in the January 8, 1996 issue of *Time*. Himmelstein, a physician in the northeast, signed up with one of the largest regional HMOs. That meant signing a contract that included what he called a gag clause. Himmelstein publicly stated that "I can't tell my patients if there's something wrong [with what] the HMO insists I do."

He was referring to his HMO's policy of awarding monetary incentives to doctors who limited referrals to specialists, emergency room use (by patients), and hospital stays.

Three days after Himmelstein appeared on the Phil Donahue Show his HMO contract was terminated.

Big Brother is awarded the power, by both patient and provider, to set the rules for treatment. To illustrate, many psychotherapists believe that a patient's ambivalence about treatment may contribute to forgetting an appointment or to canceling at the last minute. When psychotherapists believe that the patient is resisting treatment by forgetting or canceling sessions, they sometimes decide to discuss charging for missed sessions. It is generally believed that people who pay for sessions are less likely to forget them. Under managed care a psychotherapist cannot charge for missed sessions. Charging the MCO is likely to be considered fraudulent while charging the patient is likely to be prohibited by contract with the MCO. In addition, MCOs prohibit psychotherapists from waiving or decreasing co-payments. If a psychotherapist accepts $10 less on a co-payment, the MCO may view it as a $10 reduction of the psychotherapy fee. The psychotherapist can then be accused of insurance fraud for raising fees to increase third-party benefits. On the other hand, if the therapist agrees to accept a lower co-payment without informing the MCO, the therapist can be accused of collusion and violation of professional ethics. If a therapist decides that a patient is in need of treatment but cannot afford the co-payment at the time of treatment, then the psychotherapist may decide that it is in the patient's interest to allow the patient to owe the psychotherapist the co-payment. There are several issues that need to be considered. One issue is theoretical: Is it therapeutically justified to burden a patient with debt? What effect does this have on the patient–therapist relationship? On the other hand, is it ethically justified to accept the MCO directives concerning payment? Obviously, co-payment considerations are similar to the issues of fees in general. Many psychotherapists accept the compromise solution of allowing the patient to remain in debt for the co-payment amount until a later time in treatment or following termination of treatment.

Managed care also takes control from psychotherapists by producing a proliferation of forms, reports, and procedures that are often arbitrary and redundant. Many practitioners complain that for every five days of work there is at least one entire day devoted to paperwork and telephone calls. The psychotherapist absorbs the added burden and expense of billing and paperwork. The ability to navigate the system, understand its conflicts, and practice within professionally ethical guidelines has become a skill essential to running a successful managed care practice (see Part II).

One of the most troublesome impacts of managed care on practitioners may be the demise of the solo practice. In 1994 *The National Psychologist* reported that in their survey of 300 psychologists about half "felt sufficiently well positioned to maintain the status quo in their practices" (p. 1). Almost two years later in a similar study, *The National Psychologist* found that 82 percent of the respondents reported being "somewhat" or "very" concerned about continuing as a practitioner. In a chilling prediction, Robert H. Wiener (1995) wrote:

> "The independent practice of medicine and psychology will be replaced by a system dominated by a few giant, vertically integrated firms. Accountability within the system will be to corporate stockholders to maintain profits and maximize returns on investments, not to the consumers of health care." [p. 6]

Managed care employees, providers, and solo practitioners all seem to agree on this trend. Hullet (1996) talks about multi-disciplinary groups of preferred providers, while Lardiere (1996) refers to the uncertain future of a solo practitioner who tries to go against the trend. The financial analysts view professional grouping as a process necessary to compete in the new health care marketplace. Solo practitioners are looking toward networking, marketing groups, and affiliations to maintain their caseloads. Professional groups such as the American Mental Health Alliance are organizing "cooperatives" that contract directly with payers. Even provider-owned HMOs are appearing, like Island Behavioral Health (IBH), the mental health arm of MDLI (Saeman 1996). Political action advocates like Karen Shore bring professionals from many disciplines, as well as consumers, into groups that press for reform, such as the National Coalition for Mental Health Professionals and Consumers.

Working with practitioner groups, rather than individuals, helps reduce costs. Hullet (1996) observes that "micromanaging cases is very expensive." Health care cost savings were so dramatic in the beginning that the high administrative costs were often hidden. Hullet believes that the next thrust in managed care will be to cut internal costs, shifting both responsibility and administrative decisions to carefully selected providers who know the system and have been identified as both high quality and low utilizers. MCOs will contract with these practitioner groups offering less centralized administrative work, more patient referrals, and increased clinical autonomy in exchange for strict adherence to the corporation's treatment approach. Hullet predicts that this will be a temporary solution to the shift, eventually fading as cost savings naturally decrease over the life of the contract. He proposes that the future of managed care ultimately lies at the point when "the return on investment is enough to maintain the system—based on the market force of equilibrium" (1996).

It has become necessary to deal with the requirements of MCOs in the treatment room. Managed care requirements can lead to delicate conflict-of-interest problems for the therapist. For example, what does the therapist do with a patient who shows sudden manic behavior when there are no additional treatment sessions authorized? The therapist may be ethically committed to continue treatment. Failure to conform to professional standards of practice by passive agreement to termination when the psychotherapist believes active intervention will better serve the patient can be an instance of malpractice. The psychotherapist can try to negotiate a lower fee but such negotiations may violate the provider contract. What if a needy patient cannot pay? "Should one continue treatment of the patient without compensation?" asks Appelbaum (1993). "If one is expected to extend free care to this patient, how much of one's caseload must be nonpaying before it is permissible to decline to offer such services?" (p. 254).

Managed care, in its provider contracts, has increasingly placed that responsibility on the shoulders of the therapist. These conditions guarantee that the psychotherapist–managed care relationship will continue to be in tension. Hullet (1996) believes that there will be increased insistence by MCOs on placing the responsibility of decision making on the provider.

Fortunately, the legal system has begun to intervene. According to Bryant Welch, J.D., Ph.D. (1996), developments in the legal realm coupled with recent increased public attention to the managed care industry has produced a ground swell of MCO litigation in the legal field. At this point, it appears likely that psychotherapists will soon be better able to practice their profession with integrity and greater satisfaction than predicted by MCO executives.

THE PATIENT–MCO RELATIONSHIP

MCOs actually have two customers: the payer (employer or other agency) and the patient, and that duality eludes many patients. With two customers, managed care has to address the needs of both. The payers are the customers who contract with the MCO, providing billions of dollars for health services. The payers are usually employers, government agencies, or organizations of various types. All payers are not treated equally. A company with 12,000 employees gets a much better deal than a company with 12 employees.

TO THE LOWEST BIDDER . . .

According to a study by the behavioral health research firm, Open Minds, MCOs have dramatically changed who provides therapy by favoring the lowest bidder (NASW News 1996a). The study was based on a 10,000-member health plan in the southwest that converted from fee-for-service to managed care in 1994. The following chart indicates the changes in types of providers and their fees for outpatient visits before and after the advent of managed care.

	Percentage of Outpatient Visits		Average Fees	
	Before MCO	After MCO	Before MCO	After MCO
Social Workers	5%	56%	$85	$65
Psychologists	10%	33%	$100	$75
Psychiatrists	85%	11%	$150	$90

MCOs must balance the needs of the payer against the needs of the patient. If the payers do not like what they get, they can go to another MCO. Competition for payers is fierce, forcing each MCO to constantly prove its worth. In the corporate world, worth is based on how much money is made or how much money is saved. Cost containment then becomes an essential marketing tool. Obviously, this leads to serious conflicts of interest. If the MCO watches the activities of the treatment room as a representative of the payer, does that mean that the payer is entitled to access the information? If so, can this inside information be used against the patient in the workplace? If an employee has a history of depression, can that information be used to make a decision on whether or not to promote him or her? Does that violate privacy or discrimination laws? How close can one go toward violating the Americans with Disabilities Act (ADA)? It may be difficult to differentiate between discrimination and cost containment. Both the employer and the managed care company will save money by not having a person on their rolls who suffers from a chronic, costly condition. In *American Health* magazine, Joseph Anthony (1993) wrote about a man who worked in an office with only eight employees. In one year, the man's family incurred extraordinary health care expenses.

> Everyone in the office knows that the family's health problems have contributed to the group's steadily rising health care premiums. People say, "Gee, your family is so sick all the time"—as if being sick is something we were choosing to do. . . . [p. 56]

Using medical or mental health information to make corporate decisions violates an individual's privacy. But how can anyone demonstrate that in this instance Joe got the promotion over Jack because Jack's wife has panic attacks? Cost containment can have many faces.

MCOs manipulate these faces skillfully. Despite studies that support the effectiveness of psychotherapy in helping people to return to work and in reducing medical expenses, MCO executives point to selected studies to justify claims that psychotherapy may not be helpful. These executives are likely to ignore long-term gains. They want to demonstrate short-term improvement in order to sell their treatment plans and earn short-term profits. "I don't think we will ever go back to long-term therapy," predicts Mike Lardiere, M.S.W., Director of Provider Relations at GHI-BMP. "People will find more creative ways to provide services in areas such as group work, biofeedback, and hypnosis" (1996).

Pharmaceutical companies may also expose patients to unexpected breaches of confidentiality. John Riley (1996b) reports the story of an employee who innocently utilized his company's drug plan. The employee did not know that the plan was based on estimated cost, making the employer responsible for 115 percent of the amount exceeding the estimate. The employer decided to audit the plan and requested general patient information. The drug plan obliged. They compiled a list of employees who spent over $100 per month. Then they supplied the patient names and the drugs they used. Consequently, the company's chief administration officer was able to identify an employee as HIV-positive by his use of costly anti-AIDS drugs. She took this information and discussed it with two company medical officers and the chief of benefits. Eventually, the legal department advised her to keep quiet. The case ended up in court. Riley writes that the practice is not unique and reports that several pharmaceutical benefit administrators say that they share patient-specific information with employers. Some companies may provide names and prescriptions as part of their standard employer information package.

P. J. O'Rourke (1995) wrote a funny essay about health care reform. The essay is a response to Clinton's health care plan which O'Rourke criticized with rather heavy-footed humor. Unlike his criticism of the national health care proposals, however, O'Rourke's summary of the effects of managed care on health care professionals and consequently on patients revealed a penetration of issues and a wit worthy of a satirist.

O'Rourke started with the common observation that the health care system with which Clinton and the rest of us suffered was too complicated and too expensive. Noting that the Clinton plan appeared even more complicated and possibly more expensive, O'Rourke looked at what both the proposed national plans and the current managed care plans are doing to the best people in the health care professions. O'Rourke asked, "What type of person is going to become a doctor, a nurse, or, for that matter, a health insurance executive just to wind up as a bureaucratic goat or governmental hack? Students with straight A's can get more entrepreneurial freedom tarring roofs. There will come a day when you'll be wheeled in for a heart bypass operation and the surgeon will be the same fellow who's now behind the counter when you renew your car registration at the Department of Motor Vehicles" (p. 281).

O'Rourke criticized the Clinton plan especially as it related to managed health care systems. He described the effects of managed care on the health and well being of patients:

> President Clinton is attempting to convince the American voters that they're going to be able to get sick cheaply. He's right. Getting sick has always been cheap, often free. It's getting well that costs a whole lot of money. When the price of an item is fixed above market value, there is a surplus of that item—as the Arabs discovered with oil. When the price of an item is fixed below market value, that item disappears—as the Russians discovered with everything. We have here a basic law of economics. The price of health care will be fixed below market value. And we're all going to die. [p. 282]

3

Doublethink

Doublethink *means the power of holding two contradictory beliefs in one's mind simultaneously, and accepting both of them . . . it is a vast system of mental cheating.*

–George Orwell, 1984

Across the country, psychotherapists are finding comfort in discussing their profession among colleagues in networking groups. Recently, the most popular topic is managed care. The following comments are typical:

- I do not understand business ethics.
- The people who do utilization review need to protect their own salaries.
- A case manager determined that my treatment of a certain patient was not medically necessary. The manager has no medical education, no experience with psychotherapy, and no valid standards for evaluating the necessity of treatment.
- The physician who refers to me has a new capitation agreement whereby he loses income each time I see one of the referred patients.
- Of course I cannot abandon my patients for whom the MCOs are refusing payment, but if I don't make room in my schedule for patients who can pay for therapy, I will have to close my practice.

The psychotherapists in this group are grappling with doublethink concepts. While it is not likely that the new industries are intentionally confusing the professional workers as was the case in *1984*, the effect on psychotherapists is similar. They are feeling displaced and demoralized. They are looking for ways to control their lives and to protect their profession. The goals of psychotherapists and those of managed care businesses clash around the central concept of providing care. Psychotherapists are trained to provide appropriate treatment; MCO managers are trained to provide disincentives for seeking and accessing treatment. From a business point of view, MCO managers need to be responsible to their investors and refrain from criminal activities. MCOs do not have ethical responsibilities to the people seeking care. Health care professionals have refined their ethical standards over centuries of health care development and hold ethical principles central to all of their work.

Managed care doublethink has created a new assortment of clinical pitfalls that test both professional and personal values. In a 1994 national survey conducted by Tucker and Lubin (Miller 1995), 72 percent of the responding psychologists reported that managed care negatively affected the quality of treatment and 90 percent reported that reviewers often interfered with sound clinical treatment plans. "It is not uncommon for people to come up to me and say things like, 'I know what you mean by managed care problems. My mother was killed by managed care,'" says Ivan Miller. "Managed care is designed in a way that it can only harm quality" (p. 2).

The rapid change from "psychotherapist" to "provider" has triggered a global professional insecurity not found before the advent of Big Brother. The questions raised are similar to those of anyone who experiences unregulated occupational upheaval. Just as the Industrial Revolution uprooted and bewildered millions of people, the industrialization of psychotherapy is challenging the principles of private clinicians in the world of mental health. One need only read the articles and books written by experienced practitioners, attend the conferences throughout the nation, or listen to the frustration expressed by mental health professionals in order to understand the demoralizing effect of managed care.

Psychotherapists with extensive training and years of experience suddenly find themselves laid off in public sector downsizing, or taking jobs on a fee-for-service basis, or in struggling practices with too many empty hours. Patient time is often exchanged for paperwork, telephone quarrels with poorly trained case managers, and repeated rejections from closed provider panels. With de-professionalization, fewer salaried jobs, and MCOs' preference for group practices, mental health providers are getting cheaper and cheaper to employ. "Burnout thus becomes endemic and one hears more people wishing out loud they had gone into some other line of work," observes Chipman (1995). "The profits from therapists' labor go ever less into their own pockets just as the conditions of their work are dictated less by their own needs and judgment" (p. 565).

In *What Managed Care is Doing to Outpatient Mental Health* (1994), Ivan Miller wrote that managed care published some flashy examples of ways to cut expenses in outpatient mental health care including the following:

> Stop the California syndrome—stop paying for people who want to talk and grow.
> Stop the New Yorker syndrome—replace expensive treatments like psychoanalysis.
> Stop the Rich Doctor syndrome—bargain for lower fees from wealthy providers.
> Stop the Woody Allen syndrome—stop excessively long and unproductive treatment. [p. 5]

The industrialized psychotherapist has lost autonomy, social status, and income. With Big Brother in the treatment room, providers increasingly resemble employees who are being strictly observed by an overzealous supervisor. It is no surprise that many psychotherapists are "opting out," seeking alternatives to the managed care paradigm (see Part III).

Kristy Kolmansberger (1996), Network Development Specialist at CMG, disagrees with this view. "Providers are now feeling more comfortable with managed care. They have discovered that it is not a defensive relationship but more of a partnership. This is an important shift in attitude and can lead to less management. When there is a willingness between managed care and provider to work together then a lot of good things can happen" (p. 1).

Some psychotherapists are affiliating themselves with organizations that seek reform. An important example is the National Coalition of Mental Health Professionals and Consumers, whose goal is to "save ethical mental health care" (Shore 1995a). Three years ago, the group consisted of a few professionals and one consumer who met in a private home in Long Island, New York. Today it is a national organization with over 1300 members and 25 affiliated groups (Shore 1995b).

Mary Sykes Wylie (1994), senior editor of the *Family Therapy Networker*, aptly described the situation in her article, "The New Visionaries."

> Nobody knows where therapy is going, and increasingly fewer and fewer even seem to know what therapy is anymore. Never have so many therapists been afflicted with such a collective identity crisis, nor has there been a greater sense shared by members of an entire profession that they are standing on the edge of an abyss, wondering how to sprout wings in a hurry. [p. 20]

Where are those wings going to come from? Ivan Miller (1994) believes the demise of managed care is imminent. He compares the operations of

MCOs with the savings and loan scandal, where everyone was making a lot of money without being adequately informed about the field in which they were working and without caring about the effects of their own ignorance, arrogance, and misappropriation of other people's money. Miller estimates that it was fully two years between the time that the savings and loan scandal was exposed and the time that it collapsed. Miller explained that people are observing that managed care is destructive, but there is a time lag between the observation of corruption and actions to correct the corruption.

Many experts feel that legislative reform will ultimately change some of the abusive practices of MCOs. But the law moves slowly and, until then, psychotherapists must survive. Clinicians need to understand and to learn useful ways to explain to their patients the techniques used by managed care. Miller suggests that MCOs diminish both psychotherapists and mental health services by using a combination of policies and procedures that make treatment inaccessible and/or undesirable. He calls it "invisible rationing." Invisible rationing of services is not based on overt denial but on undermining the quality, quantity, and accessibility of treatment. Essentially, costs are contained by eliminating treatment sessions and changing the nature of patient-focused therapy. MCO tactics affect the patient, the psychotherapist, and the dyad, altering the emotional investment in the therapeutic process. In other words, MCOs subtly render certain aspects of psychotherapy so distasteful that the patient chooses to limit or avoid utilization. Miller identifies the following strategies as examples of invisible rationing:

1. gatekeeping,
2. developing consumer "unfriendliness,"
3. using unpopular providers,
4. restricting provider lists,
5. lowering the quality of providers,
6. preventing the treatment of personality disorders,
7. preventing a trusting relationship,
8. undermining privacy,
9. disrupting therapeutic timing,
10. judging and shaming the patient. [p. 19]

Invisible rationing occurs at two levels: one with the patient and one with the psychotherapist. Both levels are effective in discouraging treatment and thus containing costs. According to Joan Shapiro (1995), "Given the fragility of the therapeutic encounter and the stigma of mental illness, it is not difficult to see how these strategies might serve as a deterrent to an embarrassed seeker of needed treatment" (p. 445).

MCOs follow an old principle of frugality: the best way to contain costs is not to incur them in the first place. If the subscriber needs to use his or her benefits, there is a high price to be paid.

THROUGH THE EYES OF THE SUBSCRIBER

The person who seeks psychotherapy is pigeonholed before a request for services is even submitted. John J. Jannes (1996) defines the solution-focused short-term therapy patient as either "visitor, complainer, or customer." Visitors are people who come to psychotherapy just to "check it out," complainers come to "moan and groan" about their lives, and customers are looking for solutions. Therefore, customers are the only patients suitable for treatment. This quickly transforms the therapeutic dyad into a business relationship. The patient-customer is also euphemized as a help-seeker, consumer, covered life, or the particularly offensive "worried well." Managed care newspeak subtly suggests that the process of therapy is a routine fix that should be handled like any business transaction: a quick, clean contract.

Chipman (1995) draws an image of the managed care "reviewer's dream scenario." It is the patient who quickly recovers from the pain of loss or trauma, never questioning decisions made by the insurance company. When meaning has gone out of life—when an individual feels empty and hollow—the good patient numbs himself in a superficial cultural narcissism that involves material consumption and vicarious pleasure. Big Brother's well-behaved covered life asks for little, gets less, and compromises by living with chronic emotional pain. If this cannot be accomplished by the patient alone, Big Brother makes sure it is very clear when treatment is requested and authorized.

> A depressed and suicidal woman had finally left her physically abusive husband. She called her MCO for permission to begin therapy and for a referral. The request was refused. The reason given was that "domestic violence is a social problem, not a psychological one."
>
> —From the National Coalition of Mental Health Professionals and Consumers [1995]

Someone has to mind the store. MCOs use gatekeepers and case managers to do this work. Gatekeepers are primary care physicians who oversee and coordinate a patient's care. They must preauthorize any specialist referrals or hospital admissions unless there is an emergency. In contrast, case managers are administrators who match services with patients' needs (Texas Medical Association 1986). Case manager qualifications range from associate degrees to full professional training. The purpose of gatekeepers and case managers is to reduce utilization and thereby reduce costs. Primary care physicians may be encouraged to do mental health counseling themselves, even though studies like *Consumer Reports* (1995) find that mental health professionals have better results. Earl Appleby, Jr. (1995), Director of CURE Ltd., reports that many managed care companies are finally agreeing with mental health professionals that PCPs frequently fail to recognize mental illness or respond to it appropriately. However, instead of making more referrals MCOs are instituting new programs to facilitate PCPs. Some of these programs include computerized screening and treatment planning, case managers with a range of education from bachelors' degrees to doctorates, and managed care-trained therapists in the PCP office. In contrast, case managers are busy, often overworked, and privy to only a brief, superficial knowledge of the patient. They may deny treatment to a worried well patient, as the newspeak implies—someone who is seeking unnecessary treatment, without enough information.

Appleby (1995) confirms this trend by describing an experimental program that was presented at the National Managed Healthcare Congress in April, 1995. In the program the contractor uses a capitated service that sends only 15 percent of patients into traditional treatment. Mental health services for the remainder are replaced by "meeting in groups to discuss family problems; talking with helpers about on-the-job stress; or visiting PCPs for medication to help them sleep or go to work regularly. They are not told they have a mental illness." Another technique is to push self-help by distributing books. "One, called *How to Take Care of Yourself*," writes Appleby, "provides decision trees to help determine when fever or pain can be handled without medical treatment—and uses the same self-help approach for depression." A national study conducted by the Bazelon Center for Mental Health Law questions the validity of this approach (Saemon 1994). Respondents to this study felt that mental health treatment is a critical part of the health care system. Nearly 82 percent of the 800 people surveyed believe that someone who suffers from mental illness is as sick as someone who suffers from a physical illness. Furthermore, 62 percent felt that there should be parity in treatment between mental health and substance abuse and physical illness.

How does the obstacle to treatment affect the patient seeking psychotherapy? When the value of any service is minimized, it has a significant impact on treatment. The patient may become anxious, worrying about whether therapy is the right choice as well as whether it will be terminated or the insurance claims paid. Can the therapist be trusted when, at any given time, treatment can be discontinued by an outsider? These concerns can exacerbate the patient's symptoms. Fears of abandonment or authority figures may unnecessarily complicate the already abridged treatment (Miller 1995).

"Your decisions are meaningless," says John Grohol (1995), founder of *PsychCentral*, an Internet mental health page. "You see who they tell you to go see, for the prescribed amount of time they will allow you to go see them. . . . Freedom of choice in managed care systems is a moot point."

If customers still insist on utilizing their benefits they can be thwarted by not having the freedom to choose providers. This discourages them from entering psychotherapy. Although there seems to be a trend toward more point of service (POS) coverage, many managed care companies still maintain a network of psychotherapists or a staff who have contracted to follow their rules and regulations. This severely restricts choice of both modality and psychotherapist. Consumers may not be able to take referrals from trusted sources such as family, friends, schools, community associations, or religious affiliations because the name is not on the list. Clinicians know that a patient who enters treatment via a trusted referral often arrives with a far more positive attitude than a patient who gets the referral from a list. MCO executives know that, too. Impersonal lists tend to encourage greater emotional distances that mimic business deals more than psychotherapy. Patients are given the impression that their referral is one of many, not individualized for his or her needs. In addition, patients are frequently deprived of using clinicians who specialize in a specific disorder or area because they are not—and cannot get—on the list. Essentially, by controlling provider selection, managed care business procedures disempower people from the very beginning. In vulnerable patients the procedures reinforce low self-esteem, learned helplessness, and pervasive feelings of inadequacy. Newspage (1996) announced a study that supports this trend. Nearly 41 million Americans had trouble getting some kind of health care—from surgery to eyeglasses to mental health.

Mr. Krane spoke tentatively to the school psychologist about his son Bradley. He was diagnosed as ADHD with extreme difficulty relating to his peers. The school psychologist strongly recommended a local psychotherapist who specialized in children like Bradley.

"He works well with the children," the school psychologist said, "as well as the parents, the teacher, and the school."

As he was scheduling Bradley's first appointment, Mr. Krane mentioned his managed care company. The psychotherapist said he was not on the list.

"Can't you get on the list?" Mr. Krane asked.

"No," the psychotherapist replied. "I've been trying for years. It's a closed list."

Mr. Krane couldn't afford either a full or reduced fee. He never made the appointment.

If covered lives make it through the preliminary morass, they are often coerced into choices they don't want in order to secure benefits. This further infantilizes them, taking treatment out of their hands and putting it under the control of Big Brother. Edward Shapiro (1994), author, psychiatrist, and Medical Director of The Austen Riggs Center in Stockbridge, Massachusetts suggests that limitations of resources are realities in today's world of mental health. "The therapist must incorporate the management of limitations in his interpretation," helping patients to take "responsibility for financial resources" (p. 443). MCOs do the opposite, often speaking only to therapists while whitewashing benefits in consumer advertising. By prohibiting or discouraging disclosure of corporate contracts, MCOs coerce patients to relinquish control of their treatment. Once again the patient is disempowered—told to remain infantilized by the system. Another offense is carefully waged when patients find they must undergo unwanted psychiatric consults and take unwanted psychotropic medications. Both patients and psychotherapists may be against the use of these medications. When it is the only course open to a individual in pain (because psychotherapy is denied or abridged), the patient may dutifully accept Big Brother's coercion. A vulnerable patient may see Big Brother's dominance as just another validation of his or her inadequacy.

Patients need to take responsibility for their treatment, observes Robert Daly (1996), who also notes that MCOs strongly discourage patient participation in maintaining treatment.

Stripped of choice and decision-making, the worried well now face another indignity—utilization review. "An essential ingredient in psycho-

COMING OUT OF THE CLOSET

The stigma of mental illness is a powerful force in our society. Although mental illness is now seen as a disease, or brain disorder, it is still frequently associated with a failure of character. Oddly, public acceptance may depend more on where you work than who you are or what your mental illness is. "The arts and Hollywood are probably the most tolerant," writes Solomon (1996) in *Newsweek*. "Corporate America may be the least forgiving" (p. 21). Fortunately, people are becoming more willing to come out of the closet. And the more they do, hopefully, the more others will learn. Consider how coming out of the closet has changed:

Senator Thomas Eagleton is taken off the Democratic presidential ticket when he publicly confirms that he had suffered from depression and had been treated with electroshock therapy.

Betty Ford admits to her struggle with alcoholism.

Colin Powell announces at a press conference that his wife suffers from depression. "It is not a family secret," he says. "It is very easily controlled with proper medication, just as my blood pressure is."

Mike Wallace testifies on Capitol Hill about his lifelong bout with depression. "I will take Zoloft every day for the rest of my life . . . and I'm quite content to do it." (Solomon 1986, p. 22).

therapy," says Miller (1994), "is accepting a patient's feelings in a nonjudgmental, nonblaming, and nonshaming manner" (p. 561). MCOs constantly judge psychotherapeutic decisions in their utilization reviews to determine whether to continue treatment. Not only does this breach confidentiality and subsequently diminish the trust in both psychotherapy and the clinician, but it also implies that a judgment is being passed on whether a patient is worthy of treatment. This seriously dilutes the therapeutic alliance, making the patient vulnerable to the values of the MCOs. Inherent in the review process is the requirement that treatment must be medically necessary. The review process implies that patients are responsible for all of their problems (i.e., the worried well) but not sufficiently responsible, or competent, for the control of their treatment. Paradoxically, ". . . the good patient," Chipman says (1995), "is the one who puts only minimal demands on mental health services" (p. 561). The patient and the therapist are caught in a dilemma. To take control of one's life is to seek solutions to obstacles. If an individual needs professional help in finding solutions, then he or she is purportedly doing the right thing. However, in Big Brother's eyes, the opposite is true. "In today's lean and mean environment," Chipman notes, "working long and hard . . . is apt to be depreciated as the 'Woody Allen syndrome'" (p. 561). That is, in this view, those who are worried, miserable, or even depressed are considered to be suffering from a social condition. Managed care covers psychological problems, not social problems.

THROUGH THE EYES OF THE PROVIDER

The following quotation appeared on the Internet: "The HMO recognizes that a ruptured appendix can lead to peritonitis, which can lead to death. So what does it think that acute unipolar depression leads to? A bad-hair day? . . . They wouldn't argue if I were a coronary patient or a diabetic, but because I'm a unipolar, I'm treated like something on the sidewalk they wished they hadn't stepped in" (Grohol 1995).

In the mid-twentieth century, psychotherapists held a special position in America. The public generally viewed psychotherapists as having one of three characters: the erudite European-style analyst, the noble idealist dedicated to helping the underprivileged, or the earnest scientist methodically exploring the mysteries of the physiology of behavior. "What they all had in common," according to Chipman (1995), "was a commitment to relieving human suffering or ignorance, a breadth of intellectual perspective, and a proneness for raising deep questions rather than providing simple answers" (p. 443). In order to adapt to managed care these traditional characteristics of therapists must become secondary to a willingness to accept the new system. Therapists must accept changes that range from paperwork nuisances to reductions in autonomy and fees to ethical conflicts.

MCOs demand copious paperwork that follows highly specific protocols different for each MCO. In the National Psychologist Survey (Saeman 1996b), 87 percent of therapists reported that they had "more" or "much more" paperwork in the last five years. Blue Cross of California/CaliforniaCare Health Plans recently announced that they intend to convert to paperless claims by 1998. They plan to charge a handling fee for claims submitted on paper. In addition, electronic claims will be processed before paper claims. According to Larry Saltzman, M.D., president and chief executive officer of Insurance Benefit Spotcheck, Inc., paper claims can cost a provider $3–$5 each, including processing, time, and supplies (Newspage 1996e). It is another business technique that psychotherapists will have to learn in order to survive in the twenty-first century. Hopefully, these requirements will become uniform across the industry but they now represent a paperwork jungle to be painfully traversed by clinicians.

Marketing, once a business term, is now said to be another necessary adaptation. Ninety percent of psychologists in the National Psychologist Study (Saeman 1996b) said they are marketing their practices. A recent issue of *The Clinician* contains a report about MCO aggressive marketing (Chiaramonte 1995) while a New York State Psychological Association Notebook lists "Fifteen Ways to Increase Referrals from MCOs" (Polonsky 1995, p. 8). Mental health professionals need to use marketing as a way to let people know what they do. Lowman and Resnick (1994) agree, suggesting that professionals market their services constantly seeking new accounts in addition to educating existing client companies. Marketing is particularly important for the solo practitioner. "You need a marketing plan to survive in private practice," writes Polonsky (1996b) "and you need to take action" (p. 6). He firmly states that there is only one goal in creating a marketing plan—to increase referrals. This can be disturbing in a profession that only a decade ago felt that print advertising was inappropriate. Now some psychotherapists are compelled to do things to maintain visibility, such as send out brochures, letters, and other mailings, call and speak regularly to people who are referral sources, and compile mailing lists of individuals who control referrals in managed care companies. Many psychotherapists are uncomfortable with the need to sell themselves. The art and ethics of marketing require very different skills from that of a good clinician. Most clinicians would make poor salesmen, and most salesmen could never be psychotherapists.

Managed care therapists must also accept a large measure of loss of control of their work. They often feel powerless. Their frustration of being an employee with an amorphous, untouchable boss diminishes their investment in themselves and the profession. "I used to tell everyone that he or she should become a psychotherapist," says one psychologist. "I loved the field. But now I advise them to try something else that is a lot more rewarding."

The most difficult adaptations for therapists are the necessary change in philosophy and the resolution of new ethical conflicts. Providers are expected to embrace the new system, accepting that the changes are necessary to enforce cost containment. The good provider asks for little, gets less, and compromises professional ethics. In industrialized psychotherapy, this good provider knows how to work within the corporate system. It is often a struggle for the clinician to integrate the good provider and good psychotherapy. In many ways, this provider is the antithesis of the psychotherapist clinging to professional ethics. J. Shapiro (1995) argues that both patient and psychotherapist suffer in such a conflict. The patient may receive less focused treatment and the psychologist may be highly susceptible to burnout. "Managed care then becomes managed indifference. In fact, the term 'managed care' is really an oxymoron that no one notices, a euphemism for social control in the health care arena" (p. 443). The doublethink here is that therapists must keep two concepts such as "utilization review is good for managed care" and "utilization review is good for the patient" in mind at the same time and must not see any conflict between those concepts. This is a difficult adaptation to make.

DIAL 1-800-THERAPIST

Kevin Grold, a San Diego psychotherapist, decided to go national with his Southern California referral service. For a $1,000 "membership fee," Grold sells the service to a "director" (a licensed psychotherapist with malpractice insurance). The director determines how to market the referral system in his or her area. In addition, the director can choose to sign on other professionals as "subcontractors." Grold's idea utilizes a relatively untouched referral source—the general public.

When a consumer calls the 1-800-Therapist number the call is routed into the appropriate director's office. The "director" is determined by the caller's area code. Thus a call from a 212 area code would go to New York City and a call from 202 would go to Washington, DC. Grold provides support services, a newsletter, and aggressive national marketing. For example, he has a television commercial that features actress Marina Sirtis, who plays the sexy counselor Deanna Troi on *Star Trek: The Next Generation*. With only 25 percent of the 130 US area codes sold, Grold has a fertile market for expansion (Saeman 1996d).

It is no surprise that salespeople and con artists have descended upon psychotherapists with schemes guaranteed to bring instant success. Scams have begun to surface throughout the country. One "insurance company" charged a $100 "application fee" to join their panel. There were no guarantees that any referrals would be made. The offer was made nationwide. If 10,000 therapists had applied, they would have made a million dollars. A similar scam originated from a "professional group" who guaranteed referrals from the top national MCOs. They requested $75 to become a part of their network. A year or so after the fee was mailed they informed the "applicant" that he or she was denied because there were too many providers in the area.

Scams are complimented by the hustles that are found in print advertising. They feed off professional fears, making outrageous promises for success:

Is Managed Care Threatening the Survival of Your Practice?
Two Indispensable Clinical Tools That Can Save Your Neck.
Last Chance to Get Into Closed HMOs!

The advertising tells stories of providers "flooded with referrals even when the network is supposedly closed." They offer "little-known back-door secrets" and "what managed care companies don't want you to know." Many sell grandiose methods supported by testimonials from colleagues experiencing phenomenal success. ("Never mind," they counsel, "that pabulum you heard at the Managed Care Conference!")

The call for big money schemes seems to further erode a profession left shaken by MCOs. What has happened to us?

THE WAY IT WAS

"I'm so sorry, Mrs. Kant. I told them about your husband's death and your illness. They know about your psychiatric disability," Cheryl, the case manager, said. "I don't know why they refused benefits." As a CSS (Community Support System) case manager she had spent nearly three hours in the SSI office with Mrs. Kant before anyone would speak to them.

"Of course I'll go with you again," Cheryl comforted her client. "We'll try to make them listen."

Cheryl was 21 years old. She wanted to be a social worker. And the only way she could afford tuition was to work full time as a case manager. In the 1980s, being a case manager meant visiting chronic mentally ill patients, coordinating services, spending endless hours on the telephone, and becoming a regular at government entitlement offices. She carried a caseload of 70 clients.

Cheryl was paid to work 8 hours a day, with 1 hour for lunch. She usually worked 9 or 10 hours. Rarely was she able to grab lunch with her colleagues, all young girls her age struggling to pay tuition or save money for their weddings. The hours didn't really matter. Cheryl was fiercely determined to do the very best for her clients. She was a dedicated patient advocate. That was previous to the growth of MCOs and their need for case managers. Today's case manager is frequently on the other side of the fence as a gatekeeper for managed care.

The concept of case management emerged primarily from a social work generalist approach. Generalists focused on crossing the boundaries of multiple systems to provide social services. The position of case manager took hold in the '70s and '80s, the by-product of America's zeal to provide services to the needy. At that time it was popular to use federal or state funds to create programs for people with specific problems. The Department of Health, Education, and Welfare funded a series of projects that featured "systems agents" or case managers to coordinate resources. These new case managers were quickly incorporated into the NIMH project known as the Community Support System (CSS). CSS was designed to serve the high volume of people who had suddenly been thrust out into the community after the deinstitutionalization of mental hospitals. The case manager's job was to link these very vulnerable clients to resources they were unable to access by themselves.

"The CSS case managers were a formidable force," recalls a former CSS social worker. "They were young, energetic, optimistic. It was as if they carried the spent innocence of the '60s, believing they could make a difference in the system. Sadly, they have very little in common with their jaded sisters, today's managed care case manager."

Understanding the origin of case managers helps clarify why Big Brother has so efficiently incorporated them into his realm. According to Carol Austin (Austin 1993), "Case management is an idea whose time has obviously come" (p. 451). She suggests that case managers were intended to do battle with dysfunctional delivery systems. These systems, established to help people in need, have become more beneficial to "providers, funders, and professionals rather than clients" (p. 451).

In a managed care setting, the case manager usually authorizes, denies, or recommends other treatments. The Commission for Case Management Certification (1996) defines case management as "a collaborative process which assesses, plans, implements, coordinates, monitors, and evaluates the options and services required to meet an individual's health needs, using communication and available resources to promote quality, cost-effective outcomes" (p. 2).

Many MCOs hire only social workers in case management positions. "Most companies look for licensed clinicians," explains Kristy Kolmansberger, Network Development Specialist at CMG. "At CMG they must meet professional criteria for providers in the state they are practicing" (1996). Lower level employees, who don't make clinical decisions or authorizations, are not held to the same standards. "These are the intake people," Kolmansberger says, "the ones who might run the clinical screenings, or the clerical level people" (1996). Dr. Daly agrees, hiring only social workers for case manager positions in his nonprofit HMO. He believes that trained professionals are necessary in order to make treatment decisions as well as maintain a professional level of confidentiality. Unfortunately, not all MCOs follow this model. Young, inexperienced, and poorly trained people often fill these powerful positions. Many of them hold only bachelor's degrees. They listen, read, and pass judgment on assessments made by psychotherapists and physicians throughout the country. Can this new generation of case managers be expected to maintain the old professional standards?

"The medical model presupposes that there are case managers who are aware and can manage it effectively," comments Daly (1996b). "Yet many times, managed care hires people who don't."

Mike Lardiere (1996), Director of Provider Relations at GHI-BMP, strongly disagrees. "Sure, I've heard complaints," he admits. "But they usually involve a case manager not agreeing rather than not understanding." This problem has become so widespread that legislation has been introduced to require that gatekeepers and case managers hold minimum professional qualifications and "are not just high school graduates, as is sometimes the case today" (Riley 1996a, p. 31). Case managers are team players. They fit in perfectly with MCOs. "They're just doing their jobs," says Sheila Peck

(1996). "You can't really call them the bad guys because they're not the ones setting policy."

Wolk and colleagues (1994) suggest that there is a "managerial nature" in case management. The ability to service a wide range of clients using techniques such as assessment, plan development and implementation, monitoring, advocacy, tracking, and evaluation are similar to any management position; ". . . the success of case management interventions is observable and measurable because the models are generally based on observable and measurable objectives" (p. 7). In other words, they can adapt to suit clients of any kind—from social services to corporations. In managed care, the case manager's "client" has changed. It is not a human being with a face, a voice, and a personality. Instead, the managed care case manager's client is the name seen on an OTR or the central character in a story re-

ON BECOMING A CCM

A CCM (Certified Case Manager) is a credential offered by the CCMC (Commission for Case Manager Certification 1996). To get a CCM, an individual must complete the necessary application and paperwork, meet licensure or certification requirements, pass a 300-item multiple choice exam, and pay all required fees.

To be eligible, an individual must have a license or certification in an area that requires the completion of a post-secondary program in a "field that promotes the physical, psychosocial, or vocational well-being of the persons being served" (CCMC 1996). In addition, the applicant has to have at least one of the following types of work experience:

1. 12 months, full time, working under a CCM's supervision
2. 24 months, full time, with no CCM supervision
3. 12 months, full time, supervising people who provide direct case management services.

CCM is not the only certification offered by the Commission. They have a CRC (Certified Rehabilitation Counselor), CCRC (Certified Canadian Rehabilitation Counselor), and CIRS (Certified Insurance Rehabilitation Specialist), among others.

viewed on the telephone. The connection is through numbers, reports, and diagnostic codes.

Big Brother's case manager is committed to doing a job—defined by cost containment. Generally, this is accomplished through the denial of benefits and use of alternate (less expensive) treatments such as psychotropic medications and self-help groups. In this manner, the case manager echoes Orwell's (1949) "Party" in *1984*:

> A Party member is required to have not only the right opinions, but the right instincts. Many of the beliefs and attitudes demanded of him are never plainly stated, and could not be stated without laying bare the contradictions." [p. 174]

Several studies have examined the effects of this new approach to case management. Miller (1995) refers to two surveys that indicate an alarming prevalence of problems with managed mental health care: citing Hipp and colleagues who found that 64 percent of 223 Colorado psychologists reported that managed care had terminated treatment when still indicated and citing Tucker and Lubin who found that 79 percent of 718 responding psychologists reported dissatisfaction with the utilization reviewer's knowledge.

Two studies report contradictory findings. Starfield and colleagues (1994) reviewed 2024 outpatient medical records of 135 providers and found no relationships between cost-efficiency and length or quality of care. Howard and colleagues (1986) analyzed 15 studies that involved over 2400 patients in 30 years of research. Using meta-analysis, they estimated the expected benefits of time "doses" of therapy:

14 percent of patients improved before the first session
41 percent improved by the 4th session
53 percent improved by the 8th session
74 percent improved by the 26th session
83 percent improved by the 52nd session
90 percent improved by the 104th session.

Managed care discontent is growing. Consumers want a more equitable balance between cost and availability of health care. They do not like the ever-diminishing access to health care. Although employers are looking at ways to provide benefits at a reduced cost, they, too, are unsatisfied with the range of services.

DEMAND MANAGEMENT

The Orwellian metaphor for a "Party Member" describes demand management, or what some believe to be the next wave in managed care. Demand management is a cost-containment method that replaces professionals in the treatment room with case managers in the community. This is not a new idea. Case manager/gatekeepers have already replaced professionals in making treatment decisions. Demand management applies the same concept, taking it into the field.

"Demand management takes primary care medicine, combines it with behavioral care, and brings it directly to the population," says Errol Nadler (1995), managed care innovator and CEO of New Visions, Behavioral Health of New York, and OPS. Demand management emerges from the CSS model, where a case manager coordinates services for patients in the community. However, while CSS used a wide variety of resources to serve the client, demand management operates from a managed care model based on "wellness" programs and cost containment. The main focus is on three issues: assuring compliance and appropriate self-care, assuring professional cooperation, and building the best mix of product and service. Demand management depends on a rigidly defined balance between need/demand and unnecessary need/unnecessary demand. Need is defined as illness and unnecessary need is the failure to utilize preventative measures. Similarly, demand refers to requests for services (treatment, tests, etc.). Unnecessary demand refers to treatment-not-needed as well as the highly subjective failure of self-management. This is similar to the concept of "managed prevention," where employers utilize "wellness testing" to design a risk-rated benefit plan where healthy workers pay lower insurance rates than workers "who smoke, drink, or have high blood pressure or other problems" (Riley 1996b, p. 25). How does one assess "failure of self-management"? Would an individual who suffers from anxiety and does not practice relaxation techniques fit that category? Or someone with an ulcer? The final say resides with what is called a "wellness representative"—a euphemism for Big Brother's loyal representative, the managed care case manager.

"Demand management is not bad for the masses," comments one psychologist who requested that his name be withheld. "Many people with mild emotional problems can benefit from that type of treatment. But in the long run, after all these programs are set up, after all is said and done, we'll find the ones who really need help right back in our offices."

The new breed of case manager is well entrenched in the system. She is trained to fit all the requirements—espousing corporate values in a health care system. "In health care, case managers frequently have the fiscal authority to produce system change. However, questions remain—system change in what direction and to whose benefit?" (Austin 1993, p. 452).

WHO'S WHO IN HIM?

HIM, or Health Information Management, often appears like a hive buzzing with acronyms and abbreviations instead of bees. HIM workers love to design new terms that befuddle outsiders. Consider some of their systems. You can find a CIS (Clinical Information System), IDS (Integrated Delivery System), or EDI (Electronic Data Interchange). They use CPRs (Computer Patient Records) and EPRs (Electronic Patient Records), which lead to an abundance of FAQs (Frequently Asked Questions). The person who maintains these systems may be an RRA (Registered Records Administrator) or an ART (Accredited Records Technician). The difference is that an RRA holds a BS (Bachelor of Science) while an ART holds an AA (Associates) from an accredited program or an ISP (Independent Study Program). Both are certified by AHIMA (American Health Information Management Associates).

Insiders who are on the cutting edge of HIM are well aware of the TEPR (Toward an Electronic Patient Record) conference and symposium presented by MRI (Medical Records Institute) with exhibitors such as AMIA (American Medical Informatics Association), MDS (Multi-Media Data Systems Inc.) and STC (Software Technology Corporation). All of this makes NASW, APA, and *DSM-IV* seem archaic.

Imagine entering the twenty-first century with an FAQ about an EDI providing EPRs to MCOs for use in their IDS designed by HIMs with a minimum RRA credential. ASAP.

FROM THE INSIDE

Finding information on managed care has been more often a case of excess rather than scarcity. The abuses of medical managed care are appearing more and more often in newspapers, magazines, radio, and television. The drama of life-threatening situations determined by managed care are increasingly appealing to writers. A case in point is the 1995 season finale of the popular television medical drama, *E.R.* The episode concluded with head nurse Carol Hathaway, one of the main characters, "quitting" because she could no longer tolerate how managed care was dictating care. John Grisham's best-selling novel, *The Rainmaker*, is the story of how one client dies as a result of insurance company profiteering.

When the authors of this book attempted to look beneath what Ivan Miller (1994) identifies as "the veil of secrecy" into the actual work of case managers, gatekeepers, and utilization reviewers, few individuals were willing to speak. Several supervisors, managers, and other high level employees offered politically correct descriptions of the process of utilization review. Mike Lardiere, M.S.W., Director of Provider Relations at GHI/BMP (personal communication, May 1996), affirms that his company has "specific clinical criteria that case managers use as guidelines in making determinations. The criteria are used as a guide, combined with clinical experience, to make decisions." Lardiere says that these guidelines are "basic stuff" that "all large companies use" and are "shared with providers in the provider manual." He maintains that the clinical criteria are based on things such as experience, literature reviews, input from multidisciplinary staff, a panel of specialists, and an ongoing process of improving and updating clinical information.

What the case managers say in their own words might be the most revealing information of all.

"As one who served for a time in a managed mental health setting," writes Douglas Nau (1996) for Mental Health Net, "I have some insider experience." Nau speaks of some of his colleagues as being competent therapists while many others were not. "In one instance," he reports, "the utilization reviewer screamed down the hall in expletives about how stupid providers were because they kept asking for authorization to hospitalize clients. The reviewer had three answers for such requests: 'No,' 'NO' and 'Damn it, NO.'" Nau adds that in one instance, the office manager referred clients to her husband—without any "checks or balances to prevent this from happening. Case reviews were often embarrassing assaults on the abilities of the providers," Nau continues. "The lack of professionalism was sad. There was only *one* way to do therapy, and providers were often not given further referrals if they called to consult on a case or ask for more visits."

Corporate, rather than health care concerns dictate treatment, says Stephen M. Weissman (1996), a psychiatrist, psychoanalyst, and writer in Washington, DC. He suggests that "objective criteria for 'medical necessity' decisions—if they exist at all—are closely guarded secrets." He continues

> Under managed care, any and all "medical necessity" decisions by individual HCPs can be second-guessed and countermanded by clerks, accountants, or other individuals with little or no training in mental health.
>
> And corporate retribution for any outspoken mental health professional who does manage to prevail by advocating on behalf of an individual patient may be their subsequent termination from the plan (in the case of salaried doctors inside an HMO entity) or silent blacklisting (in the case of contracting doctors outside an HMO or other managed care entity).
>
> An affidavit offered last summer during the discovery phase of a lawsuit in Boston, Schiffer v. Blue Cross and Blue Shield of Mass. Inc. (Suffolk County Superior Court) by a former managed care gatekeeper describing his job provides chilling evidence of this process:
>
> "The subscribers who called were extremely upset. Many were outraged psychiatric patients who screamed and cried at me. Almost all did not want to reveal confidential information, but I was told . . . that unless they answered my questions, I could not give them a referral. . . . To make a referral and approve the visit, I had to diagnose the patient and enter that diagnosis into the computer as part of the patient's medical record. . . .
>
> "I received no clinical training at all. I had no formal education in mental health care and I had no past work experience in the mental health field. Yet I found myself fielding calls from desperate subscribers. My supervisors refused to take calls if I had problems. . . .
>
> "After a subscriber . . . answered my questions . . . I gave him or her a list of 2 or 3 providers based mainly on the subscriber's geographic area. I had no information about the provider's . . . area of expertise. . . .
>
> "I believe that [the current insurance company] systematically tried to refer subscribers to social workers in preference to psychologists for psychotherapy. For example, if a subscriber wanted psychotherapy with a psychiatrist, we told [him] untruthfully, as I was instructed by [my supervisor], that most psychiatrists were backed up for a 3 month wait. . . . [Also,] the referral assistants would ask 'Do you need medication?'

and if the answer was 'no' (which was most people's natural response), then the system automatically eliminated all psychiatrists from the list of providers. . . .

"I was instructed by [my supervisor] to talk subscribers out of wanting neuro-psychological testing, even though I had no training and did not have any idea about the clinical value of the tests. . . .

"In the [previous insurance company], the primary care doctors made the mental health referrals . . . [but now] primary care doctors could no longer make referrals because the list of providers was kept secret. Although I had such a list, I was instructed by [my supervisor] never to reveal to any subscriber or provider that such a list existed. . . .

"I was told by [my supervisor] not to refer to several providers. . . .

"[R]eferral assistants had no information about the race or ethnicity of the providers . . . so if someone wanted a black therapist we couldn't find one. . . . [M]ost black subscribers got their mental health care through hospital clinics. [My supervisor] said to me, 'Black people should go to clinics because they use drugs, have too many problems, go on forever in therapy, and you can't manage their case or they'll cry discrimination.'"

In his affidavit, the gatekeeper also made these statements:

"Subscribers would complain that they had been told they had 20 sessions available to them, that the brochure said so, or that they knew from past experience . . . about 90 percent of the subscribers . . . expected to have 20 sessions available to them and available without review. . . .

"I sat in the same area as the case managers . . . [and] I frequently heard the case managers denying sessions. . . . I often heard some case managers joking among themselves and ridiculing patients or providers as soon as they hung up. . . .

"I learned from conversations with case managers . . . [that they] were instructed to try to keep every patient to 6 sessions for the year, unless there were catastrophic issues. . . . I remember one case manager ridiculing another for having higher numbers of authorization than him. Case managers were called "patient and provider friend," and this was considered a threatening, insulting designation. . . .

"There was no clear medical necessity criteria. . . . [S]ome case managers approved more sessions for the same types of problems than did other case managers. A majority of case managers were evasive, combative, and hostile in their authorizations. . . .

"It is my impression that the primary purpose of the entire system was to discourage or prevent subscribers from using mental health benefits for which they had paid. Employees who authorized the least sessions were favored and often given more opportunity and advancement while those who were more liberal in their authorizations lost prestige, and their work situation was made extremely difficult by subjecting them to constant supervision. I am also under the impression [that] . . . employees received bonuses based on the profitability of the mental health unit. The lawsuit has not yet come to trial." [Weissman 1996, pp. xx]

4

Who's Lurking?

Whatsoever things I see or hear concerning the life of men, in my attendance on the sick or even apart therefrom, which ought not be noised abroad, I will keep silence thereon, counting such things to be as sacred secrets.

—*Hippocratic Oath, 4th Century* BCE

The social worker should respect the privacy of clients and hold in confidence all information obtained in the course of professional service.

—*Code of Ethics, National Association of Social Workers, 1980*

Psychologists have a primary obligation and take reasonable precautions to respect the confidentiality rights of those with whom they work or consult, recognizing that confidentiality may be established by law, institutional rules, or professional or scientific relationships.

—*Code of Conduct, American Psychological Association, 1992*

CONFIDENTIALITY

Since Hippocrites in the 4th century, health care professionals have observed the importance of protecting the privacy of each patient's communications. This has always led to occasional problems in balancing the needs of the patient against the needs of society. As society has become more complex and medicine has become a larger part of our social activity, conflicts have increased. The problem of confidentiality or privacy of medical records shares the same legal ground as, for example, privacy between attorney and client, and is an area of active legal debate. As Alderman and Kennedy (1995) have noted, ". . . important to an understanding of the legal right to privacy (and the crucial element missing from the debate thus far) is an understanding of other issues that may override it. Whenever an invasion of privacy is claimed, there are usually competing values at stake. Privacy may seem paramount to a person who has lost it, but that right often clashes with other rights and responsibilities that we as a society deemed important" (p. xiv).

At the present time, the privacy of communication is being especially challenged in medicine and psychotherapy. Various agencies and insurance businesses are demanding access to the records of medical professionals and psychotherapists. In the debates about the right to access patient information, an important distinction between medical records and psychotherapy records is being overlooked.

Physicians and psychotherapists record information for different reasons. Physicians share information through patient charts in order to help other physicians, consultants, specialists, and other caregivers provide the best care for the patients. Nurses check medications, specialists read histories, and other physicians avoid duplications of procedures. In addition, hospital and government organizations have access to medical records in order to assure the thoroughness and appropriateness of health care and to assess the competence of all those responsible for patient care. In general, physicians welcome access to medical records because the shared communications contribute to their ability to help patients. In contrast, for psychotherapists, the sharing of information contained in the therapy record interferes with the ability to treat patients. Psychotherapists may note material that appears in dreams or special dates that are significant for their patients. Many psychotherapists write down their own reactions to what patients say during therapy. Traditionally, psychotherapists have intended that their notes are for their own considerations, not to be shared or examined by anyone else. Thus, the purpose of keeping records for psychotherapists is different at its very basis from the purpose of keeping records for physicians.

Confidentiality is a critical component of psychotherapy that in theory is inviolate but in practice frequently is breached. In an ideal treatment situation, the psychotherapist encourages the patient to reveal his or her most intimate thoughts and fantasies in complete privacy. The psychotherapist attempts to prevent intrusions of any type. In reality it is difficult to maintain these conditions. When a child enters therapy, a parent pays for the sessions. Often a spouse will pay for the therapy of the husband or the wife. In other cases, patients are referred by schools, the court system, or are seen in clinics where confidentiality is not possible and the original one-to-one private relationship is difficult to maintain.

Brett Kahr, psychohistorian and Senior Lecturer in Psychology at Regents College, London (1996), suggests that Breuer and Freud were the first to discuss confidentiality of treatment records. After much consideration, they concluded that however critical the information, clinicians must never compromise a patient's identity. Consequently, both took great care to protect their patients. Conflicts quickly arose over the issue. Freud wrote:

> . . . the physician has taken upon himself duties not only towards the individual patient but towards science as well; and his duties towards science mean ultimately nothing else than his duties towards the many other patients who are suffering from the same disorder.
>
> . . . I was accused of giving *no* information about my patients. . . . Now I shall be accused of giving information about my patients which ought not be given. The presentation of my case histories remains a problem which is hard for me to solve. [Kahr, p. 17]

Watkins (1989) identifies two separate types of confidentiality—absolute and relative. Absolute confidentiality applies to information that is intended to be kept in the treatment room. No one is allowed access to any of this information including case records, oral discussions, or information on computers. Relative confidentiality refers to situations where breaches of confidentiality may need to be considered. Probably all therapists have encountered situations, especially ones where children are involved, in which the nature of confidentiality needs to be examined.

The introduction and acceptance of insurance into psychotherapy brought with it intensified consideration of the meaning of privacy. In private, fee-for-service therapy where no insurance is used, the patient leaves knowledge of his or her problem and diagnosis in the therapist's office and pays the bill. Traditional psychotherapists treat revelations in treatment as private material and consider privacy to be a special condition that encourages progress in psychotherapy. The introduction of insurance destroys that privacy because insurance companies require documentation of services rendered and the need for that service in order to evaluate claims and pay them appropriately. The popularity of managed care has further intensified the privacy problem because, while traditional insurers generally only want a diagnosis, MCOs generally also want a treatment plan and justification for treatment. This usually requires revelation of patient-specific, formerly confidential material.

Most insurance companies require patients to waive their rights to confidentiality as part of their coverage agreement. People who enroll in MCOs usually agree to the release of information. At the time of enrollment they are not likely to think about future problems of confidentiality. If an enrollee later seeks help for a mental health problem, the previously authorized release of information may become a major problem. As a provider, a psychotherapist must accurately submit the required paperwork to the

MCO. If the material is not submitted or if it is incomplete, the psychotherapist is failing to abide by stipulations of the contract to which he or she has agreed. In addition, psychotherapists who are MCO providers are frequently under restrictions about discussions of confidentiality and therefore limited in their ability to help the patient with decisions regarding confidentiality.

WHAT'S IN A RECORD?

Patient records are created when individuals receive treatment from health or mental health professionals. Certain records are required by law. When MCOs require detailed outpatient treatment reports, these documents automatically become part of the patient's record. Records also come from practitioners such as chiropractors, dentists, and nutritionists and from laboratories, pharmacies, employee assistance programs, and consumer questionnaires.

Consent statements to release records usually appear on the contract, the insurance claim form, or both. Frequently it reads as a general consent, release form, or blanket waiver that permits third party access. The consent, by definition, legally removes such information from the arena of privileged communications. In addition, many insurance contracts include releases to the Medical Information Bureau, a consortium of approximately 750 health, life, and disability insurers that maintains a database of 15 million Americans.

The Privacy Rights Clearinghouse (1994) writes that a blanket waiver might say the following:

> I authorize any physician, hospital or other medical provider to release to [insurer] any information regarding my medical history, symptoms, treatment, exam results, or diagnosis.

On one claim form for a managed care organization contracted to a major regional corporation, the waiver is found on the back under "Patient and Employee (subscriber) Instructions." Listed as #11 of 12 instructions, it comes under the category of "Patient's Signature." The "signature" on the face side of the claim is required for processing. The following instruction is given:

> The patient is to sign the claim form, authorizing the release of information, as provided below. If the patient is a minor, the signature must be that of the patient's parent or legal guardian.

> I hereby authorize any physician, health care practitioner, hospital, clinic, or other medical or medically related facility to furnish any and all records pertaining to medical history, services rendered, or treatment, given to me or my dependents for purposes of review, investigation or evaluation of this claim.
>
> I also authorize [employer], or its agents, to disclose to a hospital or health care service plan, self-insurer or an insurer any such medical information obtained if such disclosure is necessary to allow the processing of any claim.
>
> This authorization also permits disclosure to [employer] for purposes of utilization review or financial audit.
>
> This authorization shall become effective immediately upon execution and shall remain in effect for the duration of this claim or term of coverage of my insurance policy, including a reasonable time thereafter, until its final consummation. This authorization shall be binding upon the claimant, his heirs, executors or administration.

According to Privacy Rights Clearinghouse (1994), there is only one way to preserve confidentiality—bring a written request . . . that revokes your consent to release medical information to the insurance company and/or to your employer for that visit; you must also pay for the visit yourself rather than obtain reimbursement from the insurance company.

Records established by a provider, hospital, or facility and submitted to an MCO appear in insurance databases. Once on a system, patient records are available to all those who have access, and sometimes to others who find ways to access records. Gallo (1994) reports that in a large hospital, the average medical record is seen by approximately 77 people. In Manhattan's Columbia-Presbyterian Medical Center, a new system stores records for 1.6 million people, handling about 13,000 to 14,000 accesses per hour (Riley 1996a). According to a 1994 Lou Harris Poll, 84 percent of respondents said they were concerned about privacy (EPIC 1995). Their concerns had ample justification. Consider these examples:

> An adult man admitted to his doctor that he had experimented with marijuana when he was a teenager. The information was entered into his computer records and later used as a reason to deny him medical benefits (Nagel 1995).

A Fortune 500 corporation uses patient records to help make employment decisions (Nagel 1995).

Medicaid clerks print out patient names, addresses, incomes, and patient records and sell them to HMO recruiters (Riley 1996b).

A convicted child rapist goes through nearly one thousand electronic hospital records to get the telephone numbers of young females, one only 9 years old (Nagel 1995).

Medical records therefore may be extensive and intimate histories of an individual's physical and emotional states, his or her family's physical and emotional states, their individual and family lifestyles, and indications for their future. Much of this information is presently scattered throughout the files and databases of individuals and organizations that patients have contacted for various physical, psychological, and practical needs and may be difficult to access. As technology improves, networks and centralized databases are being connected, creating Orwellian, cradle-to-grave information for every man, woman, and child. Davidson & Davidson (1995) write about the subtle change in the nature of confidentiality of patient records. ". . . there has been a repudiation of the formerly held, tacit agreement between the clinician and client that the information shared by the client will be used exclusively for the individual's benefit. Passing information on to insurance companies has become so commonplace and pervasive that violation of confidentiality is becoming institutionalized" (p. 457).

The institutionalization of breaches in confidentiality occurs because records are handled as dehumanized commodities that do not belong to patients, according to Susan Baek (1994). She writes, "As a result, confidentiality now means making sure that those with access to patient information don't improperly share that information" (p. 52).

MANDATED ACCESS

While insurance companies violate confidentiality for business reasons, some government agencies violate confidentiality with the intention of protecting the health and well being of other members of the population. For example, according to child abuse reporting laws that exist in all 50 states, therapists who are told of physical or sexual misconduct with a child by the patient or some third party must report the alleged abuse to the authorities. As documented by Bollas and Sundelson (1995), government mandated breaches in confidentiality place the psychotherapist in the position of being a potential government informant in order to protect patients and others from harm. While psychotherapists frequently have been in the position of assessing one kind of harm as balanced against another, they are now under orders to report harm as defined by outside agencies. Thus, the problem for psychotherapists is that the required act of providing information to government agencies impairs their ability to provide successful psychotherapy.

Mandated violations of confidentiality usually involve suicidal, homicidal, or child abuses cases. Pope and Vetter (1992) found that most psychologists have repeatedly faced conflicts between their professional judgment and state mandates. While psychotherapists are involved in making clinical and ethical decisions for individual patients, MCOs are invested in complying with state laws in order to avoid potentially costly litigation. Although the positions of psychotherapists and MCOs are not necessarily adversarial, the positions often create conflict for the therapist.

THE TARRASOFF WARNING

Fundamental breaches of patient confidentiality arise from the therapist's legal duty to warn others of a patient's violent intentions or of child abuse. This is known as the Tarrasoff Warning, and it derived from the celebrated legal case of *Tarrasoff v. Regents of University of California* in 1976. Tarrasoff, a female student at the University of California at Berkeley was killed by a male student who had been dating her and who had been in therapy at the university's student health center. The girl's parents sued the university for failure to warn their daughter.

The California Supreme Court ruled that: "When a therapist determines . . . that his patient presents a serious danger of violence to another, he incurs an obligation to use reasonable care to protect the intended victim against such danger." The court added that the therapist might warn the intended victim, others who would apprise the intended victim of the danger, the police, or the therapist might take whatever steps are reasonably necessary under the circumstances.

That legal duty is also incorporated in the child abuse reporting laws that exist in all 50 states. Under the law, a therapist who is told of physical or sexual misconduct with a child, by the patient or some third party, must report it to the authorities (Bollas and Sundelson 1995, pp. 4–5).

Case Illustration

John Emmins called his managed care company, asking for help. He told the case manager that he had sexually molested his 11-year-old sister. The young man was referred to Dr. Ringoff.

Ringoff met with John and, with his permission, brought in the parents and sister. They spoke about John's problem. The family agreed to work together to prevent it from happening again. They all understood that John would enter therapy. If he made any sexual advances toward his sister, John would be reported. John was facing his problem and seemed relieved to have cooperation in setting limits on his behaviors.

The MCO case manager called and told Dr. Ringoff he had to contact Child Protection Services. "The parents are aware of the problem," Ringoff explained to the case manager. "The sister is in treatment, too, and they all agree that if John makes any sexual advances, I will be told. John is very eager to gain control of his behaviors. He understands that I will report any violation at all. The entire family has agreed to work together."

"You must call Child Protection Services," the case manager insisted. "It's state law."

"I believe," Ringoff said, "that if you violate this young man's confidentiality, treatment will be irreparably damaged."

Ringoff was concerned about his responsibility to act as a therapist rather than as an informant. However, he was as aware of the fact that he was mandated to report child abuse. Ringoff also knew that the family would deny any abuse to Child Protective Services. Before Ringoff could decide what to do, the case manager, without informing Ringoff, called Child Protective Services to report the family. They investigated the case and John never returned to treatment.

Several days later, John's mother called Dr. Ringoff. "He was crying for help," she said. "You said so yourself. Now everyone is shamed. I don't know how you could do this to him."

RECORDS AND THE LAW

The uniquely difficult confidentiality problem of psychotherapy records has been recently discussed at length by Bollas and Sundelson (1995). They note that "Lawyers still have privileged relations with clients, priests with their penitents, journalists with their sources, but therapists have allowed their privilege—equally if not more important to the practice of their profession—to be destroyed" (p. x).

Recognizing the importance of confidentiality in psychotherapy, Justice John Paul Stevens (NASW *News* 1996c) wrote: "effective psychotherapy . . . depends upon an atmosphere of confidence and trust in which the patient is willing to make a frank and complete disclosure of facts, emotions, memories, and fears" (p. 1). However, if a therapist and a patient agree to work under the scrutiny of Big Brother, these intrusions must be explored with the patient. The tacit acceptance by the therapist of the breach in confidentiality may be experienced by the patient as a lack of commitment to the therapeutic environment. Smith-Bell and Winslade (1994) summarize the situation:

> This disclosure of sensitive, sometimes embarrassing or shameful, personal information makes clients vulnerable to being harmed if unauthorized third parties gain access to such information. Clients assume or seek assurances that sensitive information will be a confidential communication to their Mental Health Plan (MHP), and unless they trust their therapist and rely on confidentiality, they are unlikely to cooperate fully in their therapy. Thus, MHPs frequently find themselves caught between clients' desires for privacy and confidentiality and third parties' demands for access to confidential information. [p. 180]

Smith-Bell and Winslade (1994) are supported by two national polls conducted in 1993 and 1994. In the 1993 Lou Harris Poll, 96 percent of the respondents believe that federal legislation should make personal medical information "sensitive" and impose penalties for unauthorized disclosure. The second poll conducted by the American Civil Liberties Union found that 70 percent of respondents reported being concerned a "great deal" or "fair amount" about insurance companies getting more information than is needed from their doctor (EPIC 1995).

In 1996, Susan Forward, a clinical social worker in California, was put on probation for three years and her license suspended for 90 days, when she revealed details of her psychotherapy sessions with Nicole Brown Simpson. During a 1994 television broadcast, Forward disclosed that Nicole had told her that her ex-husband, O.J. Simpson, had beaten and threatened her. The California Board of Behavioral Science Examiners, the state licensing board for social workers, marriage and family therapists, and education psychologists, found Forward in violation of the California Business and Professions Code and the state Civil Code. Both prohibit any unauthorized release of medical/mental health records except when there is a subpoena

PATIENT/THERAPIST PRIVILEGE UPHELD

The Supreme Court ruled on June 13, 1996 that patients and psychotherapists have the same confidential privilege as a lawyer and his client. The ruling, handed down in *Jaffe v. Redmond*, applies to both civil and criminal cases, and brings the Federal Court system into line with all 50 states which recognize some type of patient-therapist privilege. The privilege was extended to cover clinical social workers.

Jaffe v. Redmond involved a clinical social worker and her client, a police officer who entered treatment after killing a man in the line of duty. They sought to protect records of the therapy sessions from disclosure in a Federal civil rights suit brought against the police officer by the victim's family. The decision is a positive step toward protecting patients and supporting the value of psychotherapy. The majority opinion, written by Justice John Paul Stevens, notes that the privilege is "rooted in the imperative need for confidence and trust" and that "the mere possibility of disclosure may impede development of the confidential relationship necessary for successful treatment" (Greenhouse 1996, p. A1)

or search warrant. The principles of confidentiality apply for all patients—living or deceased.

In contrast to confidentiality, privilege is a legal concept. Privilege refers to how special relationships are handled in court. The concept of privilege appears related to the view that it is more important to preserve some relationships than it is to give the court access to information. The relationships covered by privilege include husband–wife, priest–confessor, doctor–patient, attorney–client, journalist–source.

John Henry Wigmore (Watkins 1989) identified four basic conditions necessary to establish a privileged communication (and subsequently avoid disclosure):

1. Communications must originate in the confidence that they will not be disclosed.
2. The element of confidentiality must be essential to the maintenance of the relationship between the parties.

3. The relation is one which in the opinion of the community ought to be fostered.
4. The injury that would incur to the relationship as a result of disclosure must be greater than the benefit gained in regard to the correct disposal of litigation. [p. 134]

Once Wigmore's four fundamental conditions for establishment of privilege against disclosure have been established, three additional rules must be met before the privilege can be claimed.

1. The relationship protected by the statute has been established.
2. The right to claim the privilege has not been waived.
3. The person who claims the privilege is the individual entitled to it under the statute. [p. 134]

Each state has licensing and regulatory statutes that deal with privileged communications. According to Jackim (1993), confidentiality is the right of the client, not the therapist. He claims that once the client waives that right, it is illegal for the therapist to refuse to share the information.

How do providers respond to these legal uncertainties and ethical conflicts?

"I don't withhold information," reports one psychotherapist, "but patients often don't understand the issues."

Another says, "I keep records that include only superficial issues, such as general goals under discussion and practical problems. I keep those records in a form that is acceptable to MCOs. In a separate notebook, I keep the information I feel necessary for treatment. That information includes confidential material, countertransference possibilities, and symbolic associations."

"I simply tell patients the truth," states another. "There is no such thing as confidentiality anymore if patients use insurance."

RECORDS THAT PREDICT

Today's problems with confidentiality may appear minor when compared with the potential problems created by the use of genetic testing to provide statistical predictions of future disease.

10 STEPS TO TRY TO PROTECT YOUR RECORDS' PRIVACY

1. ***Get your records.*** Access to your MIB (Medical Information Bureau) record is protected by federal law. Find out if there is a file on you by calling 617-426-3660 or writing MIB, PO Box 105, Essex Station, Boston, MA 02112. Check for possible inaccuracies.
2. ***Discuss confidentiality with your practitioner.*** Explain your request for privacy. Ask your practitioner to release only the essential information. Ask your psychotherapist to fill out the OTR during a session so you can have input on exactly what information is sent to the insurance company.
3. ***Know your rights.*** Privacy laws are different in each state. Make sure you know your rights. Read the federal ADA (Americans with Disabilities Act) that, among other things, prohibits employers from withdrawing a job offer based on disability, medical history, or the results of a company medical exam. Questions about your ability to perform a specific job are acceptable.
4. ***Watch what you sign.*** If you have to sign an authorization, limit the disclosure by adding your own conditions. List the names of professionals and/or organizations, insert an expiration date so the consent remains valid for a specific time period. Be aware that your changes might be rejected.
5. ***Think before you write.*** Medical questionnaires, histories, consumer surveys, company-sponsored health promotions, employee-assistance programs, and wellness groups are potential sources of information for patient records. Find out where the information is going before you agree to participate.
6. ***Watch who you speak to.*** Anything said or transacted over an 800 line can be traced back to you. Telephone surveys often ask personal questions that become part of your permanent record.
7. ***Check your records.*** Practitioners usually share their records. If they refuse, find out your state law. Most states guarantee patient access to records. If you are denied access (and your

state protects your right), get a written refusal. Complain to your state health department, the appropriate professional organization, or consumer advocate. Remember, a practitioner can charge a small fee (75 cents per page) to cover the copying expenses.

8. ***Speak to your employer.*** Ask how health insurance claims are handled, who has access, and how privacy is protected.
9. ***Know who is working for you.*** There are many resources for privacy information. Try Privacy Rights Clearinghouse, 5998 Alcala Park, San Diego, CA 92110, 800-773-7748 (in California) or 619-260-4806. E-mail address: http://www.acusd.edu/~prc/. Electronic Privacy Information Center, 666 Penn Avenue SE, Suite 301, Washington DC 20003, 202-544-9240. E-mail address: http://www.epic.org/
10. ***Avoid the risk.*** If you want complete privacy, go outside the system. Pay all expenses out-of-pocket, informing your practitioner that you want complete privacy.

In 1952, DNA was identified as the basic human genetic material, and one year later its chemical structure was mapped. The Human Genome Project was announced nearly 40 years later. It is a 15-year global effort to discover the location and exact chemical sequence of over 100,000 human genes. The goal date is the year 2005. With this information, scientists can develop genetic tests that indicate susceptibility, treatments that reverse or prevent disease, and pharmaceuticals that can alter DNA imperfections (Elmer-Dewitt 1996).

"We cannot read this entire genetic script yet," writes The Honorable Cliff Stearns (1996). "But advances in science indicate that we will be able to soon. In fact, although the Project is scheduled for completion in 2005, at its current pace, many experts believe it will be done before then. That means that we need to begin making some very difficult public policy decisions now, before those decisions are made by self-interested parties" (p. 15).

Unfortunately, the remarkable research in genetics has enormous potential for abuse. It raises serious questions concerning managed care's corporate approach. Many genetic tests now exist that statistically predict the health or behavior of an individual in the future. The person might appear healthy and normal at the time of the test. Yet the test is a double-edged sword. If a person tests positive for genes indicating a physical or mental vulnerability in the future, it may also lead to vulnerability in the present—to personal, insurance and employment discrimination. Consider some things that have already occurred.

Christine Denmark decided to be genetically tested for Huntington's Disease, an inherited disorder that destroys the central nervous system. It took nine months to get the results which in Denmark's case were positive. Unsure about whether to submit the bills to her insurance company, she confided in her boss. One month later she was fired. It appeared to investigators that the discovery of her vulnerability to the disease and the loss of her job were related.

In 1995 Dr. Francis Collins, Director of the National Center for Human Genome Research, informed the Senate Cancer Coalition that in two recent studies 100 people were identified as being denied insurance because of genetic risk, and 31 percent of surveyed families with inherited diseases were also refused coverage. Their present state of health had no bearing on the insurance company's decision ("Bias from Gene Tests Feared," Newsday 1995).

A 42-year old farmer in northern California was being treated for bronchitis. She told the doctor that her sister had died of cystic fibrosis, a genetically transmitted disease. She was tested for the gene and found to have a single copy. To develop cystic fibrosis, it takes two copies of the damaged gene. Her test results were put into her medical record. As a result, she was repeatedly denied health insurance (Gorman 1995).

The U.S. military maintains the largest bank of DNA samples in the world (Lewis 1996). The Pentagon, he says, claims that the primary purpose of the DNA is to help identify service members whose bodies have been mutilated in action. But the Pentagon has also listed other circumstances, including criminal investigations, in which these genetic indicators might be used. Where does the military get their samples? Mandatory genetic testing is required of all active service members. This 1991 policy was implemented in 1992, resulting in about one million samples of DNA. There are presently about 1.5 million people in uniform. Originally, the military planned to hold on to the tissue samples for 75 years. They recently amended that policy, announcing that samples will be destroyed at the request of the donor when he or she leaves the military. Two Marines tested the regulation by refusing to donate DNA samples. They were court-martialed.

Scientists are presently discovering genes at the rate of more than one per day (Elmer-Dewitt 1996). This process is not as straightforward as it sounds. For example, researchers have found 350 different sites where the cystic fibrosis gene mutates—with more still being uncovered. Dozens of mutations are involved in the breast cancer gene (BRCA-1) which accounts for about 5 percent of the 182,000 breast cancer cases diagnosed each year (Gorman 1995). Consequently, many of the new experimental genetic tests may only indicate susceptibility rather than a definitive future diagnosis. Many scientists theorize that the damaged genes are activated by environmental catalysts such as nutrition and chemical toxins.

Geneticists know that many questions remain in the area of genetic testing. Their rule is to be cautious, recognizing that the tests are very new and experimental. Insurance companies and employers are not as cautious as geneticists. This was proven in the 1970s when black Americans participated in a screening campaign for sickle-cell anemia. No one thought that the information would be misused. Yet people lost their jobs or were denied insurance simply because they were in the program (Gorman 1995). Today, the potential for abuse is far greater. With records open to many interested parties and centralized databases, genetic tests, whether accurate or not, can become the health care disaster of the 21st century.

Some of the most controversial research concerns relationships between genes and behavior. Although this information has immeasurable value for both patients and professionals, it can be lethal in the hands of Big Brother. Mercator Genetics has established a collaboration in Finland, Denmark, and Israel to identify the gene or genes involved in schizophrenia (NewsPage 1996b). Two independent research teams supported by NIMH (National Institutes of Mental Health) and a third by Edinburgh University are investigating at least five chromosomes involved in bipolar disorder (Asher and Weeks 1996). City of Hope's Department of Medical Genetics and associates from the Veteran's Administration Hospital in Loma Linda, CA, announced they had identified three different dopaminergic genes associated with several disorders, including Tourette's Syndrome, ADHD, conduct disorders, and stuttering (NewsPage 1996aa). Researchers have also linked a gene to "novelty-seeking" or a "love of new thrills" (Angier 1996). There are searches to link genes to alcoholism, aggression, homosexuality . . . the list seems endless. However, behavioral geneticists hotly debate research findings. Many feel that more complex behavioral disorders are caused by a combination of genes, with each having only a small effect.

Others feel that carriers may react in a multitude of ways. "So each of these disorders might be due to genes alone," writes Berkowitz (1996), "but the complexity of the genetic mechanisms might preclude a definitive finding with current techniques." Without definitive evidence, behavioral genetics may be creating a bias toward simplistic explanations. "For example, by defining any mental condition or characteristic as a 'trait,'" Berkowitz adds, "one suggests that the characteristic is somehow like Mendel's traits of wrinkled or smooth peas and thus may show a regular pattern of inheritance." The very categorization of a behavior or mental illness might distort the real effect a gene may create.

MCOs usually simplify problems rather than examining more complex issues. How much money can the MCO save by denying coverage to a person with a bad gene? If there is a mistake and the gene does not lead to the disorder, what is the penalty? MCOs carefully evaluate risks with the potential for monetary gain. Ironically, the same insurance companies that so eagerly exclude experimental or alternative medical care are clamoring to include experimental genetic testing.

Luba Shugawat (1996), President of the New Jersey Society for Clinical Social Workers, in an online communication, reported her experience in the state legislature. She observed:

> A month ago, I attended a Senate sub-committee hearing to testify on behalf of NJSCSW [New Jersey Society for Clinical Social Workers] about managed care. Prior to the testimony on managed care, a bill was discussed about legislation pertaining to genetic testing. Insurance groups are lobbying for the right to have "carte blanche" access to get genetic testing done in New Jersey. Thus, if a person is tested genetically and is found to have a predisposition towards a specific disease . . . the insurance company would be able to legally discriminate, by withholding medical coverage. Now, this really takes the phrase "pre-existing medical condition" too far, don't you think? Also, the fact that not all people necessarily get the disease to which they are, supposedly, predisposed to is of no interest, whatsoever, to these insurers. And . . . you guessed it, these companies expect access to this information without the individual's knowledge or consent.

Two weeks later the New Jersey State Senate followed the State Assembly in unanimously passing The Genetic Privacy Act. It prohibits health insurers and employers from using—or requiring—genetic testing for either coverage or employment. Life insurers, however, can use it to set premiums or deny coverage (NewsPage 1996dd). New York State, following the same national trend, passed similar legislation in two bills banning employers from denying work because of "genetic predisposition" to a disease and a creation of "safeguards to try to ensure the confidentiality of genetic tests" (Moritsuga 1996). New York, however, did not prohibit life or health insurance companies from denying coverage or raising rates. Similar measures have been proposed in the federal legislature (Stearns 1996).

Genetic privacy may become the most difficult problem in the struggle to maintain confidentiality in patient records. The result can be that even the healthiest patient, with the most impeccable lifestyle, may be at risk of insurance denial based on genetic information. The potential for such abuse is not lost in the public imagination. In a Time/CNN poll conducted by Yankelovich Partners (Elmer-Dewitt 1996), 90 percent of the 500 respondents believed that it should be illegal for insurance companies to use genetic tests to decide who to insure. On the other hand, it may be difficult to defend withholding valid information from organizations that are affected by the information. Can we expect insurance companies to provide fair rates for the general public if they do not have access to the information necessary for actuarial procedures?

TECHNOLOGY

In 1967, *Newsday* reporter Bernie Bookbinder decided to find as much information as he could on a randomly selected individual. In many weeks of searching through the archives of public agencies, Bookbinder gathered information about the man's entire life, from his early school records, to his service record in World War II. He even found the names of his dogs. Twenty-five years later it took another reporter less than two hours to gather the same information by computer.

Modern technology allows the storage of patient information in a "virtual patient record" (Forslund and Kilman 1996). Patient data is originally entered into the electronic system using a standard format. It becomes "virtual" because the record in whole or in part can be accessed and used in different ways for different purposes even at the same time.

The Medical Records Institute is an organization of people who believe that the future of health information technology lies in the creation and implementation of electronic record systems (1995). They suggest that there are five levels of organization between the paper record and the electronic record system.

Level 1: **automated records** are electronic records that still depend on their paper counterparts.

Level 2: **the computerized record system** is achieved when space and cost restraints force traditional paper records into the computer. The paper records are usually scanned into the system.

Level 3: **electronic records** represent a profound change from Level 2. Instead of being stored as complete pages of data on individual patients, medical records are broken into individual items or fields, each of which can be read separately. This accommodates automated record retrieval and data analysis.

Level 4: **electronic record systems** move beyond the computer model into a systems organization. This greatly widens the range of related information, making data available for multiple provider enterprises.

Level 5: **electronic health records** are comprehensive records that hold virtually an unlimited amount of health information within a system. This system can be likened to the proposed cradle-to-grave patient record maintained in national centralized databases (Medical Records Institute 1995).

The history of electronic claims submission to Medicare is illustrative. Since the late 1970s, the Health Care Financing Administration (HCFA) has been encouraging electronic claims submissions for Medicare. Hospitals were urged to install direct data entry terminals to submit claims. By the 1980s, many hospitals were sending claims to commercial insurance companies through claims clearinghouses which distributed claims to different payers. Practice management software offered the ability to facilitate claims submissions. By the 1990s, electronic claims became more commonplace, with 97 percent of all Part A (inpatient hospital) and 55 percent of all Part B (outpatient) claims submitted electronically to Medicare (Norman and Moynihan 1994).

More recent developments in electronic networks for medical records include the following:

In May, 1996 researchers in the United States, Europe, and Japan launched a project to set international standards for patient records that will be stored on a network linking hospitals and clinics around the world. The goal is to put the standards into practice by the year 2000 (NewsPage 1996k).

Approximately 1 out of every 7 Americans has a file in the Medical Information Bureau (MIB) national database (Anthony 1993).

Physician's Computer Network (PCN) has access to the electronic patient records of 41,000 doctors or 10 percent of office-based doctors in the United States (EPIC 1996).

Ten years ago 5 percent of all health insurance claims were transmitted and processed electronically. Today the number is over 36 percent. It is expected to increase dramatically by the year 2000 (Riley 1996a).

In 1993 the state of Maryland established the Healthcare Access and Cost Commission to reduce health care costs and increase access to health care. The goal was to collect data on all patient–practitioner contacts in the state (Whitman 1996).

Kaiser-Permanente in Colorado is computerizing 300,000 patient records, making them available to the group's 2000 health care providers at 25 different locations (IBM Healthcare 1995).

The Agency for Health Care Policy and Research made available the Nationwide Inpatient Sample (NIS) of 6.5 million patient records from 900 community hospitals in 17 states. It runs on a set of 6 CD-ROMs designed for desktop computers (NewsPage 1996h).

Twenty percent of eligible members in a voluntary group long-term care plan enrolled via the Internet according to US Care of Santa Monica, CA (NewsPage 1996g).

Jim Clark, founder of Silicon Graphics and Netscape Communications Corp. has founded a third business, Healtheon. Healtheon sells its services to insurers, using the World Wide Web to present services to employers and to register employees (Fisher 1996).

Large potential benefits drive this banking of data. Arthur D. Little, a prestigious Massachusetts consulting firm, conducted a study on the computerization of patient records (Flower 1994). They concluded that the United States could save $15 billion every year if the medical records of every man, woman, and child were put online. Other potential benefits are compelling. Researchers could conduct studies using data from large numbers of people which resides in centralized databases. Medical and mental health practitioners would have access to complete individual and family histories before a patient stepped into their offices. In emergencies, when patients are unable to give important information to providers, their records could be examined, avoiding potentially harmful treatment that may conflict with pre-existing conditions or medications. Much of this is already happening. For example, Kaiser-Permanente, one of the country's largest and oldest HMOs, scanned their database of 2.4 million Northern California members to create a registry of diabetics. They used the information to examine how diabetics were being served in this system. With their data, Kaiser-Permanente developed a program to provide better preventive care for diabetics (Hamilton 1995). In Washington, DC, the District of Columbia Coalition, a group of social service providers, uses a "CD-based multimedia Community Services Workstation" (Flower 1994). The counselor or case manager accesses information on the computer, enabling the client to get help for his or her specific problem in areas such as housing, medical care, and special programs. In Boston, the Center for Clinical Computing at Harvard Medical School and Beth Israel Hospital (Safran 1995) have built a system of nearly 3000 computers, accessible to authorized health providers, where patient information can be sent or retrieved in the hospital to improve and streamline care.

Electronic information systems can also simplify many clerical and financial transactions. Provider referrals and authorizations, eligibility requirements, claim status, and remittance information could be only a keystroke away from every office PC. Money could be transferred on time electronically. These things were actually accomplished in a pilot program called the Workgroup on Electronic Data Interchange (WEDI). WEDI was a pilot program launched in Virginia in 1992, involving federal and state governments, 30 insurance companies, 165 hospitals, and 5000 physicians (Norman and Moynihan 1994). Many of the WEDI features will appear in the paperless Blue Cross system scheduled for completion by 1998.

WHO'S LURKING?

Lurking refers to electronic voyeurism. The potential privacy problems resulting from this accumulation of data are large. As the data becomes further removed from the people it describes, the holders of the data become less concerned with its confidentiality. Kolata (1995) writes that "medical information is being sold without even minimal precautions to protect patient privacy" (p. A1). She illustrates her claim in an interview with Robert Merold, then vice president for marketing at IMS America, a company that sells, among other things, data to drug companies. Merold says that when IMS buys aggregate patient records from places like state governments, medical clinics and drugstore chains, they frequently find names included in the data. He suggests that the people who supply the data do not understand the importance of eliminating patient names. Frequently they simply pass names on along with the business transaction.

A few examples of the redistribution of information in patient records are illustrative:

In the early 1990s, a joint venture in Kentucky between The Blue Cross/ Blue Shield Association, 12 State Blue Cross plans and IBM linked with 21 private carriers and the billing offices of more than 80,000 hospitals and doctors (Bowman 1993).

The Medical Information Bureau, financed and run by the insurance industry, stores patient records of approximately 15 million Americans and Canadians with over 750 insurance firms using their services to obtain information for insurance applications.

In 1995, Equifax, one of America's largest compilers of credit information, in tandem with AT&T, announced its entry into the health care information business. Equifax already owns credit information on more than 119 million people and sells this information to other businesses.

The redistribution of this data in the private sector is presently unregulated. Medical and mental health histories are easily available to life and health insurance companies, employers screening job applicants, direct marketers, credit companies, private investigators, law enforcement agencies, forensic psychologists, and even casual viewers in company offices. If information cannot be legally obtained, then a "customer" can call one of hundreds of hackers who advertise their services online and in hacker magazines. The infamous hacker, Kevin Mitnick, is said to have broken into the North American Air Defense Computer when he was a teenager. In subsequent years he entered corporate and telephone company computers, breaking through some of the most sophisticated security systems while collecting (although never using) some 20,000 credit card numbers. With folk heroes like Mitnick, even the most secure patient records databases are vulnerable (Weise 1996).

Industry efforts to protect this information are underway. Although reluctant to admit to security problems, companies such as Citicorp, American Express, and TRW Information Systems & Services are struggling to protect their databases. TRW, which maintains credit records on nearly 180 million Americans, has spent $30 million just to update and secure its network.

Beth Israel Hospital and the Center for Clinical Computing at Harvard Medical School have developed a sophisticated security system for medical records. They established a system of computer-designed passwords which are changed every six months. Supervisors issue passwords and determine the level of authorization, restricting access accordingly. Users are told that their password is equivalent to a personal signature. Each time a record is accessed the computer registers the identity of the user. Both employees and patients can find out who accessed which records. Remote access is controlled by requiring a second password. Although the system is not completely safe, it provides important steps toward assuring greater privacy (Safran 1995).

The courts may provide some protection for medical records. In Minnesota, Attorney General Hubert H. Humphrey III announced a 17-state consumer protection settlement that ultimately affects 1 out of every 7 Americans. Medco Containment Services, Inc., a large prescription benefit company, merged with one of the world's biggest pharmaceutical companies—Merck & Co. Doctors' prescriptions submitted to Medco's mail service pharmacies were reviewed by Medco-employed pharmacists. If the medication was not a Merck product, the pharmacist would telephone the doctor with a request to change the prescription—usually to a Merck product. The class action suit alleges that the pharmacists never disclosed that they were Medco employees or that Medco was owned by Merck. They settled for a fine of $1.9 million and managed care reforms to protect consumers' privacy rights. The settlement was not an admission of guilt, only a legally enforceable court order (PRNewswire 1995).

Legislation will ultimately be needed to provide effective protection of confidential records, but progress here is also slow. The Healthcare Privacy Act, introduced in 1995, actually makes it easier to establish national databases controlled by companies that specifically collect and use electronic information. The National Federation of Societies for Clinical Social Workers (NFSCSW) has suggested on their online Web site that this legislation is rumored to be "the brainchild" of Equifax. The Healthcare Privacy Act has been opposed by many individuals and groups such as The National Coalition of Mental Health Professionals, Coalition for Patient Rights, and The Consortium for Psychotherapy. Representative Jay R. Kaufman, chair of the Massachusetts subcommittee responsible for patient and medical record confidentiality, wrote in a letter to Senator Kennedy, "In our efforts in Massachusetts, we put patient rights first. This bill puts them last" (EPIC 1995).

As public awareness of the confidentiality problem grows, other social influences will arise. The Electronic Privacy Information Center (EPIC), a public interest research center in Washington, DC, considers medical record privacy considered one of their main concerns. EPIC (1995) suggests nine essential ingredients for protection of patient records:

1. Federal legislation
2. Complete patient access to their own records
3. Criminal or civil fines for unauthorized access, disclosure, or use of records
4. Strict limitations on third-party access
5. Patient consent for inclusion in national databases. No psychiatric records are included in databases
6. Research conducted only with patient consent
7. Use of the most powerful electronic security measures
8. Social Security numbers not used to identify patients
9. After federal laws set minimum standards, state laws may be needed for additional protection.

Hopefully these efforts by business, the courts, legislators, and the general public will eventually provide security for all electronic information, especially the sensitive material in medical and psychotherapy treatment reports. As Denise Nagel, president of the Coalition for Patient Rights notes, "Technologically, we can do anything we want to do—and we can do it with fiscal as well as ethical responsibility" (Nagel 1995).

5

From the Halls of Justice

It may take five or ten years to find the right balance of managed care, physician autonomy and patient rights. . . . Our vision for health care must go beyond cutting costs, providing access, or squabbling about managed health care. Health-care reform poses the greatest political challenge to a democratic republic, because each of us is being asked to do something for all of us, and many of us feel that what might be best for all of us is not best for each of us. It's that simple. It's that difficult.

–Former U.S. Surgeon General C. Everett Koop, now medical director of Time-Life Medical, which is engaged in patient education.

In 1954, the concept of employer-paid health care was becoming increasingly popular. A survey of medical costs reported that 16 percent of American families went into debt each year to pay for treatment. President Eisenhower encouraged the private sector to strengthen health services (Microsoft 1994r). But the end of World War II was almost ten years in the past, the troops were back from Korea, the baby boom was still happening, and no one seemed terribly worried. In fact, the President's golf game was far more intriguing to the American public than health care issues.

A few years later Kennedy and Nixon are preparing to begin their classic television debates. Nixon stands at the podium, visibly worried but still able to smile. Kennedy is more polished and has the appearance of being ready to answer everything. They begin to speak and suddenly a switch occurs. Supertechnology injects today's issues into the debate. The topic is how to provide a fair and reasonable system for mental health care. Kennedy presents a case for establishing services for underprivileged populations such as children at risk for future disabilities, families threatened by the effects of substance abuse, the older population, or unemployed people. He supports government funding and government loans to students in training programs. Nixon argues for shifting control to the private sector. His ideas seem related to the ancient Chinese system of paying physicians when their patients remain healthy but not when their patients become sick. Nixon maintains that health care must be based on prevention and early detection of problems, awarding incentives for early intervention. He stresses the need for responsible management of resources by private enterprise. Kennedy counters that private enterprise will require government aid and privileged status in order to provide adequate coverage. Will private corporations be able to provide care for the very poor and the very sick? Will the middle class have to pay disproportionate rates? Would it not be ultimately more democratic and more economic to allow government participation in health care? After all, everyone agrees that what is needed is health care that can never be taken away, health care that is available for all Americans (Mitchell 1996).

Today's arguments are closely related to those of the 1960s. The questions debated by Nixon and Kennedy have become the key health care issues of the 1990s.

Looking back again: it was on February 5, 1963, that President Kennedy proposed the first major involvement of the federal government in mental health services with the establishment of the National Community Mental Health Centers Program. During the same period, the National Institute of Mental Health contributed to the availability of treatment by providing funds for the education and training of professionals in the mental health field. The goal of the federally funded programs was to provide mental health treatment to people who otherwise would not get needed services. Legitimate facilities were developed with professionally trained staffs that treated a large population of patients. The prevailing spirit of enthusiasm contributed to a sense of unlimited availability. The cost of mental health care escalated.

The idea of government health insurance entered into national debate. Special interests, such as private insurance companies and some groups in the medical profession, mounted campaigns to voice their opposition, but the more liberal voices prevailed. Voluntary cooperative or commercial health insurance programs developed that provided benefits to group or individual subscribers. Blue Cross and Blue Shield, the largest of the new insurers, sought legal avenues to become nonprofit agencies. In 1964 President Johnson persisted, signing the Medicare Act, creating the first government-operated health insurance program for Americans age 65 and older and Medicaid for low-income people. The federal government had become the single largest payer of medical care (Microsoft 1994b).

Medicare was a popular program. However, the beneficial increase in needed services brought with it opportunities for mismanagement and exploitation. It looked good on paper, but in practice the federal government was not prepared to provide efficient administration or safeguards against misuse of funds. The blank-check market increased. Public attitude appeared to move from appreciation of medical services to an attitude of entitlement. There was a growing belief that there were no limits to health services, supportive services, preventative care, funds, and even to litigation.

Paul Ellwood, Jr., who was at the time an administrator in the American Rehabilitation Institute, presented a health care plan in 1969 that provided incentives to maintain health rather than to treat illness. The new Republican president was looking for a viable alternative to the health plan of the Democrats. Nixon seized upon Ellwood's proposal, using it as the basis of his health care reform. Nixon's 1971 Health Message to Congress introduced the concept of managed health care as part of Republican policy.

The Health Maintenance Organization Act of 1973 (and subsequent amendments) reflected Republican goals. It provided the legal and financial foundation for establishing HMOs throughout the country. The new health maintenance organizations were subsidized by the federal government with the intent of creating a program of health maintenance and prevention in addition to health care. In order to qualify for subsidies, HMOs were required to provide basic patient health services, including outpatient mental health care, crisis intervention, medical treatment, and referrals for alcohol and drug abusers. Profit-making corporations were also included in the new system (Bennett 1988). The HMOs were typical of government programs. The taxpayer invested in the initial risk. When the private sector saw that there was money to be made, they took over.

Although HMOs included mental health coverage in their contracts, they instituted rigid regulations to limit these benefits. One tactic was to restrict mental health coverage to specific conditions. They excluded situations such as marital counseling, psychoanalysis, long-term rehabilitation, and chronic problems. HMOs restricted the number of visits, the number of hospital days, payment to providers, rider options, annual and lifetime maximum payments, and, of course, they restricted mental health providers to new sets of regulations.

HMOs grew steadily through the 1970s. In 1981, the United States Senate authorized $68 million to establish a National Health Maintenance Organization Intern Program to train individuals to become administrators, directors, and other types of HMO managers. After two decades of growth, HMOs leaped from an enrollment of 6 million Americans to today's 56 million (Dentzer 1996). Kenneth Abromowitz, a New York City stock analyst, suggests that there will be ten more years of turmoil in health care, with HMOs becoming the ultimate winners because they cost 40 percent less than traditional health insurance (Healthcare Systems Committee 1996a). HMO membership has been predicted to include 50 percent of Americans in group health plans by 2001 (NewsPage 1996m).

John Protos, in an article in *Smart Money* (1996), listed "Ten Things Your HMO Won't Tell You." Protos humorously exposes the hidden techniques used by various managed health care systems to save money by making it difficult to get health services.

1. The less your doctor sees you, the more he earns.
2. Your primary-care doctor is your specialist.
3. Your health is a numbers game to us.
4. Our exclusions could kill you.
5. You're not sick until we say you're sick.
6. Your ignorance is our bliss.
7. We're loose with the facts.
8. We use second-rate parts.
9. Send you to an expensive therapist? Are you crazy?
10. Unhappy? Go ahead, just try to sue us. (pp. 133–144)

The development of the HMOs occurred simultaneously with the introduction of professional accountability. In 1972, amendments to the Social Security Act created the PSROs—professional standards review organizations. This new level of accountability involved assessing the cost, quality, and appropriate utilization of services. Ten years later, the Peer Review Improvement Act replaced the PSRO program with PRO—the utilization and quality control Peer Review Organization. For the first time, Medicare providers had to submit patient data for review.

The ground rules were set. External reviewers and third-party payers now had the legal right to reduce or deny reimbursement for services. External review organizations, managed care business, and case management companies appeared overnight, demanding justification for health care services based on medical necessity. Consequently, Medicare launched a cost containment program called PPS—Prospective Payment System—using a system of classifications called diagnosis-related groups or DRGs. DRGs classified patients into more than 475 categories based on diagnosis, procedures (e.g., surgery) and co-morbid conditions. Psychiatric and drug and alcohol treatment hospitals and units in general hospitals were exempt. At the same time managed health care industries began to reduce psychiatric and substance abuse treatment benefits (Goodman et al. 1992).

Dramatic advances in medical technology and correspondingly increased medical costs were demanding more out of each American dollar. In the 1960s a patient with complaints related to a head injury would have a skull x-ray performed in an emergency room at a cost of about $35. Ten years later the same patient would have a CAT scan costing over $400. Similarly, a patient with abdominal symptoms in the 60s would have an upper GI series and a barium enema for about $200. In the 90s the patient would probably undergo upper and lower gastrointestinal endoscopy and a CAT scan of the abdomen and pelvis, costing $2000. New technology in pharmaceuticals also affected costs. Outpatient treatment of bronchitis with ampicillin in 1970 ran $10–$15, while in 1990 a second generation cephalosporin might be prescribed for $100. Psychotropic medications for mental illness have reduced inpatient treatment, shifting costs to outpatient care and, ideally, to more effective medications such as Prozac and Zoloft. The need to treat increasingly large numbers of alcohol and substance abusers also escalated mental health costs. All of this was compounded by the boom in hospital and health care facility construction, and incentives to maximize treatment, which in turn increased costs.

Instead of focusing on the cost of inefficient management, inadequate guidelines, and the effect of unregulated litigation, politicians saw only the numbers. The numbers were sobering. Between 1965 and 1992, health care went from 6 percent to 13.2 percent of the gross national product. By 1988 health care spending per capita reached $51,926. Every industrialized nation, except the United States and South Africa, had a national health care program (Microsoft 1994c). Yet health care in the U.S. was estimated to cost 40 percent more (Frank 1993).

The need for reform became a major political issue in Clinton's presidential campaign. Supporters of Clinton predicted that 1994 would be the year that the first American president would accomplish a major revamping of the health care system. In a national campaign, Hillary Rodham Clinton used town meetings, media, and an unending litany of health care horror stories to convince Americans that national reform was essential. The Clinton plan, comprising over 1,300 pages, was delivered to Congress. It called for health alliances, cost control, quality care, and universal coverage. The fighting began.

The Republicans were angry because they felt that the bill was a partisan effort. Conservatives wanted minimal change, while moderates leaned toward a coalition with centrist Democrats for broader-based reform. The Democrats were split between Clinton's bill and a Canadian-style single-payer system. MCOs fought furiously, using television and print media, to warn Americans that both taxes and health care costs would increase, while quality would decrease. Small business groups joined in grassroots campaigns. Special interest groups, such as doctors and hospitals, wielded their powerful influence. When the fight began, public opinion hovered at 50 percent for Clinton's plan and 33 percent opposed. After three months of public debate, the numbers fell to 41 percent for and 45 percent opposed. A Time/CNN poll (Church 1996) told the story:

90 percent believed Clinton's plan would make them pay more for medical care
55 percent believed they would have less choice of doctors
41 percent feared that the quality of care would go down.

By the end of 1994, hopes ended for a well-planned health care reform. MCOs rushed to fill the void with their claims for fast solutions, decreased costs, and happy family lives.

Following the rejection by Congress of President Clinton's Health Security bill, private managed health companies started their battle for the health care market. The managed care businesses fought with the marketing techniques now familiar to the public. Humorist Russell Baker (1996) responded to health care advertisements in an article called "Harry! Louise! You lied." He said:

> They told us that national health care would deprive us of the right to choose our own doctors. So we said no to national health care. . . . And they told us if we had national health care there would be government bureaucracies interfering with our medical treatment. . . . So we said no to national health care. . . . They told us that national health care would cost us billions in taxes. Leave it to the free market, they said, and it wouldn't cost us a cent to continue enjoying the best medicine in the world. . . . And that was the end of national health care. The health industry is cleaning up on Wall Street. The rest of us pray we may never get sick. [p. 19]

Members of a study group called Jackson Hole were among the advisors to Hillary Rodham Clinton. The members of the Jackson Hole group promoted the concept of *managed competition.* Jackson Hole included representatives from some of the major US insurance companies including Prudential, Metropolitan Life, Aetna, and CIGNA. The founder of the Jackson Hole group was Paul Ellwood, who in 1969 designed the plan that Nixon used for his proposal of business enterprises called Health Maintenance Organizations (HMOs).

Paul Ellwood stated in May 1996 that his objective was a health system in "which physicians had substantially greater influence and one that was organized to take better care of patients. It's true that the driving force in the changes to health care so far has been economics. However, my motivation as a doctor was trying to improve quality" (Ellwood 1996, p. 182).

GROWING UP BLUE

Blue Cross was born into a different world.

It was 1929. Sigmund Freud was still in Vienna and America was on the brink of the Great Depression. An official at Baylor University had a novel idea—he offered teachers 21 days of hospital care for $6 a year. The idea spread through Texas, Iowa, and Illinois. "Premiums" were based on the community's claim experience rather than individual subscriber conditions.

In 1933 an executive designed the symbol that would carry them through the 20th century—the blue cross. By 1935 there were 15 plans in 11 states operating as nonprofit plans under the blue cross. Enrollment grew. State medical societies decided to support prepaid plans that covered doctors' fees. By 1946 they affiliated with one another under Associated Medical Care Plans, later becoming Blue Shield.

Fifteen years later Blue Cross insured almost one-third of the United States. And in the mid-sixties, the Blues began to administer Medicare and other government plans, eventually having half of their premiums paid by the government. Monetary losses began to build as health care costs spiraled. Blue Cross and Blue Shield joined forces in 1982, hoping to weather the crisis.

Today, the managed care market has forced many Blues to go out of business, consolidate with one another, or convert to for-profit status. The twenty-first century Blues will probably look very different from their humble, egalitarian origins (Blue Cross and Blue Shield Association 1996).

WHO HAS THE JURISDICTION?

The failure of Clinton's health care plan reverberated throughout state legislatures. After nearly two years of waiting to see if they could count on Washington to solve their health care problems, the states had no choice but to address the issue.

In October 1994, Milt Freudenheim wrote prophetically in *The New York Times*: "Having worked hard in the opposition effort that led Congress to go home without action on health care, insurers and managed health care companies are braced for a flood of new state regulations. They argue that these rules would raise costs and undermine their growing managed health care business" (p. 22).

The individual states began to consider the benefits of the managed care industry. There was one major weapon that MCOs could use to win at least a part of the health care premiums, the Employee Retirement Income Security Act of 1974 (ERISA). President Gerald Ford signed ERISA into law one month after Richard Nixon resigned. The goal of the creators of ERISA was to provide federal regulation of pension funds. Because many companies had been underfunding their pension plans, employees found that when they retired, no funds were available for their retirement. ERISA corrected the problem by prohibiting, by federal law, the underfunding of large pension plans. In order to induce businesses to accept the new regulations, the promoters of ERISA agreed to provide the businesses with an important advantage—that advantage allowing ERISA funds to be exempt from all state laws (Welch 1996b).

No one foresaw that ERISA was creating a shelter destined to haunt employers and states for the remainder of the century. Instead of specifically referring to pension funds, ERISA allowed state exemption for all "employee welfare plans." It did not define the difference between employee welfare and employee insurance plans. Employers quickly took advantage, converting their health insurance policies to "self-insured employee welfare plans." A self-insured health plan is one in which a company serves as its own insurer and pays claims with its own assets. The employer can drop its conventional plan and "hire" an insurance company to manage its workers' claims, leaving it free to totally ignore state insurance regulations (Facts about ERISA 1995).

Under ERISA, MCOs could not be touched as the state passed freedom-of-choice legislation, mandates on quality health care, managed care regulations, and legal liability statutes for negligence, fraud, misrepresentation, and interference with business relationships. These self-insured companies can set up totally different health plans with virtually unregulated standards. States cannot impose taxes on premiums, cannot mandate the provision of specific health benefits, cannot require the contribution of specific amounts of money—they cannot even indicate the reporting of basic data on their costs for employee benefits (Pear 1994b).

With concerns of increased state regulations, more and more employers dropped conventional group health insurance and went to self-insured plans. Predictably, more than half of all the employees in the US found themselves working for companies with self-insured health plans (Pear 1994b). Although big multistage companies were the innovators in the changeover to self-insurance, smaller companies quickly followed suit. "As a result, states are unable to supervise or regulate the health benefits of huge numbers of people who live and work within their borders" (Pear 1994a, p. A28). The more states attempt to regulate health care, the greater an employer's motivation to change to a self-insured plan. This shift has threatened the fragile balance in insurance risk. By becoming self-insured, companies can control costs by designing plans to suit their needs, get discounts through direct negotiations with providers and hospitals, and determine, free of regulation, how to preserve the bottom line. In general, insurance companies reduce risk by spreading the cost of expensive illness into the population pool. When self-insured companies can dramatically reduce their risk through unregulated cost-containment, the cost of expensive illness gets shifted elsewhere. As a result, non-ERISA companies like Blue Cross, who insure individuals, small groups, and small businesses on a large scale, face increased risk (Freudenheim 1994).

Public advocacy groups such as the National Coalition for Mental Health Professionals and Consumers are attempting to educate the public about the need for change. In a discussion of the key issues in health care reform, coalition president Karen Shore writes, "if managed care companies continue to exist, the ERISA law must be amended to make the companies subject to state regulation" (Shore 1995c, p. 74).

State governments seeking the power to regulate ERISA plans want the law changed. However, Republicans are put in conflict between the party's support of state rights and their traditional constituency, business. Businesses do not want limits set on ERISA because they would have to pay a state tax on premiums and would have to honor state regulations that can erode profit. In another example of strange political bedfellows, labor unions support ERISA because of the protection it affords in both health and pension benefits. In 1995 three federal appeals court decisions chipped away at the ERISA block. Essentially, the message was loud and clear: the court would not allow ERISA to shield liability when an employer's decision directly affects the quality of care.

The first case was *Dukes v. US Healthcare, Inc.* Dukes, an HMO patient, was being treated for a variety of ailments by an affiliated doctor. Dukes died and blood tests revealed that he had a treatable, dangerously high blood-sugar level. The widow sued for malpractice under state law and the HMO invoked ERISA preemption, removing the case to federal district court. The HMO argued that ERISA preempted Mrs. Dukes's malpractice claim because the action could only be heard in state court, leaving her no recourse. The court found that the HMO was not actually an ERISA plan—it was only providing a benefits plan for an ERISA plan—and consequently not entitled to preemption. In other words, the court held that ERISA preemption covers only claims relating to benefits specifically regulated by ERISA, such as disclosure of the plan, withholding benefits, and rights under the terms of the plan. If a claim addresses the quality of the benefits—rather than whether they were prohibited—ERISA would not preempt state court action (Snarr 1995).

Two cases after Dukes, *PacifiCare v. Burrage* and *Rice v. Panchal*, held the same position, that "a malpractice claim does not involve the areas directly regulated by ERISA, such as the administration of plan benefits or the level of benefits promised by the plan. . . . The court therefore remanded the case back to state court, thus denying the HMO the protection from liability it sought in ERISA preemption" (Snarr 1995).

In 1996, the court continued to define ERISA protection when it related to terms of the plan and not quality of benefits provided. The U.S. Supreme Court did not allow ERISA to stand as an obstacle to protecting employee rights. Variety Corporation of Buffalo, New York, convinced employees to transfer to a subsidiary, which eventually went out of business. Variety promised that pay and benefits would remain the same. Justice Stephan Breyer wrote that companies who have benefit plans under ERISA cannot "participate knowingly and significantly in deceiving a plan's beneficiaries in order to save the employer money at the beneficiaries' expense." In other words, workers and retirees who have benefits protected by ERISA can sue if an employer gives them misleading information (Court: Benefits deceit merits trial, 1996).

In contrast, CIGNA Corporation won a battle in the struggle to control its Louisiana doctor network. Louisiana has had "any willing provider" legislation since 1993, requiring managed care panels to include any professional that meets the conditions set by the company. CIGNA argued that the state law increases costs for the entire provider network. According to ERISA, a state law cannot increase costs in ERISA health plans. The Fifth Circuit U.S. Court of Appeals agreed, denying the states' right to set up provider network rules for ERISA plans (NewsPage 1996a).

Even with these significant court decisions, Protos (1996) says that ERISA actually makes it more difficult to win lawsuits. First, they must be heard in federal court, where there are fewer plaintiff's attorneys, and there are no punitive damage awards. A lawsuit can only result in an award of attorneys fees and costs of treatment, not damages. That means if your company's self-insured health plan commits malpractice, you can't sue for damages.

Bryant Welch, J.D., Ph.D. (1996b) suggests that that position is changing. "While neither fully developed nor entirely consistent, ERISA law has evolved in a direction much more conducive to holding managed care companies responsible for their role in treatment outcomes" (p. 15). Welch suggests that ERISA plans have become more vulnerable to lawsuits, particularly when liability is assessed on the basis of "malpractice via 'ostensible agency'." Simply put, if a managed care plan has a system that provides inappropriate care, they can be held accountable for the results.

Congress is following the lead taken by the courts. In September, 1996, President Clinton signed into law the parity amendment (discussed in the following section). The measure guarantees parity between mental health and medical insurance coverage by group health plans. It is regarded as a "landmark development" by *The New York State Psychologist* (1997) because self-insured plans now must follow the new requirements, thus changing ERISA benefits.

BACK TO THE FUTURE

While states continue to be active in health care reform, Washington struggles to revive significant health care change. According to Les DelPizzo, M.S.W. (1996), Vice President of Marketing for CMHC Systems and former executive in several Pennsylvania and West Virginia mental health centers, this can have mixed benefits. "When states get too active I worry about the political process," he explains. "State government is easily accessible to the robber barons—those with money and power who work behind the scenes."

In 1996 over 400 bills affecting managed care were introduced into state legislatures. More than 30 states have taken action against HMO practices (Freudenheim 1996a,b). The American Association of Health Plans, an industry trade group, reports that it is following nearly 2000 pieces of managed care legislation in states around the country (Dentzer 1996). Federal bipartisan bills under debate in Congress would regulate the MCOs' most offensive cost-containment tactics. Most of these changes address medical managed care and would indirectly affect mental health coverage.

Tipper Gore, in a statement on mental health legislation, said "I challenge every Member of Congress, as they consider these [parity] issues, to substitute cancer or heart disease for the words mental illness. If you had a loved one with cancer, would you settle for 'another study' if the issue at hand was making sure cancer was covered by insurance? I don't think so! We have done better than 'another study' for cancer and we can, and should, for mental illness" (NewsPage 1996bb).

Proponents for or against parity have frequently crossed party lines. In 1994 both Rosalyn Carter and Betty Ford testified before a House committee pleading for mental health benefits in national health care reform. A national poll commissioned by the Bazelon Center for Mental Health Law found that 82 percent of all voters felt that someone who suffered from mental illness is as sick as someone with medical illness (The National Psychologist 1994). "Parity should be treated as a discrimination issue," suggests DelPizzo. "It should be seen as a moral issue, not a money issue" (1996).

Several groups have pooled their resources to fight for parity in The Coalition for Fairness in Mental Illness Coverage, including the National Alliance for the Mentally Ill (NAMI), National Mental Health Association, American Managed Behavioral Health Association, American Medical Association, American Psychiatric Association, American Psychological Association, Federation of American Health Systems, and the National Association of Psychiatric Health Systems. Parity demands equal insurance coverage for the mentally ill—a population that suffers greatly at the hands of MCOs. Lack of parity implies that someone with diabetes is sicker (and deserves more treatment) than someone with schizophrenia. In 1996 Senators Pete Domenici (R-NM) and Paul Wellstone (D-MN) co-sponsored an amendment for parity on the Kennedy-Kassebaum Bill. The Senate voted 65–33 for parity. There was an immediate barrage of studies and objections which confused the public. Naturally, each camp used their own numbers. To illustrate, the Congressional Budget Office (CBO) concluded from their policy research that it is possible parity may have little or no effect on health care coverage. The CBO suggested that offering a benefit does not necessarily lead to increased utilization. They estimated that insurance premiums would not increase more than 4 percent (NewsPage 1996y). In contrast, a Price Waterhouse study prepared for the business community predicted that parity would force insurance premiums up by 8.7 percent and result in 1.7 million people losing employer-sponsored health coverage (NewsPage 1996x). The National Alliance for the Mentally Ill responded by releasing analyses performed by the Lewin Group, indicating that less than 19 percent of behavioral health care claims—or between 3.4 and 5.6 percent of all health care claims—are related to severe mental illness (NewsPage 1996w).

In April, 1996 the Senate voted overwhelmingly to approve a health care reform bill that requires insurers to cover mental illness as fully as other medical problems. A House version of the bill passed a few months later, and in late September the measure was signed into law by President Clinton. The parity provision (NYS Psychologist 1997) requires health plans to specify equal annual or lifetime dollar limits on medical and mental health services. The parity requirements apply to all group health plans, including managed care plans, covering 50 or more beneficiaries. It also applies to self-insured (ERISA) plans, but not to Medicare or Medicaid. However, the law fails to address the cost containment techniques used by many managed care plans. The American Psychological Association continues to lobby for federal quality and cost-containment standards for all health plans.

In October, 1996 Gov. George E. Pataki signed into New York State law the Health Care Bill of Rights. The law, which goes into effect in two stages, includes provisions for disclosure of managed care contract details to consumers, due process protection for physicians, strengthening of utilization review (UR) procedures, and requirements that networks have enough providers to allow patients a choice of physicians.

The following provisions went into effect on January 1, 1997:

1. PROVIDER DUE PROCESS: Providers cannot be terminated from plan without being told the reasons and having an opportunity for a hearing.
2. BAN ON GAG CLAUSES: Plans cannot prevent providers from giving patients information about treatment options or advocating for approval of a patient's course of treatment.
3. HOLD HARMLESS PROVISIONS: Plans are prevented from shifting any legal liability to the provider for any of the plan's activities, actions, or omissions.

Four more provisions will become effective on April 1, 1997. These are:

4. DISCLOSURE: Comprehensive consumer disclosure requirements.
5. UTILIZATION REVIEW: UR procedures establishing personnel standards, appeal rights for denied treatment, and a prudent lay person standard for emergency care.
6. GRIEVANCE: Consumer grievance procedures.
7. ACCESS TO SPECIALISTS: Mechanisms and procedures to facilitate patient access to specialists.

The National Federation of Societies for Clinical Social Workers (NFSCSW) suggests that the parity amendment has established a new battleground with business and insurance companies fighting to repeal or modify parity before 1998, and supporters seeking to expand it (National Advocates Report 1996).

In a May 28, 1996 letter to Senators Dole, Domenici, and House Speaker Gingrich, New Hampshire Governor Stephen Merrill noted that:

> Study after study has shown that treating severe mental illness equitably in insurance is affordable. Data shows that managed care techniques effectively control costs and provide an alternative to placing individuals on Medicaid benefits. In the two years since I signed this bill (New Hampshire Senate Bill 767), this has proven to be an affordable and effective piece of legislation. [NewsPage 1996v]

Health care politics makes very strange bedfellows. Especially in health care reform. "The nation's attention" (Freudenheim 1996b), "appears to have shifted from concern about getting runaway costs under control to questions about whether managed care has gone too far" (p. 1).

Insurance companies' care went to the extreme—from not paying enough attention to cost to where cost is paramount. The media has fueled changing attitudes toward MCOs. The headlines say it all:

Patient databases have placed privacy on its deathbed (*The Washington Post*, 1993).
Who owns the patient anyway? (*Time*, 1994).
Skinned by thin health coverage (*Money*, 1994).
Medical data gathered by firms can prove less than confidential (*The Wall Street Journal*, 1994).
Medical records on sale in marketplace (*The New York Times*, 1995).

The lethal side effects of managed care (*Business Week*, 1995).
Delays by HMO leaving patients haunted by bills (*The New York Times*, 1996).
Gagging the Doctors (*Time*, 1996).

Is it time for MCOs to seek balance? Dentzer (1996) writes about a "golden age" when managed care plans compete on quality rather than "squeezing costs." Others, like Ivan Miller, Ph.D. (1994) feel that managed care faces an imminent demise, only to be replaced by another system. Whether reform or revolution, the changes will first occur in medical health care. Mental health care will hopefully follow, within its present 8–10 percent of total health plan costs (NewsPage 1996p).

It is important to understand which health care debates will affect mental health. The following is a sample of some of the other mental health issues being discussed in legislatures and by advocacy groups across the country.

WHO BELIEVES WHAT?

The Response Center, a market research firm that specializes in health care, conducted a survey that compared the responses of 286 top executives representing 40 percent of all managed care companies in the US and consumers. The results gave some interesting insights into where these two groups agree and disagree:

82 percent of consumers and 63 percent of executives feel that health care costs are too high.
70 percent of consumers and 70 percent of executives feel that coverage should be available to everyone.
54 percent of consumers and 11 percent of executives feel that experimental treatments should be fully covered.
67 percent of consumers and 25 percent of executives feel that health care costs will increase.
55 percent of consumers and 67 percent of executives feel that ailments related to chronic smoking should be covered.
67 percent of the executives agree that the industry needs a minimal amount of government involvement (NewsPage 1996r).

CONSUMER'S RIGHT-TO-KNOW LEGISLATION (CRTK)

CRTK legislation is a consumer-oriented bill introduced in Colorado in 1995. Written by a interdisciplinary committee of licensed mental health professionals, the goal is to require public disclosure of information. CRTK advocates propose that full disclosure of insurance methods, practices, and standards will enable the natural forces of the marketplace to regulate the industry. The Interdisciplinary Committee for "Consumer's Right-To-Know" Mental Health Legislation (1995) carefully spells out what information should be disclosed:

Information relevant to advertising claims of third party treatment managers.

Information about administrative expenses, the amount of treatment provided, and the efficiency of third-party managers that is relevant to the consumer making cost-versus-value decisions.

Full information about how confidential information will be handled.

Arguments against CRTK say that it will increase grievances, appeals, and lawsuits. Opponents suggest that providers with too many contracts might have difficulty tracking down the right information. MCOs do not want providers to support treatments that are not covered in the policy or make the company look bad. Gag clauses prevent providers from saying anything that may "undermine the confidence of enrollees, potential enrollees, their employers, plan sponsors, or the public" (Healthcare Systems Committee 1996b). This provision allows MCOs the freedom of choosing and limiting treatment for an uninformed consumer. Some companies actually prohibit providers from discussing alternatives they do not cover. In mental health, that can raise issues about discussing things such as long-term treatment in place of ultra-brief therapy or psychoanalytic treatment in place of solution-focused therapy. Two national health care organizations, Foundation Health and U.S. HealthCare, have already removed gag clauses from their contracts. Several states have banned gag rules and restrictions on information providers can give patients about care choices (Freudenheim 1996b).

In testimony before the U.S. House of Representatives Subcommittee on Health and Environment, William J. Osheroff, M.D., Vice President and Medical Director of PacifiCare of California, insisted that reputable managed health care organizations have no gag rules. Osheroff asserted that MCOs supported unrestricted communication between providers and patients concerning diagnosis, treatment, and other information concerning care. "That physicians may be required to discuss coverage with the health plan is not to be construed necessarily that they are precluded from discussing all possible options with the patient," explained Osheroff (NewsPage 1996u).

ANY WILLING PROVIDER

In the world of MCOs, psychotherapists are often coming up against a "closed panel." Denkers and Clifford (1994) found that 86 percent of responding psychologists had been told, at one time or another, that "the panel is closed." Forty-two percent were informed that only M.D.s were eligible and 46 percent had sent in applications and been turned down for vague or irrelevant reasons.

To illustrate, a psychotherapist found that she could get on any panel she wanted because there were only two clinicians in her zip code. Meanwhile, ten minutes away in another zip code, psychotherapists were being refused regularly. The inability to get on a panel or network often creates a decline in caseload or the breakdown of traditional referral sources. Eighty-five percent of the psychologists in Denkers and Clifford's study (1994) said that this had happened to them, while another 53 percent were forced to transfer a patient to another therapist because they were not on the list. Similarly, consumers may be unable to follow up referrals from trusted sources or see psychotherapists that specialize in a specific disorder, population, or community.

In any willing provider (AWP) legislation, MCOs must accept any professional who has appropriate credentials and is willing to follow contract terms and conditions. This would also protect psychotherapists from blacklisting based on things such as the number of appeals or managed care "good behavior." According to Freudenheim (1996), "some health maintenance organizations will exclude or expel doctors for ordering tests or consultations the health plans deem unnecessary" (p. 22). Blacklisting usually occurs without a psychotherapist's knowledge. Denkers and Clifford (1994) found that only 16 percent were notified after being dropped from the provider panel. AWP legislation would do away with closed networks that deny psychoanalysts, dynamic psychotherapists, or any other qualified professional inclusion on managed care lists. Patients would then be able to choose their own provider as long as he or she were willing to contract with their managed care company. Over half a dozen states, including Georgia and Illinois, have adopted this type of legislation.

MEDICAL SAVINGS ACCOUNTS

"Medical savings accounts are about freedom for the individual," says Karen Shore (1996), "and Americans need their freedom." MSAs offer a health care system where the consumer (employer, government, or individual) purchases a high-deductible policy and banks the difference, in dollars, between that policy and a traditional low-deductible policy. The money (up to $2000 for individuals and $4000 for couples) is placed in a tax-free account and used throughout the year to pay routine medical care and expenses. Anyone younger than 59 1/2 is penalized if the money is used for anything other than medical care. Advocates feel that MSA systems make both patients and providers responsible for health care utilization. Opponents argue that utilization review will still be used for expenses over the deductible, compromising privacy and jeopardizing choice. MSAs might not work well for people who manage money poorly. Others suggest that they will become a repository for the wealthy, as a means to avoid taxes. Presently, the standard catastrophic plans underwritten by the major MSA company have a limit of $10,000 per year for mental health—a sum inadequate for hospitalization or other intensive care (Shore 1995b).

Some critics believe that MSAs will take those who are healthy and those who are rich out of the insurance pool. As a result, risk will increase and costs will rise. This will be seen in higher premiums. Newt Gingrich, Speaker of the House, vehemently disagrees, proposing that individuals who spend their own money are much better health care shoppers than bureaucrats spending other people's money (Bowermaster 1996).

Dreyfuss and Stone (1996) offer a strong argument against medical savings accounts. They discuss in detail an Indiana company called Golden Rule Insurance. Dreyfuss and Stone accuse Golden Rule and its chairman, J. Patrick Rooney, of injecting huge amounts of money into Republican coffers to win support for Medical Savings Accounts. They found that nearly $1 million was spent in the last election cycle.

Dreyfuss and Stone paint an interesting scenario. Assume that the House and Senate agree to cut Medicare spending by upwards of $300 billion. (This is an unlikely assumption, of course, because most members of the Democratic party have opposed, and continue to oppose, such a draconian measure.) In that situation Medicare would have no choice but to reduce payments to hospitals and providers. The current fee-for-service system would collapse, forcing patients into one of two choices: (1) join an HMO or MCO that will charge patient fees in addition to Medicare, or (2) set up an MSA and run into the willing arms of its main insurer, Golden Rule.

Presently, Golden Rule cannot sell to Medicare recipients. Under Gingrich's proposals, Golden Rule "would get a crack at millions of Medicare recipients on whose behalf the government spends more than $100 billion each year" (Dreyfuss and Stone 1996, p. 24). Given those odds, Golden Rule's $1 million in GOP contributions is a good investment.

Are Dreyfuss and Stone on target? They cite the results of an investigation by the Congressional Budget Office suggesting that MSAs will fail to reduce Medicare savings and at the same time most likely increase costs by $4 billion. But who is counting?

As of January 1, 1996, MSAs began a four-year trial. Only self-employed people and employees of companies with 50 or fewer employees are eligible. According to Paul Magnusson (1996) the MSA program will initially include 750,000 policy holders, half of whom will potentially amass up to $50,000 in their accounts. The real attraction comes in later years when the MSA accounts reach peak levels. Predictably, insurance companies, banks, and mutual funds are gearing up to tap this lucrative market.

PRIVACY AND MEDICAL RECORDS LEGISLATION

One of the risks faced by legislators concerning privacy and medical records lies in identifying the significant issues rather than simply setting regulations that touch only on superficial problems. This requires a high level of technological, social, and ethical sophistication. A case in point is how the electronic systems were actually developed. The business focus was aimed at electronic records accessibility—to insurers, providers, facilities, and researchers. "When you carry this to its logical conclusion, it leads to discrimination and exclusion in jobs and insurance," says Denise Nagel, M.D., President of the National Coalition for Patient Rights, who testified before a Senate Subcommittee on The Medical Records Confidentiality Act. The problem is compounded when patients realize that what they tell their doctors is not confidential. They may then be afraid to reveal everything they know. "The irony," says Nagel, "is that people tout the research benefits from electronic records. If the patient is not telling all, or the therapist or doctor is trying to protect the patient by omitting information or upgrading diagnoses in order for patients to be certified for further sessions, you then end up doing research on pseudo-information" (1996).

Nagel suggests that electronic records must be patient-centered, based on informed consent. The patient must have the power to control the information, understanding the implications and subsequently choosing how it will be used. Technology should not be allowed to redefine privacy based on business needs, accessibility, and costs. DelPizzo states, "We must introduce an ethical component to this," stresses the VP of marketing at CHMC Systems, "to contradict economic rationality. If technology is allowed to run its own course, economic rationality will predominate."

"In some cases," writes Gina Kolata (1995) in *The New York Times*, "medical information is being sold without even minimal precautions to protect privacy" (p. A1). In a poll of psychologists in practice, Denkers and Clifford (1994) found confidentiality a serious matter. Of the responding psychologists, 90 percent said they were concerned about it, 27 percent have patients leave therapy because of concerns about it, and 32 percent have been required under managed care contracts to give company representatives access to all their patient records. "If you don't have confidentiality," says Nagel (1996), "you don't have trust and you don't have treatment." Currently, only half the states have laws giving patients the right of access to their records and only 34 states have any law protecting confidentiality—usually with severe limitations (Riley 1996d).

"With huge integrated systems," says DelPizzo (1996), "data is collected from multiple sources. The technology is sophisticated enough to consolidate the information and create 'patient profiles.' These profiles can be a tremendous asset in health care." Patient profiles can help professionals be alert to disorders before or at the onset of symptoms. They can also be part of aggregate information used for research. Of course, this only applies when patients and providers are supplying accurate information. DelPizzo (1996) warns that "when the profit motive is added to patient profiles, the problems can be very difficult to control with or without government regulation. Patients and professionals must be guaranteed both informed consent and informed knowledge."

One attempt at federal regulation, The Medical Records Confidentiality Act of 1996, falls short. The bill, being argued at the writing of this book, was sponsored by Senators Robert Bennett (R-UT) and Patrick Leahy

(D-VT). It would establish a federal right for patients to review and request corrections of their medical records, require privacy, and impose civil and criminal penalties on violators. At the same time it facilitates the establishment of large, centralized databases by overriding state laws, giving patients too little control over the use of their records, and setting weak standards for access (Riley 1996d).

Dr. Nagel (1996), representing the Coalition for Patient Rights, was called to testify before the Senate Subcommittee examining the bill. She stated her opinion that the Medical Records Confidentiality Act would ride roughshod over states that try to protect the medical privacy of their inhabitants . . . by creating both national and regional health databases without requiring the consent of the people whose most intimate details would become widely available.

When the Kennedy-Kassebaum Act was passed in the summer of 1996, consumer support groups celebrated it as a victory for health care reform. Few heard the voices of privacy advocates warning about a section on administrative simplification. According to the Center for Democracy and Technology (Policy Post 1996), administrative simplification mandates the development and adoption of standards for the exchange of electronic patient information as well as privacy rules to protect consumers.

Under the Act, the Secretary of Health and Human Services must adopt standards for:

1. Electronic exchange of a variety of health care transactions.
2. A unique health identifier for individuals, employer health plans, and providers.
3. Security.
4. Safeguards for those who maintain or transmit health information to protect the integrity and confidentiality of health information and prevent unauthorized use and disclosure.

MANAGED CARE REGULATION

Tight managed care regulation involves confronting the managed care industry in an active manner, controlling abuses in ways that eliminate the opportunity to operate just outside of the law. In addition to the legislation discussed (DelPizzo 1996) the following is a sample of abuses that need to be addressed in state and federal law:

Direct access: Patients are often forced to go through primary care gatekeepers to see specialists. Advocates want to change the system to allow direct patient access to all providers.

Utilization review: Case management and utilization review is often placed under the control of untrained, nonlicensed people who make decisions based on company protocols and cost containment. Advocates want disclosure of company protocols, simplification of case management procedures, reduction of paperwork, and qualified clinicians who will maintain professional standards and ethics.

Appeals: Crucial treatment is often denied with appeals taking months, usually resulting in a negative outcome. Advocates want to speed up and simplify the process for both consumers and providers, guaranteeing that clinicians filing appeals do not face discrimination or termination.

Long-term treatment: Patients with personality disorders and more severe mental illnesses are being dangerously undertreated or ignored. Advocates want to regulate managed care's treatment decisions concerning long-term treatment in order to service this population.

Denying access to covered treatment: Many MCOs cover a specific number of sessions on paper, but in practice only allow ultra-brief therapy. Advocates seek truth-in-advertising to cover these discrepancies, as well as public education of the limited scope of short-term treatment.

Treatment modalities: Many MCOs, in practice, will not cover treatment modalities unless they are based on brief, solution-focused therapy that addresses problem solving and symptom reduction. Advocates say that it is unsuitable for people suffering from personality disorders and other problems such as emotional and sexual abuse, physical abuse or neglect, trauma, eating disorders, depression, obsessive-compulsive disorders, relationship/marital/family problems, and many childhood and adolescent disorders. They argue that treatment that heals and cures is not always justifiable by medical necessity.

Abusive cost containment practices: Medication is often favored over therapy, cheaper medications favored over new and better drugs, alcohol and substance abuse programs thoughtlessly contracted, individual therapy replaced by group therapy against the advice of the psychotherapist, and self-help/wellness groups used to treat serious psychological problems. Advocates say treatment decisions should be made by the professional and not the company, with the patient, as well as costs, considered.

Capitation: Capitation contracts favor large groups and often incentives for non-treatment. Advocates argue that it is counterproductive to effective treatment and threatens solo practices and autonomous decision making.

Administrative inefficiency: MCOs have dramatically increased the amount of time spent on paperwork and administrative telephone calls. Advocates feel that this drains providers' income, forces them to increase their case loads (to maintain income), and exchanges clinical hours for clerical work. Electronic submissions will help alleviate this problem, but advocates feel that patient confidentiality will be further compromised in computerized records.

What really needs to happen is the restoration of truth in insurance. Patients or clients should be made aware of their policy and its limitations. Psychotherapists should be allowed to practice to the best of their abilities. Therefore, gatekeepers, used to contain costs, will be eliminated from the equation. If a patient knows he or she has $1000 to spend annually on mental health care, and the therapist understands the limitation, both participants in the dyad can work out a treatment plan. The insurance company will save money by eliminating the middlemen and all the paperwork. The patient will become an informed consumer aware of the limitations of his or her insurance coverage, and the therapist will be able to work without a manager who at any time can limit the benefits. This will eliminate the need for a specific diagnosis that meets managed care specifications as well as the need to protect that data from abuses by others.

STATESIDE

There is a long list of managed care legislation that has already been entered into law by state legislatures. Consider some of the following state laws now on the books:

Iowa allows self-employed people to take a 100 percent deduction for health insurance costs in their state taxes. The deductions are expected to cost the state over $15 million in tax revenues (Health Care Reform Newsletter 1995).

Maryland providers are required to inform Maryland Healthcare Access and Cost Commission of all patient visits, including confidential personal data—without notification or consent from patients (Shore 1995c).

Massachusetts bans "gag clauses." Health care organizations are prohibited from including any rules that limit a provider talking to patients about benefit coverage and financial incentives offered by the insurer. According to NFSCSW (1996), "gag clauses" were first publicized when Dr. David Himmelstein was terminated from the U.S. Healthcare panel after discussing problems with the MCO's gag clause on the Phil Donahue Show. Gag clauses are standard in many business contracts, but in health care they conflict with professional ethics and responsibility. Gag clauses are still legal in many states.

Minnesota allows a 50 percent tax deduction for health insurance premiums for the self-employed, limiting pre-existing condition exclusions and consenting to the creation of health purchasing pools and MSAs.

New York now prohibits managed care companies from using unidentified qualification and evaluation standards for admitting or maintaining participating providers and from terminating providers randomly or without explanation.

South Dakota requires state employees who smoke to pay $25 more a month in health insurance premiums. If their spouses smoke and are covered under the plan, their premiums will increase by $50 per month (NewsPage 1996o).

Virginia determines that health care providers own the medical records of the patients. Virginia maintains that patients do not own their records. The state clearly outlines the circumstances, procedures, and provisions for patient access. Patients can be denied access if their physician or clinical psychologist has documented that it would be harmful to them (HB 2147 1995).

Washington makes it illegal for MCOs to prohibit practitioners from contracting privately with clients (Coalition Report 1996).

In contrast, passage of federal legislation faces difficulties of partisanship, congressional gridlock, presidential veto, and intense lobbying from special interests. Frequently, laws proposed in the House are amended by the Senate, or vice versa, making it difficult to accept a revised bill that had already been approved. The power of closed-door deals with special interests and lobbyists is pervasive.

"The answer will definitely be legislative," asserts DelPizzo (1996). "But I feel that the ultimate vehicle, where the clash of values will be acted out, are the courts. However, they are reactive, not proactive. They aren't going to answer questions before they're asked. It takes a long time to get there . . ."

HERE COMES THE JUDGE

MCO's agenda is to protect the bottom line—survival of the business and accumulation of profit. State government agenda is to protect the interests of the state—economically, socially, and politically. Consumer advocates and grassroots political action committees' agendas are to protect the rights of the consumer—whether patient, buyer, employer, or all three—against the more politically and economically powerful forces in society.

The courts do the mediating. "We can't look to business to be our moral meter," says Dr. Nagel, "they operate from their bottom line. . . . We need public education so the people can take a strong position explicitly recognizing patient rights" (personal communication, June 1996).

Although Nagel was speaking about privacy issues, her remarks apply to the entire managed care empire. Ultimately, the interpretation of the law lies in the hands of the judges.

According to Gallinari (1995), the last five years have seen a dramatic increase in the number of lawsuits because of insurance industry denial for medically allowed treatment. Referring primarily to experimental bone marrow treatments used to treat cancer, she notes that many patients have been forced to resort to court intervention in order to get their treatments. In some cases, MCOs have responded by excluding specific treatments because of "insufficient medical data" to justify the expense. This touches on the oft-repeated yet unresolved debate over how to allocate medical resources. If there is a finite number of dollars—and a finite number of resources—how do we decide who gets what?

Many times, just the delay in waiting for legal interventions saves MCOs money. Managed care experts often refer to a decision-making system based on medical triage. Triage is "a system used to allocate a scarce commodity, such as food, only to those capable of deriving the greatest benefit from it" (American Heritage Dictionary 1995). If medical resources and medical dollars are not infinite, how do we make treatment choices? To illustrate, we must ask ourselves some troubling but basic questions. Should we use our limited medical resources to buy neonatal care to the exclusion or limitation of geriatric care? If an alcoholic and a nonalcoholic both need a transplant and there is only one liver, who should get it? Should physician-assisted suicide be permitted to preserve resources? If a patient is hopelessly psychotic, should we spend money on his treatment or on buying resources for dysfunctional families struggling to get better?

"Federal and state courts are not the proper vehicles to make health care policy," writes Judge Irenas in a 1993 decision in the U.S. District Court. "The pain of health care rationing must be dealt with in the political arena, not the courts" (Gallinari 1995, p. 11). But how? It seems that for every question raised, another hovers close behind. For every solution we find, another set of problems emerge. Health care rationing is MCO's lifeblood. Yet it is a highly sensitive, frequently dangerous game to play. Consequently, an integral part of health care rationing is assigning risk—who will ultimately be accountable? It is no surprise that some of the first pieces of case law were on managed care liability. These questions are similar to the problems faced by researchers engaged in developing antibiotics. When antibiotics were first launched, many people believed that we were at the beginning of a victory against the world's major infectious diseases. For a while, it seemed that way, until the bacteria mutated and became resistant to the antibiotics. And suddenly the old names like tuberculosis resurface, resistant to the original cures. MCO's only unleash a host of old—and new—problems.

When managed care first entered the scene, the courts did not fully recognize the difference between indemnity insurance and managed care. The doctor determined treatment and was considered liable. Indemnity insurance did not even get involved until after treatment. Managed care companies were originally viewed as "next generation" indemnity insurers. Consequently, insurers couldn't be liable in treatment decisions or harm (Welch 1996b).

TARGET PRACTICE

Judge Denise Cote of the US District Court for the Southern District of New York, dismissed an antitrust lawsuit filed by three anesthesiologist groups from Long Island against Aetna Health Plans. The decision found that, under antitrust law, Aetna can "set standards for its providers in its efforts to deliver high-quality, cost-effective health coverage." Cote's decision stated that the "target" of the anesthesiologists' lawsuit was the "very concept of managed care" (NewsPage 1996s).

As MCOs tightened their hold on the market, professionals found themselves in the position of being liable for the negative outcomes of treatment they were unable to control. Court attempts to assign liability for harm began in the mid-'80s. In general, the courts have gradually moved toward sharing liability between provider and Big Brother. As it became increasingly clear that insurers had become powerful determinants in medical decisions, usually as a function of health care rationing, the courts began to scrutinize intent. "Recent legal decisions," writes Paul Berman, Ph.D. (1996), "demonstrate the growing discomfort among courts when MCOs focus on cost containment and their own financial health rather than the patient's well-being" (p. 10). This represents a significant legal shift in the traditional view of the professional as holding the primary or sole responsibility for treatment. Insurance is based on risk management—pooling resources to spread or decrease risk. New cost containment methods will focus on shifting risk and administration to provider groups. The courts don't like it.

Wickline v. State of California was the first case that held managed care partially liable for treatment. It also clearly identified liability in the provider. Mrs. Wickline had been treated for various problems in her back and legs. She had undergone several operations. Her managed care company authorized ten days of hospitalization. Before the ten days were up, Wickline developed complications. The doctors requested an additional eight days and only four days were authorized. At the end of the four days she was discharged. Wickline's doctors did not appeal the decision. Nine days later Mrs. Wickline returned to the hospital. Her leg had to be amputated. Wickline sued for negligence and was awarded $500,000. The decision was overturned on appeal. The California Court of Appeals found that if a third-party payer inappropriately restricts treatment and the provider does not protest, then the legal responsibility for harm must be assigned to the provider. However, if the insurer makes the decision based on cost containment measures that when applied arbitrarily reject or ignore the provider's clinical judgment, then the insurer is liable (Berman 1996). The California Court of Appeals significantly expanded managed care liability in a subsequent case. *Wilson v. Blue Cross of Southern California* modified the Wickline decision by fully distributing the burden of liability to both provider and managed care. Wilson was diagnosed as suffering from major depression, drug dependency, and anorexia. The doctor requested three to four weeks of hospitalization. The patient was denied. After ten days, Wilson was discharged. The doctor did not appeal the decision. Three weeks later Wilson committed suicide. Initially, the case was dismissed based on *Wickline*. The Court of Appeals reversed the decision, holding the managed care company liable because they were negligent, significantly contributing to harm. They found that the case could not be dismissed based on the failure to appeal because there was no clear appeals process and no indication that an appeal would have changed the managed care company's decision. It meant that managed care and the provider shared liability (Berman 1996).

Two years later the Fifth Circuit Court of Appeals further delineated liability in *Salley v. Dupont*. Salley was a 15-year-old girl with a history of depression, substance abuse, suicidal tendencies, and self-destructive (head-banging) behavior. She was hospitalized three times and after each discharge, deteriorated rapidly until she had to be rehospitalized. During the third hospitalization, the managed care company denied additional care after thirty days. However, Salley stayed in the hospital for another three months. Eventually she was discharged and entered a school in New York State. The family sued the managed care company for terminating benefits. They won, DuPont appealed, and the court upheld the decision. They found that the managed care company agreed with part of the doctor's treatment (diagnosis), but not other "aspects" (continued hospitalization). Because the MCO did not make an independent inquiry and did not review all the records, the provider's professional judgment remained primary (Berman 1996).

If the courts are increasingly finding against MCOs, then another way must be found to soothe the sting. Some believe that one way lies in tort reform. Torts are wrongs or injuries, unlike breaches of contract, that a court can remedy through legal action (Howry 1996). They include everything from medical malpractice to product liability cases, involving some of the most sensational lawsuits in the country. In one of the most infamous cases, a plaintiff was awarded $2.9 million because McDonald's had served her a cup of scalding coffee and she subsequently spilled it in her lap (Welch 1996a). Another occurred when Proctor & Gamble had to pay $15 million to a man wrongly accused of stealing a $35 telephone (Texans for Lawsuit Reform 1996b).

In health care, torts mean malpractice litigation, where people sue for damages resulting from treatment. In malpractice cases it is the jury's job to decide whether a defendant was negligent, as well as whether the defendant held a "conscious disregard" for the patient's welfare. "Punitive damages" are determined based on two factors: the harm suffered by the plaintiff and an "amount sufficient to deter the defendant and other potential miscreants from engaging in future misbehavior" (Welch 1996a).

Tort reform is a movement aimed at reducing and/or eliminating frivolous lawsuits that clutter the court system and cost business, professionals, and consumers billions of dollars each year. For example, in 1991 the direct cost of the U.S. tort system was $132 billion (Texans for Lawsuit Reform 1996b). Tort reform does not aim to eliminate compensation for injured parties, but to cap awards and limit unnecessary litigation.

Health care has a unique position in tort disputes. Medical malpractice cases resulted in the largest award and the ten highest monetary verdicts in 1995. Yet according to John Juliano, President of the Suffolk, New York Bar Association, only 5 percent of "potential occurrences" of malpractice become claims and only 3 percent of these become lawsuits (Goldberg 1996).

The American Medical Association reported that the proportion of medical malpractice awards of $1 million or more increased from 14 percent in 1980 to 32 percent in 1994 (Littlejohn 1995).

Medical malpractice insurance is the most profitable line for insurance companies, according to A.M. Best, a company that keeps watch on the insurance industry (Aggregates and Averages 1995).

According to a study by Zeckhauser and Blackmon at Harvard University, if all states had tort reform, $14.8 billion in insurance premiums would have been saved over a three-year period (Texans for Lawsuit Reform 1996b).

In a compilation of statistics by the Columbus, Ohio Bar Association, it was found that in 845 lawsuits that have gone to trial, 43 percent of the plaintiffs lost or were awarded no damages, and only 3 percent received punitive damages (Williams 1995).

Is there really a malpractice crisis? Since 1994, nearly 40 states have passed strict tort reform laws that ban frivolous suits. West Virginia, Wisconsin, and California have caps between $250,000 and $500,000 on awards for pain and suffering. Other states, such as Illinois, have eliminated punitive damages—the award granted over and above pain and suffering that is supposed to punish the defendant. Some states like Georgia and Vermont still have punitive damages on the books (Zich 1996). A poll conducted by Texans for Lawsuit Reform (1996a) found that 91 percent of the respondents believe that lawsuits cause higher premiums and 85 percent believe that the ones who benefit the most from the system are personal injury lawyers. Only 8 percent say that no further changes are necessary in tort laws.

Yet opponents argue that tort reform is for the benefit of insurance companies, allowing them to more efficiently predict risk and, subsequently, cost. This gives them the leeway to adjust their premiums to protect their profit. Tort reform opponents believe these laws would lead to higher profit margins for insurance companies rather than lower insurance premiums (Howry 1995).

Juliano agrees (Goldberg 1996), pointing out that it simply costs too much money for a lawyer to pursue a frivolous claim. He estimates that the average case costs an attorney $35,000 in time and expenses. Physicians who testify get fees of $2500–$7500. Even the medical specialist who certifies that a claim is valid receives a whopping $1500 for his or her services (Goldberg 1996). When the vast majority of cases are taken on a contingency basis (some estimate it as high as 99 percent), why would an attorney take the risk on something frivolous?

Mental health malpractice is increasingly becoming a significant part of this scene. For example, in the well known 1994 "recovered memory" case, a California jury found that two therapists and a hospital had acted improperly by reinforcing a patient's belief that her father had sexually abused her. The plaintiff was awarded $500,000 (Shuitt 1994). In another case, a Pennsylvania jury found that a psychiatrist was negligent for not investigating and evaluating the claim of an adolescent girl that her parents had sexually abused her. The girl recanted her story, and the jury awarded the parents $213,000 and the daughter $56,000 (Schaffer 1995).

Supporters of tort reform argue that malpractice caps can help control spending in "defensive" medicine, saving as much as $41 billion over 5 years. The Healthcare Liability Alliance (HCLA) supports proposals set forth by Newt Gingrich that include: a $250,000 cap on noneconomic damages, a fair share of apportionment of liability for noneconomic damages, a cap on punitive damages set at $250,000 or three times economic damages, and a defense against punitive damages for products approve by the Food and Drug Administration (FDA). The HCLA is a coalition of physicians, hospitals, drug manufacturers, insurers, and other health care providers (Littlejohn 1996).

Ironically, the experience of the state of California has had little effect on the push for reform. In the mid-1970s, California put a $250,000 limit on general damages in malpractice cases. General damages comprise the compensation awarded for pain and suffering. There are no limits on damages for medical bills and loss of income directly related to patient injuries—although those losses must be proven. Attorneys can only receive a maximum of 15 percent on awards over $200,000 (Shuitt 1996).

California patients complain that attorneys will not take their cases. California attorneys complain that because of the costs involved in putting together a case, they are forced to make highly selective decisions on who to represent. California consumer advocates complain that the insurance industry has reaped huge profits, "paying out only 36 cents for every dollar in premiums they took in" (Shuitt 1996).

> In recent months, Californians angry with the *malpractice* system have demonstrated in wheelchairs and on crutches, dumped manure at a congressman's office, testified against organized medicine at legislative hearings in Sacramento and stuffed photos and case histories into a coffin and delivered them to a Senator's office. [Shuitt 1996]

"The managed care industry (as well as some other big business interests) obviously do not like being vulnerable to malpractice," says Bryant Welch. "If they cut corners, manipulate, deny care, and get sued for punitive damages, they stand to lose millions of dollars. They have two options. They can change their behavior or they can try to change the law. They are choosing the latter" (Welch 1996a).

Malpractice suits are the only effective defense an individual can take against Big Brother. If there is no federal regulation, if state control is hampered by ERISA, the only recourse is in the courts. Even ERISA plans are now subject to malpractice litigation. If that weapon is taken away where do we turn?

FOR THE PEOPLE

Any discussion of managed care legislation would be incomplete without reference to changes in Medicare and Medicaid. As everyone knows, the business and politics of government-supported health care is subject to many influences. At present, the government debates are moving very slowly, giving the health care industry ample time to develop strategies for taking over health care in the areas now covered by Medicare and Medicaid.

According to Joan Shapiro, C.S.W. (1995), there is a "tendency to see the private sector and the public sector as two discrete systems. In fact they are not, but are covertly, yet functionally linked" (p. 446). How? In the days of indemnity insurance, it was accepted that the high fees charged to insured patients covered the expenses of the low or no fees of the mandated poor patients. Essentially, profitability was maintained by shifting costs over to the private sector. However, this was not a one-way road. When patients in the private sector reached their limitations or began to affect the insurer's profitability, they were shifted to the public sector. MCOs have made cost shifting an art.

> Further, the private (for-profit) sector charges as much as it can in the way of premiums and co-payments from those with insurance or health plans. It then protects itself by limiting benefits when it appears that paying off will cut too deeply into its profit margin, formulating benefit contracts that allow it to disenfranchise patients whose treatment may have outlasted their profit potential. Thus taxpayers and policy-holders are charged to protect insurance company profits, yet are themselves vulnerable to becoming public-sector clients. [Shapiro 1995, p. 447]

> Ronald Gordon suffers from a serious, highly debilitating disease called Duchenne muscular dystrophy. Refusing to succumb to his illness, Gordon earned a college degree, wrote for a weekly sports newspaper, and with the help of his family, managed to remain fairly independent. When he was 27 years old, Gordon could no longer move. He was forced to rely on a ventilator. Recognizing the fragile nature of his condition, the young man turned to MetraHealth, his insurance company. In the beginning the plan paid a nurse to come to his home for 12 hours a day, 7 days a week. She made sure Gordon had no interruptions in breathing, fed him, moved and stretched his atrophied body, and was there in case of a medical emergency. Then MetraHealth decided he did not need a nurse. They said he could get by with an aide or with the family taking care of him. His insurance policy did not cover aides. Within a few months MetraHealth completely stopped all nursing care. Gordon was one of 242 New York MetraHealth patients who suddenly lost their lifelines.

Gordon, and many of the other 241 MetraHealth patients have brought the issue to court. "But while such debates rage," writes Bunis (1996), "many patients whose doctors say they require such home-nursing care have few alternatives. They can hope that a family member can step in and provide the needed care. But more likely, they say, they will end up spending all of their assets and applying to the state for Medicaid assistance" (p. A4).

Ronald Gordon is not alone. If MCOs will not pay, then the only place to turn is to the taxpayers. For example, when researchers and clinicians offered a dramatic new therapy that promised to turn the tide in the battle against AIDS, people quickly discovered that it would cost up to $15,000 a year, and insurance companies would not foot the cost. The major option open to many individuals is to "quit your job, spend down and go on Medicaid to pay for the drugs" (Garrett 1996, p. A7).

If MCOs shift costs to the public sector, why would they be interested in controlling them? Shapiro (1995) observes that managed care companies or behavioral MCOs are "courting" the public sector. . . . There is profit to be reaped from the administration of tax dollars dedicated to mental health and other health care services. "Furthermore," she writes, "there is an advantage to controlling not just one end of the continuum, but both, in order to allow for more effective leveraging" (p. 447).

The baby boomers are approaching the Medicare age. Currently, about 12 percent of the U.S. population is 65 years or older. By 2030, 20 percent, or one out of every 5 Americans, will be over 65. This is a problem for Medicare but a business boom for MCOs. According to a study by Conning & Company, an insurance consulting firm, MCO enrollment is expected to jump by over 80 percent before the turn of the century, and most of those new covered lives will belong to Medicare and Medicaid. "The aging of the U.S. population and congressional reforms favoring HMO delivery of Medicare are a potential economic boon for HMOs over the next five to ten years," reports Conning (NewsPage 1996a).

Medicaid is right behind. In a national survey assessing state Medicaid agencies, Integrated Healthcare Services found that 76 percent of the 38 responding states contract with managed care. Of these states, 86 percent contract with HMOs that assume full risk and 79 percent have mandatory managed care enrollment (NewsPage 1996cc). It has been estimated that a total of 44 states offer some form of Medicaid managed care (Bacha 1995). HMO services to Medicare recipients (Kilborn 1996) are financed through grants from the Federal Healthcare Financing Administration (HCFA). The HMO receives from HCFA approximately 95 percent of what it "would typically pay to cover a beneficiary." The numbers are drawn from local health care costs. For example, in Tucson, Arizona, HMOs get $438.58 per month per patient. The grants, plus volume, when complimented by strict cost containment measures, leave room to maximize return. "The companies," reports Kilborn, "say profits range from 2 to 5 percent in Arizona" (p. A1).

Buying up federal health care contracts shifts the MCOs' marketing strategy. The managed health care customer is no longer the corporation—it is the Medicare recipient shopping for the best medical care bargain. "The environment is so competitive here [Arizona] for the business of the elderly," writes Kilborn (1996), "that HMOs are behaving like banks giving away toasters" (p. A1). This also changes the approach to cost containment. Medicare contracts will only be secured if MCOs promise—and deliver to individuals—rock-bottom prices with adequate care. This is what Big Brother does best. He simply adjusts the profit margin in exchange for volume. MCOs have also reduced payments to providers who are part of the MCO network and willing to treat Medicare or Medicaid patients. Using this "supermarket" approach, huge profits can be made from the tiniest of co-payments. Of course, quality-of-care issues also plague the system, including hospital and nursing home discharge disputes, denial of benefits, limited access to specialists, difficulty of appeals, and such. However, it is a small price to pay for such a lucrative market. And managed care across the country has already set the lures. Here are some of the advertising headlines:

- What are you doing the rest of your life? Vytra Medicare wants to know.
- What are you doing about Medicare?
- Wouldn't you like to pay no monthly plan premium?
- Why settle for just a plan when you can get a relationship, too?

The New York Times, Sunday, April 21, 1996

Ironically, MCOs may find controls in ways not afforded to corporate customers. For example, the Department of Health and Human Services (McBride 1996) has tightened regulations on managed care providers who see Medicare or Medicaid patients. The new rules limit the penalties that managed care plans place on physicians for referring patients to specialists. In addition, providers who have specific "referral incentive" arrangements must disclose that information to the appropriate Medicare or Medicaid regulating agency as well as to patients requesting that information. Noncompliance results in sanctions, ranging from fines to cancellation of Medicare/Medicaid contracts. This places Medicare and Medicaid recipients in the position of potentially having the most regulated managed health care in the country.

Any discussion that involves Medicare or Medicare must be couched within the context of politics. It is ultimately the politicians who will de-

> "It's Really True! The U.S. Healthcare Medicare Plan Offers $0 Premium Plans And Prescription Benefits, Too!"
> *If you're Medicare-eligible, you're invited to join us for a cup of coffee and complete information on U.S. Healthcare Medicare.*
> Our comprehensive, no-deductible plan can provide significant cost savings and more benefits than Federal Medicare plus many supplemental/gap plans combined! Benefits include:
>
> - •Zero premium options (You must continue to pay your Medicare Part B Premium)
> - •Prescription drugs covered with a $10 co-payment ($1000 annual maximum)
> - •New carryover privilege—any unused portion of Rx allowance, up to $500, for one calendar year
> - •Wide choice of network primary care physicians in private offices, with visits for as little as $5
> - •Full coverage for referred hospitalization and home health care
>
> *Newsday*, April 10, 1996

cide their fate. Cuts in funding will decrease the financial burden on government and possibly force more recipients into managed care. Those same funding cuts could potentially decrease the value of each contract and/or the number of eligible recipients, sending less money as well as fewer bodies to MCOs. Politicians must rely on their constituents to elect them to office. Senior citizens have an extremely high turnout in elections. Seniors also do not support cuts in Medicare. In contrast, the lobbyists employed by MCOs carry the power of political contributions and favors. Politicians devoted to business, reducing federal spending and power, and lowering taxes may quickly find themselves in an ideological paradox. The solutions for managing managed care are difficult and involve far more than professional integrity. They encompass intricate legal, governmental, professional, and health care issues.

II

Inside the Treatment Room

6

Look Before You Leap

Forced to conform to the requirement (of managed care) . . . the analyst . . . must expend a great deal of energy both to assure that benefits continue and to maintain the integrity of the treatment situation. He must manage his own reactions to the intrusions, demands, and undermining of his professional role, while remaining available to understand and respond to the needs of his patients.

–Beth Meehan, C.S.W., B.C.D. "From Comfort to Chaos" (1996)

Whether we like it or not, managed care has, for the moment, gained the upper hand in the world of psychotherapy. In the years ahead, managed care organizations (MCOs) will undergo many changes. Some will come as a result of challenges in the American judicial system. Others will be mandated by legislation. Protocols will be revised and practices redefined. The ultimate system may be quite different from what we have today.

One must realize that there is victimization on both sides of the managed care equation, company and provider alike. Although the government, the American Psychological Association, and other interested groups have developed guidelines, there has been no standardization. In the meantime, psychotherapists and case managers alike are confused about how to adapt their knowledge, and perhaps their values, to a new system of mental health care. That will mean learning new concepts, new rules, and even a new language. Some may find the system an affront to their intelligence, training, and beliefs. Others will adapt to the new rules and attempt to make the necessary changes and compromises to fulfill managed care's objectives, which focus on cost containment rather than quality of treatment. Cost containment is the managed care organizational objective. That goal also includes control of prices, the need for services, and uniformity in treatment.

It is difficult to imagine just how powerful some managed care organizations have become. Wellcare of New York, a growing MCO, told providers at a public meeting that although the package sold to participants stated they could have up to twenty mental health sessions, that did not mean they were entitled to twenty. The therapist is forced to act as the gatekeeper. Providers were openly threatened by Carmel Gold, vice president and clinical director of the managed care organization, who warned that therapists who consistently used more than seven sessions would be flagged and would receive fewer referrals. Providers who showed good outcomes in less than seven sessions would receive more referrals.

Providers were also told that group practice is the wave of the future. Preference would be given to psychiatrists, psychologists, social workers, nurses, and others who joined together under one roof to provide centralized services. The goal is to save money for the MCO by consolidating service and billing. This represents another way of containing costs, because it now falls on the provider to figure out the complicated group billing system and distribute funds to group members when payment for services arrives. Solo practices will not survive in the future of managed care organizations, the director predicted. The providers themselves were encouraged to join the MCO for their own health care coverage. In essence, the audience was told that the way to a "fat practice" is to keep sessions down, join a centralized group practice, and switch personal insurance coverage to the MCO. Providers were warned that sessions that are billed by accident will not be paid, but will be deducted from the patient's available sessions. In other words, if a therapist sees a patient in an initial session and does not realize it has not been precertified, the therapist will not be paid. Thereafter, even if seven sessions are authorized, the patient will only be entitled to six. In essence, the session is taken out of the provider's pocketbook, and also out of the care-seeker's allotment. Managed care wins both ways. The negative impact on the audience was obvious, but no one stood up and complained.

The same company gave providers a small raise in 1995, but in actuality the co-payment was increased as well, requiring the patient to pay more for therapy. Meanwhile, the insurance company calculated that the increased co-payment would deter consumers from using their benefits. In 1996, Wellcare's behavioral managed care component was taken over by Merit Behavioral Care Corporation, the nation's largest behavioral health company serving over 17 million subscribers. MBC is partially owned by Kohlberg Kravis Roberts & Co., the leveraged buy-out (LBO) specialists.

The emergence of managed care caught many psychotherapists unprepared. Some regarded it as a temporary phenomenon that would run its course and disappear as suddenly as it had arrived. Others were unsure of the consequences of becoming a participating provider and wary of the possible compromises in their personal convictions that might be required. Change is seldom welcome and is regarded with uncertainty and suspicion. But those psychotherapists who hesitated too long found they were frozen out. When they finally decided to jump on the bandwagon, it was gone. Managed care companies had quickly processed a wave of applications, filled their requirements, and closed the lists. As Joseph Hollett, vice president of Value Behavioral Health (1996) explained: "We're not worried about recruitment. There will always be an ample supply of psychotherapists willing to work at reduced fees. What we really need are therapists who will take the shortest possible time to reduce patient symptoms. This is about reducing maladaptive behavior, not mental health."

While many participating providers are voicing complaints about their new managed care partners, many psychotherapists on the outside are now eager for the chance to sign up. They are willing to accept reduced fees for services, loss of professional autonomy, and compromised confidentiality for promises of patient referrals that will hopefully boost their practices. Those outsiders who want to be on an MCO provider list will find that persistence pays off. However, given their current power, MCOs are getting more particular about the providers they select. Those practitioners who have taken brief-therapy courses or workshops, or are trained in alcohol and substance abuse counseling or other specialties, will have a definite edge (see Part III).

Short-term therapy will remain the choice of managed care organizations for obvious reasons. The sessions are severely time-limited, and focus on a measurable, empirical problem. The patient is taught more effective ways to deal with a problem, then returns to his or her life armed with a new skill. There is no consideration of such things as the unconscious or transference to muddy the waters. It's all straightforward, simple, and hopefully cost-effective. Typical of the process is the deShazer and Berg Solution-Focused Interview (deShazer and Berg 1988). The interview is focused on instilling an awareness that treatment is time-limited and aimed at a specific problem (Hoyt 1995) without a once-and-for-all cure. Words such as "treat," "resist," "defense," "cure," and "insight" are out. They have been replaced by words such as "solution," "facilitate," "expand," and "partner." Based on an interview (deShazer and Berg 1988), patients are categorized as "complainers," "visitors," or "customers." Customers are seen as viable clients or consumers.

Shectman (1986) points out that "Necessity is thus not only becoming the mother of invention, but of intervention as well" (p. 521). However, in actual practices, should managed care be the creator of psychotherapy? Or is managed care one more aspect to be considered in the search for a viable solution to the mental health problems of today?

Merit Behavior Health's clinical philosophy is based on "assessing the total biological, social and psychological needs of the patient, with a focus on improving the patient's daily functioning" (Merit Behavioral Care Corporation 1996). "Our goal is to optimize patient functioning. In order to fulfill this goal, our clinical delivery system provides individualized treatment for every one of our patients, regardless of the type or complexity of the presented problem."

The MCOs of the future will be more highly organized, and may look toward group practices rather than solo caregivers. There have been suggestions that managed care organizations will pare down their provider lists, retaining only those providers who have demonstrated a performance pattern that is consistent with managed care goals.

It should be noted that managed care companies are actively keeping statistics on providers and their performance. They want to know about a good track record of brief therapy that can be documented. CVs should be rewritten to highlight what they are looking for: training in brief therapy, alcohol and drug abuse counseling, or other specialties. Many universities and institutes currently offer the necessary courses leading to a certificate. It might well be worth the investment. Keep abreast of what is happening in today's health care environment. The larger, more successful managed care organizations systematically buy up the smaller companies. Laws governing managed care services appear to be in constant flux.

If the door remains closed, all is not lost. Consider building a practice around the growing managed care drop-outs (see Part III). Think about establishing a sliding fee scale for those patients who do not want to participate with Big Brother, want one-on-one confidentiality, and are concerned with mental health rather than symptoms. There are probably quite a few people that fall into this category. As Blanck and Blanck (1992) pointed out in the New England Educational Institute Workshop on Ego Psychology, many psychotherapists believe that only structural change—from the inside out—is permanent. Time will tell what impact short-term therapy programs will have on the participants. Often, managed care subscribers faced with new problems return to brief focused treatment in search of new solutions. No one has yet researched the cost of this recidivism.

Before you leap, understand what it is about. The managed care industry includes at least three basic types of organizations: health maintenance organizations (HMOs), preferred provider organizations (PPOs), and employee assistance programs (EAPs). All are managed care organizations. HMOs are closed systems in which members can be treated only by health care providers approved by the HMO. Subscribers pay a flat monthly fee for all care plus a minimal co-payment fee for each approved visit. Practitioners operate semiautonomously, at reduced fees under a cost-effective protocol enforced by HMO case managers. Two of the largest HMOs in the country are the Health Insurance Plan (HIP) of New York and Florida, and the Kaiser-Permanante Medical Care Program. There are more than 35 HMOs in New York state alone.

PPOs have a preferred provider network, where providers are chosen because of their credentials and, usually, a history of successful short-term treatment. Some companies still manage their own PPOs. A pilot program by Value Behavioral Health focused on ten PPOs to determine if they can contain costs without caseworkers acting as gatekeepers. The elimination of case managers would cut a major cost component from the managed care organization system. At present, most managed care companies have a formulary, based on diagnosis, which dictates how many sessions a patient should receive. The number of authorized sessions is limited in order to cut down the cost of case management. For example, a patient with dysthymia may be authorized 10 treatment sessions according to the insurance company's formulary. If treatment is not completed in that time frame, the case is sent to formal review.

EAPs were originally developed in response to the growing problems of alcoholism and drug abuse on the job, and now have expanded to other mental health areas. An EAP manager, employed by the employer or union, is responsible for referring the employee to an approved provider for brief focused therapy. As with PPOs, providers receive a reduced fee, which is augmented by a small co-payment by the union member.

Some managed care organizations have now developed point-of-service programs, which provide free choice of any credentialed practitioner, even if he or she is not a plan provider. However, payment is usually limited to 50 percent of the usual fee for service and is limited in total amount to the same level, or less, than the no choice plan. Many patients are happy with the idea of free choice in a system where choices are usually limited or nonexistent. They fail to recognize this option as another way to cut the cost of care and make money for the company and its stockholders.

Managed care organizations are dedicated, to one degree or another, to the concept of utilization review (UR), which often requires the practitioner to provide a detailed written justification for treatment, a regular submission of specific treatment plans, an evaluation of progress toward treatment goals, and an estimate of the expected duration of treatment. In some cases, these reports can be telephoned or faxed by the practitioner directly to the case manager. They are evaluated for medical necessity by the case manager who may be a mental health clinician but does not have to be. Based on the review, and the specific insurance policy, additional treatment sessions are authorized or denied. Once the approved sessions are used, the authorization process starts all over again.

MEDICAL NECESSITY

Medical necessity, severity of illness, and intensity of service are critical parameters in the managed care system's clinical protocol. Medical necessity is a term that effectively limits treatment to those services that the patient clinically requires. Treatment intended solely for self-improvement or for normal life stress reactions is not considered medically necessary. For example, if a patient comes to treatment because a close family member has died and the patient exhibits the normal range of symptoms associated with mourning, he or she would not be eligible for treatment. However, if the patient's grieving symptoms are outside the normal limits, the patient is eligible for treatment. How reliable is medical necessity as an indicator of required treatment? Essentially, it creates a situation in which a third party uses the therapist's narrative to evaluate someone else's grief. Is the evaluation of the grief or of the therapist's skill as a storyteller?

The reviews to determine medical necessity can be performed by a physician, psychologist, social worker, nurse practitioner, substance abuse counselor, or a utilization review professional. Because not all MCOs use the same standards, it is best to know the company and its specific requirements. It also helps to know the level of the "professional" on the other end of the telephone.

The appropriate level of care is based on severity of illness and intensity of service. Severity of illness for a given level of care is represented by signs, symptoms, and functional impairments that require treatment at a specified level at a given point in time. The intensity of service must match the patient's dysfunction.

Value Behavioral Health (VBH), one of the more successful managed care organizations, published a checklist to help clinicians understand medical necessity. (VBH Clinical Manual 1995). The checklist is divided into three sections: (1) general considerations, (2) risk assessment, and (3) special considerations.

General considerations apply to all patients, and include such things as reasons for treatment, level of functioning, diagnosis, goals, length of treatment to reach those goals, a specific treatment plan, services required to support the treatment plan, and how the plan will enable the patient to be most rapidly reintegrated into family and community. Of particular concern are treatment plans that are so indefinite or ambitious that treatment could be interminable.

Risk assessment involves the details of suicidal ideation, suicidal attempts, and homicidal potential. Special considerations are specific to each patient and cover the details of such items as the patient's strengths and limitations, Global Assessment of Functioning (GAF) score, eating disorder, substance abuse, and dual diagnoses. The GAF scale (American Psychiatric Association 1994) is a tool for assessing a patient's mental health. A patient's level of functioning is rated on a continuum from 0 to 100. Usually, insurance companies consider a GAF of less than 55 as a situation too extreme for psychotherapy and more amenable to psychopharmacology or hospitalization. They also consider a GAF of more than 70 as too high for psychotherapy.

This is an abbreviated version of the GAF Scale.

100–91	Superior functioning. No symptoms.
90–81	Absent or minimal symptoms. Good functioning.
80–71	Symptoms are transient and expectable reactions to psychosocial stressors.
70–61	Some mild symptoms, but generally functioning pretty well.
60–51	Moderate symptoms or impairments in social, occupational, or school functioning.
50–41	Serious symptoms of impairments in social, occupational, or school functioning.
40–31	Some impairment in reality testing or communication.
30–21	Behavior considerably influenced by delusions or hallucinations, or serious impairment in communication or judgment.
20–11	Some danger of hurting self or others, occasionally fails to maintain minimal personal hygiene.
10–01	Persistent danger of hurting self or others, inability to maintain personal hygiene, serious suicidal act with clear expectation of death.
0	Inadequate information.

VBH states that it does not exclude any treatment model from possible consideration for patient care. Their guidelines reflect the belief that time and cost are legitimate parameters of effectiveness. Medical necessity requires that treatment be delivered in the most cost-effective manner consistent with quality outcome. Quality treatment can be considered a treatment reasonably expected to improve the patient's illness, condition, or level of functioning, and is safe and effective according to the nationally accepted, standard clinical evidence generally recognized by mental health or substance abuse care professionals or publications. Specific goals for change should be behaviorally referenced.

Many people seek treatment at a time of life stress because they are developmentally unprepared to make the necessary adaptation to deal effectively with a problem. The goal of focused treatment is to restore or enhance its abilities to find solutions. In such an approach, it is accepted that the patient may not implement significant or permanent positive change until some time after his or her treatment sessions have concluded.

It is recognized that the return to problem-focused treatment to deal with another conflict may be a logical outcome. New life problems require new life solutions.

Brief Outpatient Therapy, for patients with a GAF of less than 70, is limited to ten sessions or less over a period of sixteen weeks. The patient must demonstrate adequate judgment and responsibility for behavioral change. One focal conflict must be identified by patient and therapist as the main therapeutic issue. Intermediate outpatient therapy, for patients with a GAF of less than 60, may be appropriate for patients who have shown significant improvement in brief outpatient therapy, or may be initiated at the inception of treatment if brief therapy is considered clinically unrealistic.

Therapeutic stabilization is the name given to treatment of a patient who requires scheduled or intermittent contact with a clinical professional to maintain his or her level of functioning and to preclude the need for more intensive, and more costly, care. These patients usually have a GAF of less than 60. Sessions may be scheduled no more frequently than every other week. Up to 26 sessions may be authorized over a period of one year.

Case managers operating under formulary guidelines are responsible for authorizing treatment sessions and the number of sessions normally authorized may differ from one organization to another. Nevertheless, all managed care organizations operate with the implied (if not actual) promise that early, successful patient discharge from treatment will result in additional referrals. Conversely, there is always the threat that providers who usually handle complex cases that require in-depth treatment will receive few referrals or be dropped from the provider list. For example, insurance companies do not want to deal with personality disorders, which by their very nature require long-term treatment.

The primary mission of the insurance companies is to keep costs down. Ultimately, everything must be translated into the common denominator of cost. Managed care organization reports are written in behavioral language that focuses on targeted impairments, time-critical interventions, and scheduled results. The system is completely cost oriented. Yet the National Association of Social Workers (Landers 1996) advises clinicians to use *DSM-IV* diagnostic language in managed care organization reports. *DSM-IV* is required by managed care organizations as the basis for diagnosis. Ironically, it is the one remaining element that ties the system to the now fading language of dynamic psychotherapy. The diagnosis must still be translated into "newspeak" for the managed care organization. That puts practitioners in a double bind. They need to learn the language in order to mediate the system. The professional language of the practitioner now has to be reduced to behavioral terms so that insurance companies can make medical decisions about what the therapist can or cannot do with a patient. In spite of this, practitioners should not lose sight of the fact that their allegiance belongs to their professional code of ethics.

One managed care organization provider tells of treating a patient with a multiple diagnosis of Generalized Anxiety Disorder (300.02) and Eating Disorder (307.50).

> The patient was a divorced mother of two small children. Her ex-husband was an alcoholic. She and her live-in boyfriend moved into a new community and bought a house that neither of them could afford alone. The boyfriend subsequently lost his job and abandoned the patient and her children, leaving her with the house expense. She knew no one in the neighborhood, and had no friends or family to turn to for support. Acting out her anger, the patient began fighting with her children and thinking more and more about suicide. The managed care organization authorized six sessions of every-other-week therapy. The provider was told that in ten weeks, he could apply for family sessions, but that no further individual therapy would be granted.
>
> The therapist, concerned about the welfare of the patient, applied for a peer review under the terms of his contract with the managed care organization, only to be told that the patient would have to be referred to an alcohol evaluation clinic or be denied any further sessions at all. The therapist reiterated that the patient had been abstinent since entering therapy. Under stress, the patient relapsed, drank one too many, and became frightened by the memory of what alcohol did to her ex-husband and vowed never to drink again. The case was referred to the Level II Appeals Committee, where the case manager's decision was confirmed. The therapist considered a Level III appeal, which includes a comprehensive written review. This process requires a new outpatient treatment report plus all the progress notes from each session. Frustrated by the thought of the overwhelming paperwork and the lack of privacy, the therapist decided against Level III appeal and agreed instead to see the patient privately at a reduced fee. The therapist recognized that the patient was in crisis and needed to be protected from the intrusion and humiliation of going to an alcohol clinic for evaluation. The therapist also felt the patient required weekly rather than bi-weekly treatment to support her abstinence. Two months later, the thera-

pist received a telephone call from the managed care organization announcing that the Appeals Committee had revised their decision. The patient was authorized for weekly treatment. The surprised therapist never understood how or why the case went to the third appeals committee, since the required paperwork was never completed. A new OTR would be required only if circumstances changed significantly or treatment could not be completed within a revised time-frame. The patient has since completed treatment. Her anxiety is under better control and her eating problems have diminished. She is struggling with difficult financial circumstances, but remains strongly committed to her vow not to drink again. One wonders what could have happened if the provider had accepted the original decision to see this patient every other week.

Missed sessions represent another difficulty. Pay-for-service patients who are charged for missed sessions quickly learn to keep their appointments. However, most managed care contracts forbid the clinician to charge the patient for missed sessions. The provider is forbidden to bill the managed care organization for them as well. As a result, managed care patients whose resistance prevents them from looking at their problems can miss sessions and not be held responsible, leaving the provider with no recourse.

Each participating provider must sign a contract that carefully defines the relationship with the managed care company. Although each contract differs, they contain common elements, such as fees, precertification procedures, and reporting protocols. Many of the contracts also prohibit the provider from disclosing the inner workings of the managed care organization to any third party, including the patient. In addition, most contracts contain a "hold harmless" clause designed to provide the managed care organization with legal immunity for their policies and procedures, placing the responsibility solely on the participating provider in the event of patient litigation. The participating provider has the primary responsibility for providing the covered mental health services to the plan subscribers. By signing the contract, he or she agrees that the managed care organization's referral, quality assurance, utilization review procedures, and protocols shall not affect the practitioner's obligation to provide treatment that conforms to usual and accepted medical standards. Coverage and payment determinations under the plan shall in no way absolve the practitioner from the responsibility to render these services to subscribers.

This can place the provider at risk because the professional code of ethics requires that service to patients cannot be precipitously ended without appropriate referral to another therapist when treatment is incomplete. When authorizations have been denied, some practitioners resolve the dilemma by continuing to provide services to the patient without hope of payment, or refer the patient to either a low-cost self-help group or an agency with a sliding fee scale. The options are diminishing because many of these agencies are now in a financial crunch as they adapt their operations to the realities of managed care. Typical of the dilemma created by rising caseloads and reduced funding is a local methadone clinic at a small town in New Jersey. The director recently announced that the clinic had only two weeks of financial resources left to treat 192 drug patients. What happens if they are forced to close and the patients go untreated?

Whether or not a subscriber will be certified or re-certified for treatment under the plan depends on the definition of medical necessity. Many of the decisions are made by relatively inexperienced clinicians using a general formulary based on patient diagnosis. The case manager will only know the patient through verbal or written reports. MCOs usually have an appeal process—sometimes even provisions for a second or third level of appeal. The process is time-consuming and frequently frustrating; and, of course, there is no compensation to the psychotherapist for the time spent.

7

The Managed Care Practice

> *. . . transformations (in mental health care) have created a practice environment which is increasingly hostile toward psychodynamically oriented clinicians who value meaningful psychotherapeutic treatment of the individual; as opposed to amelioration of a symptom fragment.*
>
> *–James Barron and Harry Sands (1996),*
> Impact of Managed Care on Psychodynamic Treatment (*p. xiv*)

Initial contact with a patient is usually in the form of a telephone call requesting an appointment. Most callers voluntarily identify themselves, the source of the referral, and the reason for seeking therapy. Some may explain that they have insurance coverage or ask about the fee schedule. An appointment time is usually arranged at this point. Most psychotherapists expect the patient to know whether or not precertification is required before he or she enters therapy. However, therapists should raise the issue of precertification if the patient mentions insurance coverage. Always ask who referred the patient. The answer may reveal a clue about insurance or managed care coverage.

In the initial phone call, the therapist should be empathic yet professional. If there are any indications that this is an emergency, the patient must be seen as quickly as possible. If the therapist is not available, the patient should be sent to a hospital emergency room or referred back to the managed care organization caseworker. Managed care organizations usually do not look favorably on therapists who repeatedly send patients back unseen. It is a good idea to telephone the case manager to explain the problem. If it is not an emergency, the therapist should set up a mutually agreeable appointment. The telephone call is not a substitute for an initial session and should be limited to the bare details. Remember that the first call sets the stage for future sessions.

The initial visit is usually dedicated primarily to a structured or semi-structured interview to determine the patient's demographics, history, and presenting problem. The interview may indicate a clear-cut or preliminary diagnosis. The psychotherapist has the opportunity here to outline for the patient the ground rules and the limited nature of patient–therapist confidentiality in today's environment. That would include both legal and MCO reporting mandates.

Although he or she might well mention the fragile nature of confidentiality in the MCO environment, the therapist is often bound by contract not to divulge the extent of MCO reporting requirements, the potential leaks in confidentiality, or the potential nonprofessional use of patient records. However, if applicable to the patient's presenting problem, the therapist should briefly explain his legal responsibility in regard to suicide, harm to others, and child abuse, without sounding too legalistic. If there is any suggestion of suicide or homicide, the therapist should see the patient quickly or refer the patient to an appropriate agency.

Usually the MCO patient will have been referred by a primary care physician or the case manager. If the patient has MCO coverage and has not applied for precertification, the therapist must telephone the managed care organization for the necessary approval. Know the protocol for the managed care organization. Some will require precertification, while others may allow three to five sessions for evaluation. Still others regard three to five sessions as enough time to perform effective solution-focused therapy.

In the first session, make insurance forms available for the patient to sign. Although some companies have their own forms, most will accept the standard HCFA form. Copies of the HCFA form are available, preprinted with the therapist's name, address, and PIN number, from a number of business form companies listed in the Appendix. (For guidance in filling out a standard HCFA form, please see page 183.) Usually the patient's signature on the completed form accomplishes two functions: (1) approves payment directly to the psychotherapist, and (2) authorizes the therapist to provide the required patient records to the managed care organization.

It is not unusual to discover that the patient has little or no understanding of the extent of the information required by the MCO or the impact of that information on the number of future sessions the therapist will be assigned to deal with his problem. At this point, patients are upset and concerned with their problems and the potential cost of therapy. Although cost is a real issue, it should be remembered that they will agree to almost anything to get out of emotional pain. When a patient signs up with any managed care organization, part of the contract usually includes authorization for release of patient records. Therefore, in a sense, the patients have already signed away their rights to confidentiality from the very outset. Nevertheless, an approved consent form is a good idea, and will provide an extra measure of safety (see Form A in the Appendix).

> The story of Mr. Alle highlights the patient's limited understanding of confidentiality. Mr. Alle was a well-known politician preparing to run for reelection. He was well liked in the community, and donated large sums of money to local projects. But behind the scenes his home life was a shambles. His wife moved out of their bedroom and became involved in an affair with a younger and more attentive man.
>
> Mr. Alle was referred for help with his interpersonal relations to Dr. Davis by a colleague with whom he served on a local hospital board. When the therapist attempted to establish the usual ground rules of treatment, Mr. Alle proudly announced that he was insured by a managed care organization, and his co-payment was only $15 a session. Dr. Davis attempted to explain to his patient the realities of confidentiality, the extent of the MCO reporting requirements, and the pitfalls for the patient, especially a politician, if his records ended up in the wrong hands.
>
> "Don't be ridiculous," the patient responded. "My life is an open book. If it's the paperwork that bothers you, I'll get my secretary to help you."
>
> Dr. Davis patiently explained the benefits of putting the MCO coverage aside in favor of entering private therapy. Mr. Alle would be required to pay a full fee but the record of his treatment would not be divulged to anyone. The patient proudly announced that, "When I can, I save a dollar. That's why I'm a millionaire." If this high-functioning patient failed to understand the implications of what he might be sacrificing to save a few dollars, how can we expect lower-functioning patients to understand?

There is another problem here as well. Dr. Davis may have violated his contract with the MCO. Many contracts prohibit the therapist from charging the patient privately for services. If the patient reported the incident, the therapist may well have been dropped from the provider list.

PATIENT FILES ON PAPER

Under state law, a therapist is required to maintain basic patient records. In addition, a common managed care organization contract provision covers the availability of patient records to the MCO for utilization review and quality control purposes. Most managed care companies reserve the right to inspect a psychotherapist's files, and expect to find a basic level of data. That makes the maintenance of comprehensive patient files more important than ever.

In addition, a systematic approach to the files will ease the burden of filling out updated outpatient treatment reports (OTRs) for managed care organizations. Many therapists use one of the many computerized help programs now available that facilitate record-keeping, as well as the printing of acceptable billing HCFA forms. Whether computerized or not, patient files should include basic data, as well as treatment progress notes. A typical patient file must include demographics, diagnosis, psychosocial history, and progress notes (see Form B in the Appendix). We have included in the file the MCO protocol or the specific step-by-step requirements necessary for that MCO. It is well worth the time and effort to establish a basic Payment and Session Monitor (see Form C in the Appendix) with each managed care organization's requirements. This form, designed by the authors, combines all critical information in one place, including the name of the case manager, the number of sessions authorized and used, authorization numbers, and co-pay amounts. It also shows patient debits, credits, and balances. The form can be set up in your computer or can be handled manually and kept in a looseleaf book. It only takes a few minutes per week to review the forms for each patient. Yet it can save you hours of unnecessary phone calls and paperwork as well as lost payments. Some MCOs require telephone certification before an initial patient visit. Others automatically allow a limited number of sessions before certification is required. Some require written reports, while others accept OTRs by telephone or fax. Still other MCOs provide their own forms that must be filled out. The requirements include the critical date when an update OTR must be filed for the authorization of continuing treatment.

In addition to the Payment and Session Monitor, separate patient files should also be organized and include Progress Notes, Consent Forms, and OTR Reports. (Form D in the Appendix is a Confidentiality Statement for use with OTRs that are faxed to the managed care organization.) Please note that facsimile transmission is probably the most unreliable way to deliver an OTR to the managed care organization, since one can never be sure who is receiving the document and where it will end up. Although mail appears more secure, there are no controls that assure the report will be seen only by the case manager to whom it is addressed.

DIAGNOSIS: DSM-IV

An easy and effective guideline for patient evaluation, as required by most OTR reports, is the Diagnostic and Statistical Manual (*DSM-IV*) Multiaxial Assessment System, which offers an overall picture of various mental disorders and general medical conditions, psychosocial and environmental problems, and the patient's level of functioning. A diagnosis is coded numerically on five axes. A listing of specific codes is beyond the scope of this book. For detailed diagnostic information and coding please consult the *Diagnostic and Statistical Manual of Mental Disorders* (see References).

The following is a listing of the general categories included on each axis.

Axis I: CLINICAL DISORDERS and OTHER CONDITIONS THAT MAY BE A FOCUS OF CLINICAL ATTENTION

(These are broad categories only. See *DSM-IV* for descriptions and coding.)

Please note that certain psychiatric disorders (i.e., cognitive and mental disorders, delirium and amnesia, schizophrenia) are usually considered by most MCOs as not amenable to psychotherapy. In addition, many of the substance abuse-related disorders are referred to the insurance companies' clinics, AA, or NA, instead of to individual therapists.

Disorders Usually First Diagnosed in Infancy, Childhood, or Adolescence (Excluding Mental Retardation, which is diagnosed on Axis II)

- Delirium, Dementia, and Amnesia and Other Cognitive Disorders
- Mental Disorders Due to General Medical Condition
- Substance-Related Disorders
- Schizophrenia and Other Psychotic Disorders
- Mood Disorders

Somatoform Disorders
Factitious Disorders
Dissociative Disorders
Sexual and Gender Identity Disorders
Eating Disorders
Sleep Disorders
Impulse Control Disorders Not Elsewhere Classified
Adjustment Disorders
Other Conditions That May Be a Focus of Clinical Attention
Unspecified Mental Disorder (non-psychotic)
No Diagnosis on Axis I
Diagnosis deferred on Axis I

Axis II: PERSONALITY DISORDERS and MENTAL RETARDATION

Please be aware that many, if not most, Axis II disorders are not considered treatable by managed care since they require long-term treatment which is inconsistent with managed care's short-term focus. Managed care's goal is to return patients to normal functioning as quickly as possible.

Personality Disorder
Schizoid Personality Disorder
Schizotypal Personality Disorder
Antisocial Personality Disorder
Borderline Personality Disorder
Histrionic Personality Disorder
Narcissistic Personality Disorder
Avoidant Personality Disorder
Dependent Personality Disorder
Obsessive-Compulsive Personality Disorder
Personality Disorder NOS (Not Otherwise Specified)
Mental Retardation
No Diagnosis on Axis II
Diagnosis deferred on Axis II

Axis III: GENERAL MEDICAL CONDITIONS

Although Axis III diagnoses cannot be recorded as the primary diagnosis, they can be used in conjunction with an Axis I diagnosis of Adjustment Disorder with Medical Problems.

Infectious and Parasitic Diseases
Neoplasms
Endocrine, Nutritional, and Metabolic Diseases and Immunity Disorders
Diseases of the Blood and Blood-Forming Organs
Diseases of the Nervous System and Sense Organs
Diseases of the Circulatory System
Diseases of the Respiratory System
Diseases of the Digestive System
Diseases of the Genitourinary System
Complications of Pregnancy, Childbirth, and the Puerperium
Diseases of the Skin and Subcutaneous Tissue
Diseases of the Musculoskeletal System and Connective Tissue
Congenital Anomalies
Certain Conditions Originating in the Perinatal Period
Symptoms, Signs, and Ill-Defined Conditions
Injury and Poisoning
None
Deferred

Axis IV: PSYCHOSOCIAL and ENVIRONMENTAL PROBLEMS

All IV-code diagnoses can be used only with a primary diagnosis on Axis I. For example, you can use 300.4 (Dysthymia) in addition to a problem with a Primary Support Group; or a 300.02 (General Anxiety Disorder) in relation to financial problems. Axis IV is actually a reality problem in conjunction with an Axis I diagnosis, but will not be covered as a diagnosis on its own.

Relational Problems:
Relational Problem Related to a Mental Disorder or General Medical Condition
Parent–Child Relational Problem
Partner Relational Problem
Sibling Relational Problem
Relational Problem NOS

Problems Related to Abuse or Neglect:
Physical or Sexual Abuse, or Neglect of Child (Code 995.5 if Focus of Attention is on the Child)

Physical or Sexual Abuse of Adult (Code 995.81 if Focus of Attention is on the Victim)

Additional Conditions That May be Included for Attention:

Non-Compliance with Treatment
Malingering
Adult Antisocial Behavior
Child or Adolescent Antisocial Behavior
Borderline Intellectual Functioning (This is coded on Axis II)
Age-Related Cognitive Decline
Bereavement
Academic Problem
Occupational Problem
Identity Problem
Religious or Spirituality Problem
Acculturation Problem
Phase of Life Problem

Axis V: GAF–GLOBAL ASSESSMENT OF FUNCTIONING (See GAF Scale in *DSM-IV*)

Note: A GAF of under 50 or over 70 is usually unacceptable and will automatically unjustify further visits.

Axis V is actually an estimated score given to the patient's level of functioning. (See page 181.)

DIAGNOSIS: THE LANGUAGE OF IMPAIRMENT

In order to work effectively with MCOs, psychotherapists must learn a new language. Terms like unconscious, transference, resistance, free association, and many others have no place in the world of managed care. Even patient and therapist may be obsolete titles.

Patients are members, clients, care-seekers or covered lives. Psychotherapists, psychologists, social workers, nurse practitioners, and psychiatrists are care-providers (or just providers) who report to a case manager. Certifications and authorizations refer to the number of sessions for which the provider may see the client. The member's problems are described in terms of impairment that are simple, nontechnical, behavioral descriptions of maladaptive behavior. Interventions, once the verbal interpretation by the therapist designed for structural psychic change, now are aimed specifically at changing the member's maladaptive behavior. That may include homework, written exercises, relaxation exercises, outside support groups, or referral to a psychiatrist for medication. Those psychotherapists familiar with behavior management techniques will find most of the terms in that vocabulary. However, others must learn the new vocabulary of behavioral medicine.

Each year, more and more books are published to help therapists learn the new language. Goodman and colleagues (1992) should be given recognition for the term "target impairment," which is now standard behavioral terminology for most dysfunctions. In most cases, the language of these books have been simplified for the understanding of nontrained case managers. The authors of the books aim to help in matching diagnosis to behavioral treatment. The managed care system has become an administrative nightmare with problems for all participants, providers and case managers alike.

THE TREATMENT PLAN

The specificity of the managed care treatment plan may pose a problem for psychotherapists who are not trained in behavioral management, the language of impairment, and short-term therapy. The treatment plan is only one component of the comprehensive outpatient treatment report (OTR), which includes a *DSM-IV* multiaxial diagnosis, a nontechnical description of the patient's behavioral problems, treatment goals, short-term objectives, a plan to meet those objectives, and an estimate of how long treatment is expected to last.

The language of the treatment plan is impairment. Impairment describes the patient's maladaptive behavior, consistent with *DSM-IV* diagnostic criteria, that will be the focus of treatment. Each of the impairments should also receive a severity rating. Although no standard severity rating system has been established, it is reasonable to follow the simple *DSM* system, which uses "mild," "moderate," and "severe" as specifiers.

Each treatment plan should include the specific interventions designed to meet the OTR's short-term objectives. Some sample treatment plans for selected impairments are included in Form E in the Appendix. Assistance with treatment plans is also available in book form and on computer disk from *Therascribe* (see Resources in the Appendix). However, therapists are cautioned against using canned reports that will come across in the presentation as insincere or plastic. The treatment plan can be used to help the patient. It is a nuisance to develop and record, but if one gets angry, and it comes across to the case manager, the plan can be misinterpreted. Because it is all very subjective, the best approach is to meet the case manager where the case manager is. Be accurate and succinct. They may be reading the same books you are. At present, we are all victims of a crude system designed to insure patients, make money for the insurance companies, and provide limited treatment without scientific measurement or a way to provide privacy for the patients. For example, one MCO requested an OTR on a four-year-old child.

> Dr. Leiter, a family therapist in northern Florida, submitted the paperwork. She reported that the four-year-old boy had been seen in six sessions with his mother. She diagnosed him as having a conduct disorder and reported that considerable progress had been made in initial therapy sessions. Requesting the authorization of further treatment, Leiter wrote that the child needed further services due to conflict in the home. No more sessions were authorized.
>
> Six months later the mother changed jobs. Her new employer had contracted with a different managed care company. The new company sent a letter to Dr. Leiter reporting that the family had applied for new coverage. It was denied because of the child's conduct disorder.
>
> Leiter wrote back that the diagnosis was mild, primarily the result of problems in the family, which the mother had reported were resolved. Under those conditions, Leiter said, the child's risk status was reduced to "normal" relative to his peer group.
>
> The insurance company still denied coverage.
>
> The mother wrote a carefully worded letter to Dr. Leiter. "I do not blame you for this terrible situation. I know you have done everything possible to help us. However, you can be sure that when it comes time to switch policies again, I will conveniently forget our association with you."

Not all experience with managed care has been negative. One Chicago psychologist (*The National Psychologist* 1996) saw the handwriting on the wall back in the early 1980s. He tried to position himself to take advantage of the imminent changes in mental health care. Dr. Richard Chaifetz began, in 1982, to offer employee services to a small number of Chicago-based companies. Today, he operates the largest privately held employee assistance program (EAP) managed health care company in the country.

"Psychologists need to be open minded to new systems and approaches to mental health," Dr. Chaifetz says, "and not be so arrogant as to believe that their way, or the way we were trained, is the only way that can or will work in the future" (p. 7).

HOW TO WRITE AN OTR

Managed care organizations are dedicated to the reduction of medical costs. Their preferred model of care is brief psychotherapy, which means the reduction of symptoms and the resolution of patient problems in the shortest possible time. Medical necessity is the overriding principle in managed care. Medical necessity refers to the condition being treated. The condition must have an *ICD-9* or *DSM-IV* diagnosis in order to be considered medically necessary. Be aware that a case manager might refer a patient with presenting problems such as anxiety, depression, or job problems. If the psychotherapist uses these terms as a diagnosis the managed care organization will not approve the treatment and consequently not pay for it. The psychotherapist *can only use* the codes in the *DSM-IV* or *ICD-9* for diagnoses.

The psychotherapy must relate to the diagnosis. Each step in the therapy must be directed to the diagnosis. The types of therapy also have codes. These can be found in the *Current Procedure Terminology* (CPT) (AMA 1996). Medicare has issued revised fee schedules and service codes for 1997. G0073 is the "G" code for individual psychotherapy, insight-oriented, behavior modifying and/or supportive, in an office or outpatient facility, approximately 45–50 minutes face-to-face with patient. G0079 is the "G" code for individual psychotherapy, interactive, in an office or outpatient facility, approximately 45–50 minutes face-to-face with patient (The Medicare News Brief 1996).

New 1997 HCPCS Codes

Health care procedure codes, required on all HCFA forms, have been revised for 1997. Although these codes went into effect on January 1, 1997, the older codes will be accepted by Medicare until April 1, 1997.

G0071	Individual psychotherapy, insight-oriented, behavior modifying and/or supportive, in an office or outpatient facility, approximately 20–30 minutes face-to-face with patient
G0072	G0071 with medical evaluation and management services
G0073	G0071 approximately 45–50 minutes
G0074	G0073 with medical evaluation and management services
G0075	G0071 75–80 minutes
G0076	G0075 with medical evaluation and management services
G0077	Individual psychotherapy, interactive, in an office or outpatient facility, approximately 20–30 minutes face-to-face with patient
G0078	G0077 with medical evaluation and management services
G0079	G0077 45–50 minutes
G0080	G0079 with medical evaluation and management services
G0081	G0077 75–80 minutes
G0082	G0081 with medical evaluation and management services
G0083	Individual psychotherapy, insight-oriented, behavior modifying and/or supportive, an in inpatient hospital, partial hospital, or residential care setting, approximately 20–30 minutes face-to-face with patient
G0084	G0083 with medical evaluation and management services
G0085	G0083 45–50 minutes
G0086	G0085 with medical evaluation and management services
G0087	G0083 75--80 minutes
G0088	G0087 with medical evaluation and management services
G0089	Individual psychotherapy, interactive, in an inpatient hospital, partial hospital, or residential care setting, approximately 20–30 minutes face-to-face with patient
G0090	G0089 with medical evaluation and management services
G0091	G0089 45–50 minutes
G0092	G0091 with medical evaluation and management services
G0093	G0089 75–80 minutes
G0094	G0093 with medical evaluation and management services

The code modifiers for clinical psychologists is AH and for clinical social workers is AJ.

A typical OTR includes the following elements:

1. Patient demographics
2. *DSM-IV* Multiaxial diagnosis with severity specifier
3. A list of impairments that will be addressed in treatment
4. A brief psychosocial history that describes the nature, severity, and duration of the symptoms or behavior
5. A list of the short-term objectives of treatment
6. A treatment plan, including specific interventions designed to meet those objectives
7. Target dates to meet goals and an estimated date when treatment will end.

All OTRs should be short and to the point (see sample OTR, Form E in the Appendix). MCOs are interested only in symptom alleviation, described in behavioral terms, with measurable outcomes. It may be easy to measure the outcome of a panic attack and its demise, but far more difficult, if not impossible, to measure the outcome with most emotional disorders. In the treatment of depression and anxiety it is more cost-effective to use psychotropic drugs with 15–minute evaluation sessions monthly by a psychopharmacologist than it is to authorize ongoing weekly talk therapy. If psychotherapists decide medication is not needed, they should state their reasons. The following examples are generally acceptable:

1. Mr. A. has a job requiring alertness that may be impaired by medication.
2. Ms. B. cannot tolerate the side effects of the medication.
3. Mr. C's anxiety is related to conflicts that can be addressed without medication.

The OTR must reflect behavioral health outcomes in the language of impairments, targeted goals, and specific interventions used to meet those goals in a specific time frame. It should include a short psychosocial description and, in follow-up sessions, a paragraph describing treatment progress. Although the time frames may be extended in the next OTR, it is better to work within a realistic frame right from the outset.

Target dates for meeting stated goals and estimated termination dates represent other pitfalls in preparing managed care OTRs. When the insurance company has authorized ten sessions, Browning and Browning (1993) suggest working with the patient as though only six sessions have been authorized. They justify their suggestion by claiming that patients "take their clues from the therapist" (pp. 75–76). The idea is that if patients think they have less time, they will use the time they actually have more productively. However, in order to help a patient, psychotherapists must be honest and maintain allegiance to a professional code of ethics. To do anything otherwise leads to a lie therapy that is degrading and ultimately helps no one. Termination dates are difficult for everyone. It was once possible to indicate that termination was "impossible to estimate at this time," but that is no longer acceptable. Simply estimate a reasonable target date and try to achieve it. If other symptoms emerge and treatment is delayed, add these developments to the next OTR with a revised termination date. One company may routinely grant six sessions, while another may have different levels of care and different time expectations. At present, MCOs have established formulas that determine how they mete out office visits. These are usually closely guarded secrets. As a simple rule of thumb, request six to ten sessions for brief therapy, ten sessions for intermediate cases, and twenty sessions for long-term treatment. In intermediate and long-term cases one should not, and perhaps cannot, ask for all the sessions at once.

When filing an OTR by telephone it is advisable to follow the prepared OTR format. The case manager will have the patient file in front of him or her, and the therapist should also have the file available. Remember, speaking from prepared notes makes the conversation go quicker and easier.

A few examples may help put the OTR in perspective. First, we will present a short scenario, then look at what needs to be included in the OTR. You will remember Mrs. Brook from an earlier story in Part II.

Scenario I–Ellen Brook

Ellen Brook was a 34-year-old divorced school teacher and mother of two small children, Sarah, 4, and Margaret, 6. Her ex-husband was an alcoholic. She moved from the city to accept a job teaching history at a suburban high school. Her boyfriend moved in with her and together they rented a small house that was within their combined means. Within a short time, her boyfriend lost his job and the family was thrown into financial crisis. Unable to find employment and disillusioned by the family bickering over money, he moved out on his own, leaving her to face the financial problems alone. The patient, who was dysthymic, began drinking occasionally and one night experienced a frightening blackout. She arrived at the next session committed never to drink again. She also began binge eating, and was gaining weight. Her children began acting out at home. This was the situation when the patient sought treatment for depression and support of her abstinence.

Beware. Some managed care companies do not consider psychotherapy a viable approach to alcohol or substance abuse, and will not approve further sessions without a drug evaluation from one of their specified clinics. At least one major company will approve up to 60 sessions as long as the patient is actively involved with a support group such as AA. However, that policy is now being reviewed and it may no longer be a viable solution. Most MCOs do not recommend treatment of substance abuse by private practitioners.

OUTPATIENT TREATMENT REPORT

GENERAL INFORMATION:	Date: December 10, 1996
Provider:	**MANAGED CARE ORGANIZATION:**
Address:	**Address:**
City, State, Zip:	**City, State, Zip:**
Lic/Cert #:	**Case Mgr.:**
	Phone:
	Fax:

PATIENT DATA:	
Patient's Name: Ellen Brook	**Date of Birth:**
Address:	**SS#:**
	Y#:
Member #:	**Initial Date of Service:**
Telephone:	**Authorization #:**
Insured's Name: Same	**No of Sessions:**
Address:	**Date Effective:**
Employee SS#:	**Total Sessions to Date:**
Group #:	**Release Signed:** [x] **Date:**

DIAGNOSIS:	
AXIS I: Primary: 300.40	Secondary: 307.50
AXIS II: V71.9	**AXIS III:** Sinus Problems (Headaches)
AXIS IV: (Stressors) Financial, Partner, Environmental	
AXIS V: (GAF) Current: 55	Highest Past 12 Months: 55

DESCRIPTION:
Document nature, severity ,and duration of symptoms/behaviors:
Depression is moderate and reactive to environmental problems. Eating disorder is also reactive to stressors. Pt. was physically and sexually abused as a child.

CURRENT MENTAL STATUS:
Describe mood, judgment, dress, memory, intelligence, and risks of suicide or violence:
Pt. alert and oriented, with no risk of suicide or violence.

SUBSTANCE ABUSE:
[ ] None Abuse Dependence [x] Remission
Identify Substance and Specify Quantity/Frequency: Pt. has gone out on a couple of occasions and experienced blackouts. She is now abstinent, and has agreed to consider AA or an alternate group if she cannot stay in remission.

BRIEF PSYCHOSOCIAL HISTORY:
Provide short history of central life role functions related to symptoms/behaviors:
Pt. is employed as a teacher. Her major problems are money and relationships. She is divorced from AA+ husband and is raising two little girls (4 and 6) by herself. Her boyfriend recently moved out, leaving her with bills she cannot afford on her own. Her social support network is poor, since she teaches all day, tutors at night, and has two children to raise.

TARGET IMPAIRMENTS:		
List all impairments/symptoms/problems. Rate Severity: 1 = Mild; 2 = Moderate; 3 = Severe. Specify Duration: 1 = < a Month; 2 = 1–6 Mos; 3 = 7–11 Mos; 4 = > a Yr.		
Impairments:	Severity:	Duration:
1. Depression	2	4
2. Eating Disorder	2	4
3. AA	1	1

GOALS OF TREATMENT:
Describe the improved or adjusted behaviors that will result from treatment:
1. Pt. will deal with anger/depression more appropriately.
2. Pt. will avoid triggers for bingeing and AA relapse.
3. Pt. will develop viable sources of support.

INTERVENTIONS: (Methods of Achievement)
1. Help pt. recognize and express anger appropriately.
2. Explore with pt. better methods of coping with depression.
3. Use behavioral modification to help pt. deal with eating disorder.
4. Develop appropriate response system for urge to drink.
5. Help pt. explore potential sources of support.

TARGET SCHEDULE:	
Symptom:	Target Date(s):
1. Depression	2–3 months
2. Anxiety	2–3 months
3. Eating Disorder	5 months
4. AA	Immediately
5. Proposed Termination Date:	(e.g., 5 months from report date)

PROPOSED TREATMENT MODALITY:				
[X] Ind.	Medication Monitoring	Group	Family	Collateral
Community Resources		Self-Help		

MEDICATION:			
[X] None	Psychiatric	Medical	
Specify Dosage:		**Frequency:**	
Prescribing Physician:			**Telephone:**
Psychiatrist	Other MD		

Clinician's Signature:__________________________ Date: __________

Scenario II–John Patterson

John Patterson is a 38-year-old New York City housing worker and recovering alcoholic, in remission until he was injured in a job-related accident that left him with significant visual loss. An adopted child, he suffered serious learning disabilities while in school, and would probably meet the criteria for a diagnosis of ADHD. He was enrolled in a special high school for children with learning disabilities and emotional problems. Eventually he left school and worked for a New York City agency. He performed well on the job and got along satisfactorily with his fellow workers. However, the patient's recreational drinking got out of control and he was referred to AA for treatment. Following immersion in a 12-step program, his alcoholism was in effective remission. Faced with diminished visual acuity and unable to work, the patient became severely depressed and began thinking of suicide. He became anxious over the possibility of relapsing into alcoholism. The patient sought psychotherapy to cope with these problems. He was having problems with daily flashbacks of the accident. The court eventually ordered treatment for post-traumatic stress disorder.

OUTPATIENT TREATMENT REPORT

GENERAL INFORMATION:	Date: December 14, 1996
Provider:	**MANAGED CARE ORGANIZATION:**
Address:	**Address:**
Cty, State, Zip:	**Cty, State, Zip:**
Lic/Cert #:	**ATT:**

PATIENT DATA:	
Patient's Name: John Patterson	**Date of Birth**
Address:	**SS#:**
	Initial Date of Service:
Member #:	**Authorization #:**
Telephone:	**No of Sessions:**
Employer:	**Date Effective:**
Address:	**Total Sessions to Date:**
Employee SS#:	**Release Signed:** [x] **Date:** 12/3/96
Group #:	

DIAGNOSIS:	
AXIS I: Primary: 309.81	Secondary: 303.90 Unstable Remission
AXIS II: V71.9	**AXIS III:** 369.90 - Visual Impairment
AXIS IV: (Stressors) Occupational Problems	
AXIS V: (GAF) Current: 50 Average: ? Highest Past 12 Months:	

DESCRIPTION:
Document nature, severity, and duration of symptoms/behaviors:
Post-Traumatic Stress Disorder creates serious emotional problems for this patient. He was injured at work, and suffered visual loss. Pt. is a recovering alcoholic and is concerned about relapsing into alcoholism in response to his problems

CURRENT MENTAL STATUS:
Describe mood, judgment, dress, memory, intelligence, and risks of suicide or violence:
Pt. is depressed with suicidal ideations (no active plans or history).

SUBSTANCE ABUSE:
[ ] None Abuse Dependence [x] Unstable Remission
Identify Substance and Specify Quantity/Frequency:
Pt. relapsed immediately after accident, but is now in remission.

BRIEF PSYCHOSOCIAL HISTORY:
Provide short history of central life role functions related to symptoms/behaviors:
Pt. was an adopted child, and has had difficulty with learning disabilities. Probably can be diagnosed as ADHD. He found a niche for himself as a housing cop. As a result of the visual loss related to the accident, he has gone into a depression.

TARGET IMPAIRMENTS:		
List all impairments/symptoms/problems. Rate Severity: 1 = Mild; 2 = Moderate; 3 = Severe. Specify Duration: 1 = < a Month; 2 = 1–6 Mos; 3 = 7–11 Mos; 4 = > a Yr.		
Impairments:	Severity:	Duration:
1. Post-Traumatic Stress Disorder	3	4
2. Depression	3	4
3. Suicidal Ideations	1	3
4. AA—Unstable remission	1	4

GOALS OF TREATMENT:
Describe the improved or adjusted behaviors that will result from treatment:
1. Lessen effect of post-traumatic stress disorder.
2. Find alternative employment where visual loss is not critical.
3. Deal appropriately with feelings of hopelessness; eliminate suicidal ideations.
4. Improve social skills.
5. Attend alcohol support group.

INTERVENTIONS: (Methods of Achievement)
1. Help patient deal with flashbacks and triggers of depression by gradually reliving the accident experience with desensitization techniques.
2. Encourage pt. to actively explore occupational alternatives.
3. Together with pt. develop life goals consistent with his reality.
4. Develop with pt. a plan to spend more time in supportive social groups to counteract the urge to drink and improve his social skills.
5. Help pt. look at positive cognitive/behavioral solutions to improved relations with his wife and daughter.
6. Encourage pt. to attend alcohol awareness support group.

TARGET SCHEDULE:	
Symptom:	Target Date(s):
1. Post-Traumatic Stress Disorder	3–6 months
2. Depression	3–6 months
3. Suicidal Ideations	1 month
4. AA	1 month
5. Proposed Termination Date	6 months

PROPOSED TREATMENT MODALITY:				
[X] Ind.	Medication Monitoring	Group	Family	Collateral
Community Resources		[x] Self-Help		

MEDICATION:		
[X] None	Psychiatric	Medical
Specify Dosage:	**Frequency:**	
Prescribing Physician:		**Telephone:**
Psychiatrist	Other MD	

Clinician's Signature:____________________________ Date: __________

Scenario III–John McIntyre

John McIntyre is a 45-year-old man who was raised in a dysfunctional family. His brother was serving a prison sentence for burglary and his sister had unsuccessfully attempted to commit suicide by slashing her wrists with a razor blade. His father, father-in-law, and stepfather had all died of cancer. Now his wife was diagnosed with lymphoma and started on radiation treatment. The patient became depressed and anxious over his wife's condition and began overeating. By the time he sought treatment for depression, he had gained 25 pounds over a short period of time. His wife's family often resorted to physical violence and from time to time were involved in street brawls. She refused psychotherapy.

OUTPATIENT TREATMENT REPORT

GENERAL INFORMATION:	Date: April 8, 1996
Provider:	**MANAGED CARE ORGANIZATION:**
Address:	**Address:**
City, State, Zip:	**City, State, Zip:**
Lic/Cert #:	**Case Mgr.:**
Phone:	
Fax:	

PATIENT DATA:	
Patient's Name: John McIntyre	**Date of Birth**
Address:	**SS#:**
Member #:	**Initial Date of Service:**
Telephone:	**Authorization #:**
Insured's Name: Same	**No of Sessions:**
Address:	**Date Effective:**
Employee SS#:	**Total Sessions to Date:**
Group #:	**Release Signed:** [x] **Date:**12/21/95

DIAGNOSIS:	
AXIS I: Primary: 300.4	Secondary: 300.02/307.50NOS
AXIS II: V71.9	**AXIS III:** V61.9—Related to wife's illness
AXIS IV: (Stressors) (1) Wife has lymphoma and is undergoing radiation; (2) Sister is depressed and has attempted suicide; (3) Dysfunctional family, acts out, overtly aggressive.	
AXIS V: (GAF) Current: 65 Average: 60 Highest Past 12 Months: 65	

DESCRIPTION:
Document nature, severity, and duration of symptoms/behaviors:
Depression—Moderate to Severe
Anxiety—Moderate to Severe
Eating Disorder—Moderate to Severe

CURRENT MENTAL STATUS:
Describe mood, judgment, dress, memory, intelligence, and risks of suicide or violence:
Pt. alert and oriented. No risk of suicide. Possible low risk of violence.

SUBSTANCE ABUSE:			
[X] None	Abuse	Dependence	Unstable Remission
Identify Substance and Specify Quantity/Frequency:			

BRIEF PSYCHOSOCIAL HISTORY:
Provide short history of central life role functions related to symptoms/behaviors:
Pt. is married to wife with lymphoma. Pt. has lost father, father-in-law, and stepfather to cancer. He comes from dysfunctional family—brother in jail, sister suicidal, and family prone to physical acting out and domestic violence.

TARGET IMPAIRMENTS:		
List all impairments/symptoms/problems. Rate Severity: 1 = Mild; 2 = Moderate; 3 = Severe. Specify Duration: 1 = < a Month; 2 = 1–6 Mos; 3 = 7–11 Mos; 4 = > a Yr.		
Impairments:	Severity:	Duration:
1. Depression	2–3	3
2. Anxiety	2–3	3
3. Eating Disorder	2–3	4
4. Problems with family	2	4
5. Wife's medical problem	2–3	4

GOALS OF TREATMENT:
Describe the improved or adjusted behaviors that will result from treatment:
1. Reduce anxiety and depression.
2. Implement an eating management plan.
3. Recognize and avoid dysfunctional family relationships.
4. Improved attitude toward wife's illness.
5. Participation in Cancer Care or alternative group.

INTERVENTIONS: (Methods of Achievement)
1. Help pt. separate past and present experience with cancer.
2. Help pt. recognize and express anger appropriately.
3. Explore with pt. better methods of coping with depression.
4. Use relaxation techniques to deal with eating disorder.
5. Suggest and encourage participation in Cancer Care group with wife.

INTERVENTIONS: (Methods of Achievement)
1. Help pt. recognize and express anger appropriately.
2. Explore with pt. better methods of coping with depression.
3. Use hypnosis to help pt. deal with eating disorder.
4. Develop appropriate response system for urge to drink.

TARGET SCHEDULE:	
Symptom:	Target Date(s):
1. Depression	2 months
2. Anxiety	2 months
3. Eating Disorder	2 months
4. Proposed Termination Date:	3 months from report date

PROPOSED TREATMENT MODALITY:				
[X] Ind.	Medication Monitoring	Group	Family	Collateral (Cancer Care)
Community Resources		Self-Help	(Family refusing therapy)	

MEDICATION:		
[X] None Psychiatric	Medical	
Specify Dosage:	**Frequency:**	
Prescribing Physician:		**Telephone:**
Psychiatrist	Other MD	

Clinician's Signature:______________________________ Date: __________

Scenario IV–Cynthia Keane

Cynthia Keane is a 43-year-old divorced nurse and mother of a 22-year-old homosexual son who lives on his own. She has been through two marriages and at least three subsequent relationships that have ended in disaster. She is emotionally and sexually obsessive, and terrified of being alone. Following a stormy argument and breakup of her fourth recent relationship, she started drinking. While driving to visit her son, she was involved in a minor traffic accident and charged by the police with DWI. The charge was later reduced to DWAI, and the patient was mandated to attend a DDP group. She was granted a restricted conditional license. Following the break-up of her fourth recent relationship, she began going out, picking up men and bringing them home. Although she reported suicidal ideations, the patient insisted that she was too frightened to act on them.

OUTPATIENT TREATMENT REPORT

GENERAL INFORMATION:	Date:
Provider:	**MANAGED CARE ORGANIZATION:**
Address:	**Address:**
City, State, Zip:	**City, State, Zip:**
Lic/Cert #:	**Case Mgr.:**
	Phone:
	Fax:

PATIENT DATA:	
Patient's Name: Cynthia Keane	**Date of Birth**
Address:	**SS#:**
Member #:	**Initial Date of Service:**
Telephone:	**Authorization #:**
Insured's Name: Same	**No of Sessions:**
Address:	**Date Effective:**
Employee SS#:	**Total Sessions to Date:**
Group #:	**Release Signed:** [x] **Date:**12/21/95

DIAGNOSIS:	
AXIS I: Primary: 300.40/305.00	Secondary: 305.00 Prov.; 303.90 Prov.
AXIS II: 300.30	**AXIS III:** None
AXIS IV: (Stressors) Problems with primary support group, social, legal.	
AXIS V: (GAF) Current: 55 Average: 60 Highest Past 12 Months: 60	

DESCRIPTION:
Document nature, severity, and duration of symptoms/behaviors:
1. Depression—non-active suicidal ideations, no plan.
2. Obsessive-Compulsive Traits—long-term.
3. Fear of being alone.

CURRENT MENTAL STATUS:
Describe mood, judgment, dress, memory, intelligence, and risks of suicide or violence:
Pt. alert, oriented, and well-motivated. Non-active suicidal ideations without plan.

SUBSTANCE ABUSE:
[ ] None [ ] Abuse Dependence [x] (Unstable Remission
Identify Substance and Specify Quantity/Frequency : Alcohol. DWAI charge.
Now abstinent.

BRIEF PSYCHOSOCIAL HISTORY:
Provide short history of central life role functions related to symptoms/behaviors.
Pt. arrested for DWAI following breakup with boyfriend. In denial re AA+ and refuses to attend AA. Divorced twice and unable to sustain meaningful relationship. Sexually and emotionally obsessive. Depressed over latest breakup with boyfriend.

TARGET IMPAIRMENTS:		
List all impairments/symptoms/problems. Rate Severity: 1 = Mild; 2 = Moderate; 3 = Severe. Specify Duration: 1 = < a Month; 2 = 1–6 Mos; 3 = 7–11 Mos; 4 = > a Yr.		
Impairments:	Severity:	Duration:
1. Depression	2–3	4
2. Obsessive-Compulsive Traits	2–3	4
3. Fear of being alone	2–3	4

GOALS OF TREATMENT:
Describe the improved or adjusted behaviors that will result from treatment:
1. Pt. will be medicated to control drinking.
2. Will comply with medication requirements.
3. Alcohol abuse vs. dependence will be determined.
4. Pt. will attend AA or alternate self-awareness group.
5. Pt. will recognize obsessive behavior as source of relational problems.
6. Depression will be lessened.

INTERVENTIONS: (Methods of Achievement)
1. Refer pt. to MD for medication; monitor and evaluate compliance.
2. Teach pt. to recognize and express anger appropriately.
3. Encourage participation in self-awareness group.
4. Help pt. recognize and deal with obsession/depression.
5. Use relaxation techniques to help pt. deal with eating disorder.

TARGET SCHEDULE:	
Symptom:	Target Date(s):
1. AA	2 months
2. Depression	2 months
3. Obsessive-Compulsive Disorder	6 months
4. Proposed Termination Date:	(6 months from report date)

PROPOSED TREATMENT MODALITY:
[x] Ind [x] Medication Monitoring Group Family Collateral
Community Resources [x] Self-Help

MEDICATION:
[x] Recommended [x] Psychiatric [x] Medical
Specify Dosage: Maltixon recommended Frequency: TBD
Prescribing Physician:
[x] Psychiatrist Other MD

Clinician's Signature: ____________________ Date: __________

Here are some suggestions for completing OTRs:

1. *Diagnosis*—Be familiar with *DSM-IV* and fill out all five axes.
   a. If there is more than one Axis I diagnosis, include each specific numerical *DSM-IV* code.
   b. If the patient does not have an Axis II disorder, but does have some Axis II personality traits, note them on Axis II. (Although sometimes there is no choice, managed care organizations usually frown on personality disorders. If there is another presenting problem on Axis I, list personality disorders as a trait, if possible.) If there are no Axis II disorders, the code is V71.9.
   c. If the patient is allergic to, or has severe side effects from medication, or has a chronic illness or learning disability, this should be noted on Axis III to alert the case manager that treatment issues are more complex and may justify an extended period of care.
   d. Axis IV—Severity of Stressors. The nature of the stressors should be included in the OTR either under history, current symptoms, or the treatment plan.
   e. Use the Global Assessment of Functioning (GAF) chart in *DSM-IV*. A GAF of 55–60 is usually a clear indication that the patient needs treatment. A GAF of 70 or higher, however, will usually require special justification of medical necessity for continuing treatment. If the GAF does not improve from one OTR to the next, the reason should be addressed because a patient can be unjustified for not making progress and using treatment appropriately.
2. *Current Symptoms*—Please note the symptoms or state that there are none. (Describe them in behavioral terms as best as possible.) Remember, add or subtract symptoms on future OTRs.
3. *History, Treatment Goals, and Treatment Plan*—Behaviors that demonstrate functional improvement or deterioration should be described. It is important to note past psychiatric and/or chemical abuse history and treatment, as well as significant traumatic events. Check for congruence in the History, Treatment Goals, and Treatment Plan.
4. *Treatment Modality*—To assist the review process, it is often helpful to clarify which treatment modality is being used to address

specific diagnostic concerns. If the patient is on medication note the dosage, frequency, and response to date.

5. *Adjunctive or Collateral Treatment*—If adjunctive or collateral treatment has been suggested to the patient, mention that such treatment is under consideration. Include plans to implement or note why.
   a. If a major stressor is a family problem and the patient is not in family therapy, please indicate why. Often, adjunctive and collateral therapy are sequentially added to the Treatment Plan. Case Managers want assurance that all relevant treatment modalities have been considered. (Although family therapy was once excluded from insurance coverage, most companies now recognize this modality as a viable cost-saving option. The sessions are usually billed under the name of the designated patient.)
   b. Substance abuse review should also address collateral therapy. Indicate whether patient is attending or not attending self-help groups. (Case managers tend to look favorably on self-help groups and, in fact, often regard self-help groups as the treatment of choice for addictive problems.)
6. *Frequency/Duration of Visits*: The usual frequency for outpatient treatment is once a week. Reasons for more than once-a-week therapy may include:
   Crisis Intervention.
   Symptoms (identify) cannot be managed with once-a-week therapy.
   More frequent sessions would avoid hospitalization or day treatment.
   More frequent sessions are needed to step down from hospitalization or day treatment.
   More frequent sessions are needed because patient is contacting therapist outside of appointment times.
   More frequent sessions are needed in the medication adjustment phase.
   The patient is attending individual as well as group therapy in one week, or weekly individual therapy and monthly medication management treatment with another provider.
7. *Some Further Hints*: A few years ago, most cases were reviewed every three months. Now some managed care organizations review cases every three weeks. Clear congruence between Treatment

Goals and Session Frequency is important. An expected termination date of "indefinite" will often trigger a review. When working with another therapist in the treatment of a patient, or if another clinician is managing the patient's medication, managed care organizations require that regular communication between therapists is maintained and documented.

GETTING PAID

Although managed care companies have reduced the fee schedule for health care providers, most psychotherapists do not consider the reduction critical. Health care providers must routinely accept modest fee adjustments and write-offs for bad debts. Providers are therefore usually willing to accept the discounted fees for services in exchange for a steady patient flow and a simple and reliable method of getting paid. Problems arise when providers find themselves accepting a new kind of bad debt write-off in the form of denied claims.

MCOs deny provider claims for payment for many reasons. One common reason is simply sending the form to the wrong address. It's easy to do. Many MCOs have changed location as the result of expansion or merger. In other cases, the company or address to which a claim must be directed for payment may be different from the company that precertified the treatment.

Sometimes a provider may submit a claim form with a minor error or omission. Despite the fact that the MCO has the information on file, they may consider the claim incomplete and return it unpaid.

An additional caution about precertification may be in order. Precertification of a claim does not mean that the claim will be paid, even when the provider fulfills all the requirements of his or her contract. The patient must be eligible for coverage at the time of service and the claim must be filed within a specified time period. The patient's coverage may be cancelled for nonpayment of premium. Neither the patient nor psychotherapist may know about the cancellation until some later time. A psychotherapist who is treating several patients for precertified conditions or impairments may be dropped from the MCO provider list without explanation. Although the MCO no longer accepts responsibility for payment, the provider remains ethically and legally responsible for continuing to care for the patients.

Another frustrating issue is the delay of payment by MCOs. Alpert (1996) reported the investigation of the payment policies of the Wellcare Management Group, an MCO based in Kingston, New York. Although Wellcare is one of the smaller publicly traded MCOs, it dominates health care coverage in the Hudson Valley region of New York state. Wellcare was a Wall Street favorite, with prestigious accounts such as IBM and the Archdiocese of New York. Alpert documents complaints that Wellcare became a chronically late payer after the company went public. Wellcare and State Insurance Department documents suggest that Wellcare's slow pay tactics may have resulted in the appearance of an inflated financial position. Although it is not illegal to withhold payments to health care providers, investigators are looking at the possibility that the intention was to provide potential stockholders with a false picture of the company's financial health. Wellcare has now been taken over by Merit. The possible impact of the acquisition on procedures and reduced payment delays is still uncertain.

With a few exceptions, the standard Health Care Financing Administration (HCFA) claim form is accepted by all insurance companies, including managed care. The HCFA form includes spaces for 33 entries, and Medicare has cautioned therapists that claims will not be processed unless *all* of the information has been provided. Although largely self-explanatory, the form can pose problems for the uninitiated. Let's take a fast look at some of the information requested. (If you're not familiar with it, a copy of the HCFA-1500 (12/90) form is included on page 184.)

At the outset, it should be noted that Items 1 through 13 may not refer to the same person if the patient is not the insured. The top half of the form is divided vertically into patient data (left two columns) and insured person's data (right column). Some practitioners find it helpful to fill in the right side of the form before inserting the patient data, especially if the patient is covered under someone else's policy (e.g., husband–wife, parent–child). Whether you tackle the form from right to left or left to right, you should be aware that the patient is not always the insured.

Box 1 seems pretty straightforward, but could be confusing if one organization administers the program for another (e.g., Blue Cross/Blue Shield and Medicare). More often today, insurers do not administer their own programs. Check off the insurer, not the administrator. Usually the box under the word *other* is the appropriate choice. Box 1a requests the insured's ID number, frequently the same as that person's Social Security number.

PLEASE DO NOT STAPLE IN THIS AREA

ANY MANAGED CARE INSURANCE

APPROVED OMB-0938-0008

CARRIER

PICA **HEALTH INSURANCE CLAIM FORM** PICA

1. MEDICARE (Medicare #) MEDICAID (Medicaid #) CHAMPUS (Sponsor's SSN) CHAMPVA (VA File #) GROUP HEALTH PLAN (SSN or ID) FECA BLK LUNG (SSN) OTHER (ID) X

1a. INSURED'S I.D. NUMBER (FOR PROGRAM IN ITEM 1): 315-11-3076

2. PATIENT'S NAME (Last Name, First Name, Middle Initial): JUAN ALICIA

3. PATIENT'S BIRTH DATE MM DD YY — SEX M ☐ F X

4. INSURED'S NAME (Last Name, First Name, Middle Initial): JUAN DON

5. PATIENT'S ADDRESS (No., Street): 7 SEVENTH AVENUE

6. PATIENT RELATIONSHIP TO INSURED: Self ☐ Spouse X Child ☐ Other ☐

7. INSURED'S ADDRESS (No., Street): 7 SEVENTH AVENUE

CITY: NEW YORK — STATE: NY

8. PATIENT STATUS: Single ☐ Married X Other ☐; Employed ☐ Full-Time Student ☐ Part-Time Student ☐

CITY: NEW YORK — STATE: NY

ZIP CODE: 10004 — TELEPHONE (Include Area Code): (212) 214 1996

ZIP CODE: 10004 — TELEPHONE (INCLUDE AREA CODE): (212) 214 1996

9. OTHER INSURED'S NAME (Last Name, First Name, Middle Initial):

10. IS PATIENT'S CONDITION RELATED TO:

11. INSURED'S POLICY GROUP OR FECA NUMBER: 1012JT

a. OTHER INSURED'S POLICY OR GROUP NUMBER:

a. EMPLOYMENT? (CURRENT OR PREVIOUS) ☐ YES X NO

a. INSURED'S DATE OF BIRTH MM DD YY: 01 02 65 — SEX M X F ☐

b. OTHER INSURED'S DATE OF BIRTH MM DD YY — SEX M ☐ F ☐

b. AUTO ACCIDENT? ☐ YES X NO — PLACE (State)

b. EMPLOYER'S NAME OR SCHOOL NAME: BUSTER INDUSTRIES

c. EMPLOYER'S NAME OR SCHOOL NAME:

c. OTHER ACCIDENT? ☐ YES X NO

c. INSURANCE PLAN NAME OR PROGRAM NAME: DOGG

d. INSURANCE PLAN NAME OR PROGRAM NAME:

10d. RESERVED FOR LOCAL USE

d. IS THERE ANOTHER HEALTH BENEFIT PLAN? ☐ YES X NO *If yes,* return to and complete item 9 a-d.

READ BACK OF FORM BEFORE COMPLETING & SIGNING THIS FORM.

12. PATIENT'S OR AUTHORIZED PERSON'S SIGNATURE I authorize the release of any medical or other information necessary to process this claim. I also request payment of government benefits either to myself or to the party who accepts assignment below.

SIGNED: SIGNATURE ON FILE — DATE: 05 01 96

13. INSURED'S OR AUTHORIZED PERSON'S SIGNATURE I authorize payment of medical benefits to the undersigned physician or supplier for services described below.

SIGNED: SIGNATURE ON FILE

PATIENT AND INSURED INFORMATION

14. DATE OF CURRENT: ILLNESS (First symptom) OR INJURY (Accident) OR PREGNANCY(LMP) MM DD YY: 05 01 96

15. IF PATIENT HAS HAD SAME OR SIMILAR ILLNESS. GIVE FIRST DATE MM DD YY

16. DATES PATIENT UNABLE TO WORK IN CURRENT OCCUPATION FROM MM DD YY TO MM DD YY

17. NAME OF REFERRING PHYSICIAN OR OTHER SOURCE: GOSHEN MEDICAL

17a. I.D. NUMBER OF REFERRING PHYSICIAN: 262

18. HOSPITALIZATION DATES RELATED TO CURRENT SERVICES FROM MM DD YY TO MM DD YY

19. RESERVED FOR LOCAL USE

20. OUTSIDE LAB? ☐ YES ☐ NO — $ CHARGES

21. DIAGNOSIS OR NATURE OF ILLNESS OR INJURY. (RELATE ITEMS 1,2,3 OR 4 TO ITEM 24E BY LINE)

1. 309.28
2. 291.5
3.
4.

22. MEDICAID RESUBMISSION CODE — ORIGINAL REF. NO.

23. PRIOR AUTHORIZATION NUMBER

24. A DATE(S) OF SERVICE From MM DD YY	To MM DD YY	B Place of Service	C Type of Service	D PROCEDURES, SERVICES, OR SUPPLIES (Explain Unusual Circumstances) CPT/HCPCS	MODIFIER	E DIAGNOSIS CODE	F $ CHARGES	G DAYS OR UNITS	H EPSDT Family Plan	I EMG	J COB	K RESERVED FOR LOCAL USE
1 05 22 96	05 22 96	11 (office)	1	90844		1,2	90 00	01				
2 05 29 96	05 29 96	11	1	90844		1,2	90 00	01				
3 06 14 96	06 14 96	11	1	90844		1,2	90 00	01				
4												
5												
6												

25. FEDERAL TAX I.D. NUMBER: 115 30 0050 — SSN X EIN ☐

26. PATIENT'S ACCOUNT NO.: 131300993

27. ACCEPT ASSIGNMENT? (For govt. claims, see back) X YES ☐ NO

28. TOTAL CHARGE: $ 270 00

29. AMOUNT PAID: $ 0 00

30. BALANCE DUE: $ 270 00

31. SIGNATURE OF PHYSICIAN OR SUPPLIER INCLUDING DEGREES OR CREDENTIALS (I certify that the statements on the reverse apply to this bill and are made a part thereof.)

Sondra M. Tuckfelt, PhD

Sondra M. Tuckfelt, PhD

SIGNED 06 18 96 DATE

32. NAME AND ADDRESS OF FACILITY WHERE SERVICES WERE RENDERED (If other than home or office)

33. PHYSICIAN'S, SUPPLIER'S BILLING NAME, ADDRESS, ZIP CODE & PHONE #

SONDRA M. TUCKFELT, PH.D.
56 SLEEPY VALLEY ROAD
WARWICK
NEW YORK 10990
Phone (914)986-7777 Provider # 3254

PHYSICIAN OR SUPPLIER INFORMATION

(APPROVED BY AMA COUNCIL ON MEDICAL SERVICE 8/88) *PLEASE PRINT OR TYPE* FORM HCFA-1500 (12-90) FORM OWCP-1500 FORM RRB-1500

FORM 9487 COLWELL SYSTEMS CHAMPAIGN IL

BECAUSE THIS FORM IS USED BY VARIOUS GOVERNMENT AND PRIVATE HEALTH PROGRAMS, SEE SEPARATE INSTRUCTIONS ISSUED BY APPLICABLE PROGRAMS.

NOTICE: Any person who knowingly files a statement of claim containing any misrepresentation or any false, incomplete or misleading information may be guilty of a criminal act punishable under law and may be subject to civil penalties.

REFERS TO GOVERNMENT PROGRAMS ONLY

MEDICARE AND CHAMPUS PAYMENTS: A patient's signature requests that payment be made and authorizes release of any information necessary to process the claim and certifies that the information provided in Blocks 1 through 12 is true, accurate and complete. In the case of a Medicare claim, the patient's signature authorizes any entity to release to Medicare medical and nonmedical information, including employment status, and whether the person has employer group health insurance, liability, no-fault, worker's compensation or other insurance which is responsible to pay for the services for which the Medicare claim is made. See 42 CFR 411.24(a). If item 9 is completed, the patient's signature authorizes release of the information to the health plan or agency shown. In Medicare assigned or CHAMPUS participation cases, the physician agrees to accept the charge determination of the Medicare carrier or CHAMPUS fiscal intermediary as the full charge, and the patient is responsible only for the deductible, coinsurance and noncovered services. Coinsurance and the deductible are based upon the charge determination of the Medicare carrier or CHAMPUS fiscal intermediary if this is less than the charge submitted. CHAMPUS is not a health insurance program but makes payment for health benefits provided through certain affiliations with the Uniformed Services. Information on the patient's sponsor should be provided in those items captioned in "Insured": i.e., items 1a, 4, 6, 7, 9, and 11.

BLACK LUNG AND FECA CLAIMS

The provider agrees to accept the amount paid by the Government as payment in full. See Black Lung and FECA instructions regarding required procedure and diagnosis coding systems.

SIGNATURE OF PHYSICIAN OR SUPPLIER (MEDICARE, CHAMPUS, FECA AND BLACK LUNG)

I certify that the services shown on this form were medically indicated and necessary for the health of the patient and were personally furnished by me or were furnished incident to my professional service by my employee under my immediate personal supervision, except as otherwise expressly permitted by Medicare or CHAMPUS regulations.

For services to be considered as "incident" to a physician's professional service, 1) they must be rendered under the physician's immediate personal supervision by his/her employee, 2) they must be an integral, although incidental part of a covered physician's service, 3) they must be of kinds commonly furnished in physician's offices, and 4) the services of nonphysicians must be included on the physician's bills.

For CHAMPUS claims, I further certify that I (or any employee) who rendered services am not an active duty member of the Uniformed Services or a civilian employee of the United States Government or a contract employee of the United States Government, either civilian or military (refer to 5 USC 5536). For Black-Lung claims, I further certify that the services performed were for a Black Lung-related disorder.

No Part B Medicare benefits may be paid unless this form is received as required by existing law and regulations (42 CFR 424.32).

NOTICE: Any one who misrepresents or falsifies essential information to receive payment from Federal funds requested by this form may upon conviction be subject to fine and imprisonment under applicable Federal laws.

NOTICE TO PATIENT ABOUT THE COLLECTION AND USE OF MEDICARE, CHAMPUS, FECA, AND BLACK LUNG INFORMATION
(PRIVACY ACT STATEMENT)

We are authorized by HCFA, CHAMPUS and OWCP to ask you for information needed in the administration of the Medicare, CHAMPUS, FECA, and Black Lung programs. Authority to collect information is in section 205(a), 1862, 1872 and 1874 of the Social Security Act as amended, 42 CFR 411.24(a) and 424.5(a) (6), and 44 USC 3101;41 CFR 101 et seq and 10 USC 1079 and 1086; 5 USC 8101 et seq; and 30 USC 901 et seq; 38 USC 613; E.O. 9397.

The information we obtain to complete claims under these programs is used to identify you and to determine your eligibility. It is also used to decide if the services and supplies you received are covered by these programs and to insure that proper payment is made.

The information may also be given to other providers of services, carriers, intermediaries, medical review boards, health plans, and other organizations or Federal agencies, for the effective administration of Federal provisions that require other third parties payers to pay primary to Federal program, and as otherwise necessary to administer these programs. For example, it may be necessary to disclose information about the benefits you have used to a hospital or doctor. Additional disclosures are made through routine uses for information contained in systems of records.

FOR MEDICARE CLAIMS: See the notice modifying system No. 09-70-0501, titled, 'Carrier Medicare Claims Record,' published in the Federal Register, Vol. 55 No. 177, page 37549, Wed. Sept. 12, 1990, or as updated and republished.

FOR OWCP CLAIMS: Department of Labor, Privacy Act of 1974, "Republication of Notice of Systems of Records," Federal Register Vol. 55 No. 40, Wed Feb. 28, 1990, See ESA-5, ESA-6, ESA-12, ESA-13, ESA-30, or as updated and republished.

FOR CHAMPUS CLAIMS: PRINCIPLE PURPOSE(S): To evaluate eligibility for medical care provided by civilian sources and to issue payment upon establishment of eligibility and determination that the services/supplies received are authorized by law.

ROUTINE USE(S): Information from claims and related documents may be given to the Dept. of Veterans Affairs, the Dept. of Health and Human Services and/or the Dept. of Transportation consistent with their statutory administrative responsibilities under CHAMPUS/CHAMPVA; to the Dept. of Justice for representation of the Secretary of Defense in civil actions; to the Internal Revenue Service, private collection agencies, and consumer reporting agencies in connection with recoupment claims; and to Congressional Offices in response to inquiries made at the request of the person to whom a record pertains. Appropriate disclosures may be made to other federal, state, local, foreign government agencies, private business entities, and individual providers of care, on matters relating to entitlement, claims adjudication, fraud, program abuse, utilization review, quality assurance, peer review, program integrity, third-party liability, coordination of benefits, and civil and criminal litigation related to the operation of CHAMPUS.

DISCLOSURES: Voluntary; however, failure to provide information will result in delay in payment or may result in denial of claim. With the one exception discussed below, there are no penalties under these programs for refusing to supply information. However, failure to furnish information regarding the medical services rendered or the amount charged would prevent payment of claims under these programs. Failure to furnish any other information, such as name or claim number, would delay payment of the claim. Failure to provide medical information under FECA could be deemed an obstruction.

It is mandatory that you tell us if you know that another party is responsible for paying for your treatment. Section 1128B of the Social Security Act and 31 USC 3801-3812 provide penalties for withholding this information.

You should be aware that P.L. 100-503, the "Computer Matching and Privacy Protection Act of 1988", permits the government to verify information by way of computer matches.

MEDICAID PAYMENTS (PROVIDER CERTIFICATION)

I hereby agree to keep such records as are necessary to disclose fully the extent of services provided to individuals under the State's Title XIX plan and to furnish information regarding any payments claimed for providing such services as the State Agency or Dept. of Health and Humans Services may request.

I further agree to accept, as payment in full, the amount paid by the Medicaid program for those claims submitted for payment under that program, with the exception of authorized deductible, coinsurance, co-payment or similar cost-sharing charge.

SIGNATURE OF PHYSICIAN (OR SUPPLIER): I certify that the services listed above were medically indicated and necessary to the health of this patient and were personally furnished by me or my employee under my personal direction.

NOTICE: This is to certify that the foregoing information is true, accurate and complete. I understand that payment and satisfaction of this claim will be from Federal and State funds, and that any false claims, statements, or documents, or concealment of a material fact, may be prosecuted under applicable Federal or State laws.

Public reporting burden for this collection of information is estimated to average 15 minutes per response, including time for reviewing instructions, searching existing date sources, gathering and maintaining data needed, and completing and reviewing the collection of information. Send comments regarding this burden estimate or any other aspect of this collection of information, including suggestions for reducing the burden, to HCFA, Office of Financial Management, P.O. Box 26684, Baltimore, MD 21207, and to the Office of Management and Budget, Paperwork Reduction Project (OMB-0938-0008), Washington, D.C. 20503.

Box 2 is for the patient's last name, first name, and middle initial.

Box 3 calls for the patient's birthdate in MM/DD/YY form and the patient's gender.

Box 4 switches to the insured's last name, first name, and middle initial.

Box 5 reverts to patient data, and requests the patient's address and telephone number.

Box 6 asks the patient's relationship to the insured. Be careful.

Box 7 requests the insured's address, which may not be the same as the patient's address and telephone number. If the *insured* is the *patient*, just write *same*.

Box 8 deals with the marital and employment statuses.

Box 9 requests the last name, first name, and middle initial of an other insured. For instance, if the patient is a child, he or she could be covered under the father's policy *and* a possible separate policy that insures the child's working mother. The mother is then the other insured. Most of the time, the therapist should just leave this blank, unless he or she is certain that the information is correct and that the information for Boxes 9a, b, c and d, that request additional information about the *other insured* is also correct.

Box 10 asks if the patient's condition is related to (10a) employment, (10b) automobile accident, or (10c) other accident. 10d is usually left blank. Again, be careful. If the psychotherapist is certain that the patient is being covered by worker's compensation or no-fault then go ahead with the information requested. Otherwise, check the entries for *no*.

Box 11a through 11c switch once again to the insured's data. 11a requests the insured's policy or FECA number, 11b the insured's date of birth and gender, 11c the name of the insured's insurance plan or program. Again, if the patient is the insured person, leave the boxes blank, except for 9a where *same* is entered. Box 11d is really a cross reference to Boxes 9a through 9d. Usually it is safe to leave this blank.

Box 12 is a standard release statement authorizing the release of medical and/or other information necessary to process the claim. It also requests payment of government benefits to the insured or the therapist, who accepts assignment by checking Box 27. (The implications of accepting assignment are explained in detail on the back of the HCFA form and partially summarized under Box 27 below.) It is important to have the patient sign on the line that is there and to sign another HCFA form periodically to be safe. Include the date.

Box 13 authorizes payment to the undersigned therapist who has provided the services. Even if this in on file, ask the patient to sign another form about every four months.

Box 14 calls for the date of illness (first symptom), injury (date of accident), or pregnancy (likely month). The date that psychotherapists need to enter is usually the date that the patient experienced the symptoms with sufficient severity that he or she called for an appointment.

Box 15 asks if the patient has had the same illness or a similar illness and the first date of that illness. This entry is not required for psychotherapists. Leave it blank.

Box 16 is for the dates in MM/DD/YY form that the patient was unable to work in his current occupation. Unless this form is being filed for worker's compensation or for cases considered in accident reports, write *NA* for *not applicable.*

Box 17 is for the name of the referring physician. Again, entry is not necessary but the name of a referring physician may be included if relevant.

Box 18 requests the dates in MM/DD/YY form of the patient's hospitalization related to the services listed in Box 24. Unless this form is for a hospitalized patient there is no need for a psychotherapist to fill in any dates.

Box 19 is reserved for local use and usually left blank.

Box 20 is for outside lab tests. Not applicable.

Box 21, line 1 is for the patient's primary diagnosis in *DSM-IV* code. If the patient has more than one diagnosis, the secondary diagnosis is entered on line 2. These are related to Box 24E below. Watch these entries, please. These are the most important lines on the form. This part is *not* comparable to multiaxial diagnoses required on OTR forms. On this form, use the Axis I diagnosis codes that are appropriate, *one* code on a line. For example:

1. 309.30
2. 316.00
3. 346.20

Please note that line 3 is a physical disorder that is affected by the psychological condition, but is not the disorder being treated by the psychotherapist. The codes for physical disorders are in *DSM-IV*, Appendix G, page 813. Further explanation for the use of these codes can be found in La Bruzza (1994).

Box 22 asks for the Medicaid resubmission code and the original Medicaid reference number. If the patient is not on Medicaid, leave this entry blank.

Box 23 requests the patient's prior authorization number sometimes provided by managed care organizations before treatment.

Box 24 has space for 11 separate entries from A through K. Box 24A is for the date of service in MM/DD/YY form. (If the entry covers just one office visit, the dates will be the same for "from" and "to.") Box 24B is for the place of service code, usually 3 for psychotherapy services performed in the therapist's office. Common service codes include:

1–Inpatient Hospital,
2–Outpatient Hospital,
3–Doctor's Office,
4–Patient's Home,
7–Nursing Home,
8–Skilled Nursing Facility, and
0–Other Locations.
A–Psychotherapists may not get paid for services provided in a patient's home. It is advisable to check with the insurance company. When the insurance company representative provides a response, record the representative's name, title, exact words, and date. Ask for a written statement regarding this response and any other responses. If the written response is sent, photocopy it and attach a copy to subsequent forms.
B–Ambulatory Surgical Center
E–Comprehensive Outpatient Rehabilitation Facility
F–Independent Kidney Disease Treatment Center

Box 24C lists the numerical code for the Type of Service performed, typically 1 for medical psychotherapy or 3 for consultation. Type of Service Codes include:

1–Medical
2–Surgery
3–Consultation

Box 24D lists procedures, services, or supplies in CPT format. G0073 or G0079 are the new "G" codes for a 45–50 minute session of psychotherapy. The procedure code for a 30 minute session is G0071 or G0077. Some companies may require a different code. Check each MCO contract for the correct codes to use. The modifier for a Clinical Psychologist is AH and a Clinical Social Worker is AJ. The modifiers are not required at this time by Medicare. Do not enter the codes unless they are required. Psychologists are presently reimbursed for psychological testing if the correct codes are used. Codes are listed in the current CPT, but psychotherapists need to check with Medicare at least once every six months.

Box 24E refers to the diagnostic code (Box 21) treated. It is not necessary to repeat the *DSM-IV* code. Just enter the number, usually just 1 and 2 from Box 21.

Box 24F is the amount billed for your services. That sounds pretty simple, but can be a problem. The psychotherapist should enter his or her full and usual charge for the service, even if it is known that the insurer will not pay that amount. The insurance carrier will take it from there. If you know that the insurer's approved fee for that service, and issue a claim in that amount, the carrier might use that fee to determine the usual and customary fees for the provider and the profession. Be assured that it is highly unlikely that there will be an overpayment.

Box 24G refers to the number of days or units covered by the charges in 24F. For instance, if on 24A you had listed multiple dates of service, 24G is where you can qualify how many office visits were involved. It may be safer to list one office visit per line at 24A and code 24G as 1 than to risk possible misinterpretation by the carrier.

Box 25 is for the therapist's Federal tax ID or Social Security number. Use only one or the other.

Box 26 provides space for the patient's account number. If the therapist does not assign account numbers to patients the space can be left blank.

Box 27 is for you to accept or reject assignment. By checking the assignment box the therapist agrees that the payment will be sent to him or to her. (The small print on the back of the HCFA form explains, among other things, that the information from claims and other related documents may be given to various government and private agencies and organizations, including the Department of Veterans Affairs, the Department of Health and Human Services, the Department of Transportation, the Department of Justice, the Internal Revenue Service, Congressional Offices, and private collection agencies and consumer reporting agencies.) Note well: although the psychotherapist, by contract, has agreed to accept assignment of payment, the insurance organization, especially Medicare, does not pay the therapist directly unless this box is checked.

Box 28 lists the total of the charges covered by this claim form on lines 24–1 through 24–6.

Box 29 is for the amount paid and may be left blank if there is any question about the amount. Box 30 asks for the amount due and should be completed.

Box 31 is where the psychotherapist signs and dates the form. Include degrees or credentials.

Box 32 is provided to list the location where the services were performed if they were not performed in the office (Box 33). This is almost always left blank. Box 33 asks for your name, address, phone number, and PIN number. Write carefully the provider number assigned by the MCO or by Medicare. If the number is omitted, the resulting EOB might read *provider unknown.*

It is suggested that the psychotherapist make at least one copy of the form with Boxes 1–21 completed to keep on file. Medicare patients, and perhaps others, would have an easier time with secondary payers if they have a copy of the entire form, Boxes 1–33, for their records. After having a copy of Boxes 1–21 on file, it is all right to write *signature on file* for entries 12 and 13.

HCFA forms can be purchased with your name, address, phone number, and carrier-assigned provider identification number (PIN). A list of vendors is included in the Appendix. Acceptance of the standard form greatly simplifies what once was a billing nightmare. That doesn't mean that the monthly billing process is not tedious and time-consuming. Therapists with sizable practices will find solace in computerization. Most computer programs on the market today will automatically print out a HCFA billing form once the required data is entered. If the monthly billing cycle is a horrendous chore, we recommend trying the electronic route. Not only will computerization help with the bills, but it will provide a new level of organization for all patient files. Some computer programs even provide the capability to track managed care organization sessions and alert the therapist to the imminent need for filing on OTR. One word of caution: make sure computer specifications match the program requirements. Limited RAM (random access memory) will considerably slow down the process when working with large interactive patient files.

For those of us who are computer-phobic, all is not lost. A form for Payment and Session Monitoring is included in Form C (see Appendix), which can be used with the computer or filled out by hand. It will provide all the information needed to track sessions and payments. It also indicates when to call or write for further authorization or check on copayment amounts or member status. It even contains a section that summarizes the specific managed care organization data and protocol. Another alternative is to hire an experienced billing company or secretary. In those cases, the issues of competency and confidentiality must be thoroughly considered.

Shelley Malin, a medical billing specialist (see Resources in Appendix), cautions that psychotherapists need to make sure that the person doing the billing and the psychotherapist agree on what is meant by confidentiality. Most billing administrators have experience billing for physicians, which is a situation that is very different from billing for psychotherapists. The key to getting paid on a timely basis by managed care organizations is to make sure authorizations are current and OTRs are filed on time in printed form or by fax. From there on, accuracy is critical. If an HCFA form contains errors or missing data, expect the managed care organization to disqualify the entire bill, no matter how simple the error may appear. The claim will be rejected, and the form will have to be corrected and refiled. The managed care organizations make errors, too. It is important to check all codes on the benefit statements provided by managed care organizations and follow up any discrepancies or errors promptly by phone or mail.

Electronic billing may be a source of hope for therapists who are inundated with billing paperwork, or it may create more problems than it solves. That depends on how computer literate you are. A few managed care organizations have followed the lead of Medicare in accepting patient billing by computer modem. This number will be dramatically increasing in the future (see Chapter 4). The required software may be different in each case and, of course, the patient billing data must still be entered into the program, but the process is fairly simple and easy once learned. Electronic billing has another benefit as well—it takes the companies considerably less time to process the electronic claims and you'll get the check faster (maybe).

For therapists who have not made the transition to computer, Medicare now has a Telephone Claim Entry system (MTCE) for inputting claims directly into Medicare's computer system. It is necessary to enroll in the program before you can use it, but there's no charge for telephone submission. Medicare also has an Automatic Response System for therapists to request information on a specific claim directly by touch-tone phone. The system is handy for checking claims, patient status, deductibles, and pricing information.

If your experience with managed care is especially abusive, there *is* something you can do about it. Form F (see Appendix) includes an Insurance Abuse Report for documenting your experience. The report should be sent to The National Coalition of Mental Health Professionals and Consumers, P.O. Box 438, Commack, NY 11725. Phone/fax: 516/424-5232; e-mail: NCMHPX @ aol.com. Copies should also go to your state and federal legislators and the state insurance commissioner. Contact the League of Women Voters in your area for the address of the appropriate officials.

Dr. Robert Langs (1988) warned therapists a decade ago that when insurance is used to enable patients to pay low fees or no fees, meaningful therapy is impossible. He pointed out that the simple divulgence of the patient's name and diagnosis brings a third party into the treatment room and destroys the intimacy required for any form of therapy. With managed care we don't bring a third party into the room, we invite a gang of clerks, case managers, computer operators, peer reviewers, and CEOs. At a London conference in 1993, Langs said it would take a hundred years for people to fully understand what he meant by upholding privacy in the treatment room. Unfortunately, only a decade later, we are now faced with understanding more than we want to. Timing and economy have become big problems for managed mental health care. Translating cost containment into good treatment while maintaining professional integrity may be the most difficult terrain we will ever have to cross. We may not want managed care, but we can't afford to reject it. Patients' lives and the mental health of the United States are being challenged. If good therapists are bought or brainwashed by insurance investors or drug companies interested only in profit margins, what will the future of our world be like? Behavioral change is the mode of the day and, for the moment, we cannot ignore that trend. However, truth through interpretation (Bail 1981) is honesty in the managed care arena. Bail said:

> Truth through interpretation is love, is comfort for despair, is security against terror, is growth in the face of death, is friendliness in the face of

> loneliness; it is, in short, the summoning up of the most virtuous qualities developed by humanity in the course of its history. [p. 64]

For faint-hearted therapists to desert the battlefield, leaving patients in the hands of managed care alone, would be an unthinkable crime. Although this book has focused on how to get along with Big Brother, it is important to remember that ultimately it is up to the provider to deliver quality treatment.

8

Computerizing Your Practice

One way to adapt to the increased recordkeeping demands of a modern psychotherapy practice is to computerize the process. The following article by Carolyn Colwell, CSW, appeared in *Nassau Newsnotes* (1996):

❑ ❑ ❑

Managed care would be impossible without computers. And it's those cyber-powerhouses that enable managed care companies to inflict such burdensome paperwork requirements on practitioners. Without . . . computers to help carry the paperwork load, therapists are going to have a hard time keeping up.

There are a number of practice management programs that will streamline your client billing, insurance forms, outpatient treatment reports, progress notes, assessments, treatment plans, and referral databases. Some have the added benefits of providing Rolodexes, mail merging for form letters, tracking systems for telephone contacts, graphing of client progress or percentage of practice by client type, and calculation of profit/loss statements. One software vendor, Therapist Helper, estimates that computerizing all this work saves its users about $4800 a year or five hours a week.

These computer bells and whistles can then have additional practical marketing uses that can help you build your practice. For example, a full-scale practice management package might enable you to pinpoint the months you are most busy in your practice and where most of your referrals come from during those months. Then you can target those sources next year just before that same time period with a mailing via a form letter that's addressed from a mailing list in the program's Rolodex. All of this can easily be generated from data that you've already inputted for each client—the same data that has driven the billing and insurance forms. By hand it's a major project.

The barriers to jumping into this computer age appear to be cost and the complexity of the choices. Bare-bones billing programs start for as little as $99 and full-fledged packages that include scheduling and electronic billing can total close to $1,000. And there is also the question of whether by going the budget route you may be dollar-wise but pound foolish in terms of reaping the efficiency and marketing benefits of computerization in this highly competitive time. So this is not a decision to be made lightly.

But there are a number of ways to "partialize" the process. The first is to take a quick survey of what's out there so that you won't settle for an expensive program that lacks many of the additional features included in another program for about the same price. Many of the most popular programs advertise in the *NASW News* as well as other professional publications. But if you can go on-line, the World Wide Web Page Mental Health Net's Professional Resources' *Computer Billing and Office Management Programs* (http://www.cmhc.com/guide/pro24.htm) will give you a comprehensive list with a thumbnail sketch of how they will help you manage your practice. In addition, Wiley & Sons' new *Managed Behavioral Healthcare* guide is scheduled to include a section on computers and software (1-800-879-4539).

The second step is to order some demo disks and try out various software packages to get the feel of what you will be buying. Some demo disks are free; others require a small charge but then often include a full manual which spells out exactly what the program will do and how. After you've run a couple of demos, call back the sales offices or technical assistance lines and make sure you have all your questions answered. Some general questions you may want to ask vendors when assessing how useful a practice management program may be to you are: the availability and cost of upgrades (e.g., to Windows 95); the cost and ease of access to technical support; the completeness of the program or whether add-ons at further expense are necessary to do all your necessary tasks; the degree of professionalism in the graphic display of printouts, such as bills; and the compatibility to other programs you may be using, such as *Quicken.*

It also may be helpful to check out whether customizable reports or forms are available and at what charge. Also, if you have a special need, as for example you see a lot of children with divorced parents, you might want to ask about how the program handles that particular billing situation. Almost all the programs will fill out a HCFA claim form, but not all of them provide electronic claims filing.

Finally, you might want to check how long the software vendor has been in business. Will they be there when you have a problem three years from now? How happily and easily the vendor answers questions like these may tip you off to how accommodating they will be after you've bought your program.

A third step is to consider whether you want to buy a whole program or go with a company that allows step-by-step additions to its package. For example, *Touched* comes in two stripped-down versions (*Billing* $275 or *Lite* $160) that allow later upgrades to a full package. As a fourth step, you might want to consider how worthwhile electronic billing is because it is an add-on for many of the programs. Providers generally submit at least 40 insurance claims a month to reap cost efficiency from an electronic billing program. Applied Computing Services estimates that its Electronic Media Claims option can save its customers $1,126.41 a year for 50 claims a month.

The fifth step is to weigh whether any trade-offs make it worth choosing a program that has a time-payment program, such as *The Cure*, a DOS-based program which charges zero percent interest. And finally, if you are happy with whatever system you already have for billing and insurance forms, you may want to consider whether a program that computerizes only clinical records may be helpful. There are three major ones on the market, *Sisyphus Software* ($275), *Therascribe* ($345), and Owen Consulting's *Social Work* ($249). *Therascribe*, which is Windows-based, will generate treatment plans and outpatient treatment reports based on the behavioral criteria that are required by managed care. It also streamlines mental status exams via a quick checklist. *Social Work*, which has been developed by a Long Island company, also is Windows-based. Its owner, Jeffrey Smith, has plans to make it compatible with a billing program and Microsoft *Scheduler*. Among the advantages of *Social Work* is that it can be used for hospital-based practices and case management. It allows users to build a database of community referral sources. *Social Work* allows users to start out with a basic $99 version for just case management with minimal reporting features and then upgrade.

There are at least a dozen major practice management programs available. Here's a look at a few of them which run on IBM-compatible machines and in one case on Apple equipment. Prices listed are for solo practice versions and are subject to change. The best-known practice management program appears to be *Therapist Helper*, a $595 Windows-based package that provides a scheduler for an additional $99 and an "insurance connector" for $200 if purchased at the same time as the original package. It has a "starter version" for $99 that can handle up to 12 clients and the company will apply that $99 to a later purchase of the full package. The advantages to this program include the long-standing viability of its producer. *Therapist Helper* advertises that it's been endorsed by a number of professional organizations, including the National Federation of Societies for Clinical Social Work. One disadvantage is that there is a $125-a-year charge for technical assistance and upgrades after the first six months. Calls are not toll-free. *Therapist Helper* has a three-month payment option.

Other Windows-based programs are *Touched* and *$umTime*. One advantage of *Touched* is that it bills from a scheduling program that is included in its $475 full package rather than being a $99 add-on as the scheduler is with *Therapist Helper*. An electronic billing add-on is $99. Consequently, *Touched* is a significantly less expensive choice. It also has a graphing feature that enables you to use some statistical measures to chart client progress, data which may be appealing to managed care companies. But its graphing capacity (based on a review of the demo) does not look as complete as the one offered by *The Cure*, which still is a DOS-based program that is not as agile to use as *Touched*. *Touched* allows you to computerize the HCFA 1500 insurance form and it also will allow you to correct your own forms from a template with a limited number of choices. Technical assistance for *Touched* is free via a toll-call.

$umTime ($399) has the advantage of coming in both agile Windows and Mac versions. An electronic claims filing package is $49. Technical support is free for three months and available for the balance of one year for $49 including upgrades. Thereafter maintenance contracts are $129 a year. *$umTime*, as many other programs, exports data to *Quicken*. This vendor will make customized modifications to its program for $20–$60. The demo will let you work with it for five clients for five activities for a month as a test.

Delphi may have the most friendly marketing, sales, and technical assistance. *Delphi* estimates that its program will cut billing time by 75 percent. Its hallmark is its one-price, one-package approach, which includes unlimited technical assistance via an 800 number, and all upgrades based on client requests and needs. *Delphi* is DOS-based, though plans are in the works for a Windows or graphical interface version, but will not be ready until next year at the earliest. The full package price is $895 and a 30-day working demo with manual is available. There is a 10 percent discount for buying within the 30-day demo period. One of the disadvantages of *Delphi* is its scheduler which cannot be billed off and appears only in half-hour increments.

The *Therapist*, a DOS-based program, may be one of the bargains out there. At $247 it offers many of the features of *Delphi* at much less cost. It has a working demo that will let you take it for a test ride for a month. The market for these programs is changing rapidly. The addresses and phone numbers of major vendors are listed in the Appendix.

❑ ❑ ❑

Although the computer packages offer help with the paperwork, there are tasks they cannot perform. No computer package can check your Explanation of Benefits (EOB) for missing sessions or missing payments. Omitted sessions and payments occur frequently. When examining an EOB, it is necessary for the practitioner, or someone hired to do this job, to actually examine each date and payment and check this information against the actual information submitted to the managed care organization. It is possible that the MCO received a statement for six sessions but paid for only five. In order to verify the discrepancy, one has to check prior bills, co-payments, deductibles, and submission dates.

All the computer packages can save time. This is especially true if the mental health professional has computer expertise and the time to spend in entering data and creating databases. Many psychotherapists were hopeful that computer programs would help them resolve the conflicts about managed care. There is no way, however, that a software package can extend the number of sessions that have been allocated for a particular patient or follow up when a claim is delayed or relieve the practitioner of the responsibility of informing patients of the limitations of their coverage. The software package cannot even inform the psychotherapist about how many sessions are left unless the psychotherapist is willing to turn on the computer and check. In order to take advantage of what the package can provide, the user has to know how to access the desired information and be consistent in the use of it.

9

Time-Limited Psychotherapy

Short-term psychotherapy includes an array of modalities and techniques that are compatible with today's managed care environment. These range from short-term dynamic psychotherapy (STDP), which incorporates many techniques from long-term psychoanalysis, to the popular cognitive-behavioral modalities. Brief time-limited therapy, cognitive therapy, and rational-emotive therapy are included here as the treatments of choice for MCOs. Other short-term therapies or techniques are included in Part III. This chapter will review the historical development of brief therapy and the highlights of the major theories and techniques.

The following article, "Brief Therapy and Psychoanalytic Technique," originally appeared in the *International Journal of Communicative Psychoanalysis and Psychotherapy*, *8*(1): 105–108 (1993), and is reproduced here in modified form with the permission of the author, Irving Weisberg, Ph.D., and the International Society for Communicative Psychoanalysis and Psychotherapy.

❑ ❑ ❑

INTRODUCTION

In 1919, Freud wrote the following about the distinction between psychoanalysis and other more solution-focused therapies whose emphasis was on problem-solving and symptom relief: ". . . the large scale application of our therapy will compel us to alloy the true gold of analysis freely with the copper of direct suggestion . . ." (Freud 1919, p. 168).

Earlier, at a lecture delivered at Vienna's Doctors' College (December, 1904), he differentiated psychoanalysis from those treatments where the therapist was more actively involved in indirect suggestion:

> With these other therapies, the concern is not with the origin, strength, and meaning of the pathological symptoms, but with the symptom itself.

Analytic concern is with the factors related to the early genesis of the symptoms and to bring out these factors during the analysis.

Psychoanalytic exploration does not indicate speedy results, and should not be attempted when the speedy removal of dangerous symptoms is required.

Psychoanalytic technique for uncovering the origins of an illness and helping to remove its manifestations is fraught with difficulty and should not be practiced without training.

Psychoanalysis is based on the recognition that the unconscious nature of certain mental processes is causally related to the pathological symptoms.

Psychoanalytic treatment is conceived as a re-education to remove roadblocks. [Freud 1905]

With the sudden and ubiquitous cost-cutting by managed care, limiting financial coverage to a short-term (4 to 20 sessions) form of therapy, many psychoanalysts feel they are in crisis. The dialectic nature of the arguments is clear. On the one side, the thesis is presented as follows:

"It is important at this time when psychoanalytic therapy is under attack as 'non-cost effective,' when there is a rush to drug therapies and more manifest and conscious psychotherapies, that we solidify our sense of who we are, of what we do best, of whom we serve, and where our ethics lie."

On the other side sits the antithesis: "Of what value are ethics if we do not survive? Ethical considerations often seem to mask our fear of altering and expanding our approach and validating its effectiveness—not so much to satisfy managed care, but rather to meet the changing needs of those seeking therapy. If we fail to do so, we shall surely become a white elephant."

Perhaps from these seemingly antithetical arguments we can forge a new hypothesis.

DESCRIBING GOLD AND DEFINING COPPER

For psychoanalysts interested in working with patients in brief contact, it is important to illuminate the most effective analytic techniques, and where necessary, parameters. Kurt Eissler (1953) introduced the term *parameter* to describe modifications and alterations in technique—as well as additions required by specific dysfunctions of the patient's ego. Movement from the expected baseline of appropriate technique, for whatever reason, must be justified, the nature of the baseline constantly kept in mind, and the patient's unconscious perception of the changes monitored. In other words, we need to note the sacrifices inherent in varying the conditions of treatment. Though brief therapy can be dynamic and uncovering, it departs from classical analysis in a number of distinctive ways:

The brief nature tends to stifle the process of regression essential to the release of unconsciousness material.

The introduction of a fixed time limit sets in motion a number of action thoughts in both the patient and the therapist.

The face-to-face nature of the contact also tends to foster the presentation of manifest material, inhibiting the discharge of unconscious material.

The intense focus on specific conflicts sometimes leads to a problem-solving, symptom relief approach in order to achieve speedy closure.

The increased activity of the therapist often consists of non-adversarial confrontation, persistent interpretation, and, again, a discouraging of regression. This is contrasted with the more reflective and contemplative role of the analyst. To achieve completion within the agreed upon number of sessions, the brief therapist's stance commonly appears relentless and hurried.

Yet, as with psychoanalysts, one sees among brief therapists the same divisions that separate those who focus on intrapsychic conflicts and internal coping capacities, and those who stress the intereffecting, reenacting nature of significant relationships. The former group emphasizes ego functions, particularly those defense functions regulating the drives and coping with external stress. The latter highlights the triangle of interaction with present significant others, then with the therapist in the transference relationship, and, finally, linking the presenting symptoms to their roots in the interactions with the earliest significant others when traumatic messages about self and other were first internalized.

Despite differences between brief therapy and psychoanalysis, and the divisions within each group, they share a number of major goals:

Relief of symptoms and a removal of impediments blocking a continuation of the process of growth.

A desire to make the connection between symptoms and influencing circumstances.

To be aware that these early developmental conflicts set in motion ego mechanisms: dynamics, interpersonal operations, and reenactments.

For after the completion of the therapy, providing patients with a useable understanding of the therapeutic process so that they can continue the dynamic exploration of residual conflicts and the interpersonal context within which they take place.

To summarize the nature of brief dynamic psychotherapy: it is a treatment modality where a single conflict, fundamental to the patient's presenting symptoms and complaints, is highlighted and emphasized in active, face-to-face contact during once-a-week sessions, usually numbering 4 to 20 (maximally 45). Psychoanalytic theory is employed to identify and illuminate the central conflict, and to trace its unconscious origins. The dynamics and interpersonal patterns of the transference–countertransference relationship, where they relate to the central conflict, are identified and confronted directly.

HISTORICAL ROOTS OF BRIEF THERAPY

Mentions of brief therapy go back to the archives of earliest recorded history. There are chronicled accounts, from Egypt and Greece, of what might be considered short-term therapy. Transcribed in ancient documents are elaborate ceremonies to heal the afflicted, to provide relief to the troubled, and to ease the distress of the suffering. Among interventions described are rituals leading to emotional catharsis, interpretations of dreams and fantasies, persuasive suggestion, trance incantations, and even bodily manipulations.

In more recent times, brief dynamic therapy is rooted in the beginnings of the psychoanalytic tradition. Most of Freud's earliest patients were short-term. Emmy von N. was seen 15 times, and the Rat Man lasted 11 months (Jones 1955). The orchestra leader Bruno Walter was successfully treated by Freud for cramps in his conducting arm in six sessions in 1906 (Walter 1940). The composer Gustav Mahler was relieved of an impotence problem in one four-hour session with Freud in 1905 (Jones 1955). And Freud's many training analyses rarely lasted more than six months.

Of the number of early analysts who indicated concern for the ever-lengthening duration of psychoanalytic treatment (Freud 1937), the first to specifically raise the issue of shortening the length of treatment, and address modifications in technique toward that end, was Sándor Ferenczi. He wrote on a more active role for the therapist (Ferenczi 1920) more than 75 years ago, dealing with many of the issues faced by brief therapists today. Ferenczi's explorations of active measures was to move patients past their resistances and anxieties in stymied therapies.

Otto Rank, who worked with Ferenczi on reducing the length of analytic therapy (Ferenczi and Rank 1924), approached the problem from a different vantage point. His emphasis was on the need for a time limit. Rank's belief in the trauma of birth (1924) anticipated by several decades the studies of symbiotic attachment and subsequent separation from the mother by Spitz (1965) and Mahler (1969). Though it was Ferenczi who first advocated an active role for the therapist, it was Rank who initially presented the idea of setting a fixed time limit for therapy. He felt that the time limit would help mitigate the patient's separation anxiety. It is interesting to note how Rank's views of the original trauma of birth and the resultant terror or separation in the transference has so influenced the contemporary time-limited advocate, James Mann (Mann and Goldman 1994). It is Mann who uses the conflict of separation, experienced at the termination of treatment, as the central dynamic in his technique of brief (12 sessions) therapy.

Over 20 years after the pioneering explorations of Ferenczi and Rank—with almost nothing written in between—a Hungarian émigré to the United States studied brief therapy. Franz Alexander (Alexander and French 1946) published research done at the Chicago Institute of Psychoanalysis. Though openly acknowledging that the work was a continuation and realization of ideas first proposed by Ferenczi and Rank, Alexander introduced a new curative factor—

the corrective emotional experience, the results of identifying with and internalizing aspects of the therapist—to go along with interpretation as a treatment tool to be used in curative reconstruction.

RECENT CONTRIBUTIONS

To understand the present state of brief dynamic psychotherapy, one must review the output of the major contributors who followed Alexander: David Malan (1976), who worked with the Balints at the Tavistock Clinic in London, Lewis Wolberg (1965) at the Postgraduate Center in New York City, James Mann from Boston University (Mann and Goldman 1994), Peter Sifneos (1972) of Harvard University in Cambridge, and Habib Davanloo (1992) from McGill University in Montreal.

David Malan's efforts (Malan 1976) grew out of efforts begun with Michael and Enid Balint at Tavistock. Central was their selection process that involved assessing a potential patient's capacity to integrate and react to a trial interpretive intervention during an evaluative interview. More recently, Malan has incorporated the techniques of Davanloo. Regarding the more active role of the therapist and methods to more directly handle resistance, Malan (1980) writes:

> In the early part of this century, Freud unwittingly took a wrong turning, which led to disastrous consequences for the future of psychotherapy. This was to react to increasing resistance with increased passivity—eventually adopting the technique of free association on the part of the patient, and the role of 'passive sounding board,' free-floating attention, and infinite patience on the part of the therapist. The consequences have been strenuously ignored or denied by generations of analysts and dynamic psychotherapists, but are there for all to see. The most obvious effect has been an enormous increase in the duration of treatment—from a few weeks or months to many years. A less obvious development is that the method has become, to say the least, of doubtful effectiveness. [p. 13]

Of the different models, Malan's (1976) seems to work most assiduously toward an initial assessment of appropriateness for brief therapy. A panel studies the evaluative material, then develops vignettes specific to the patient that would show the likelihood of either no change, change restricted to the main symptoms and complaints, some change in the fundamental causal unresolved conflict, marked resolution of the causal conflict, or cure, implying resolution, as well, of additional conflicts related to the fundamental one.

Lewis Wolberg and the group at the Postgraduate Center in New York City first explored brief therapy as a form of crisis intervention. Their psychoanalytic focus was clearly influenced by Heinz Kohut and self psychology. Wolberg's emphasis was on the value of the therapist's ability to "experience and communicate" an empathic interest in the patient (Wolberg 1965, pp. 52–53). The flow of brief therapy is divided into phases: (a) the establishment of a working alliance through offering empathic support; (b) experiencing the patient's personality with an awareness of its connection to the presenting disruption; (c) helping the patient to select new coping mechanisms, change interactive roles and patterns; and (d) consolidating therapeutic gains, providing new knowledge and new approaches dealing with stress. Wolberg is easily the least rigid and most eclectic of the brief therapists, using elements from every model.

Few theorists of brief therapy are as philosophically interesting as James Mann (Mann and Goldman 1994), proponent of a pre-fixed, time-limited psychotherapy. Strongly influenced by Otto Rank, Mann attempts to diffuse the trauma of separation and differentiation by introducing a fixed end-point at the outset. He made a particular point that the essential task of maturation is to accept the finite nature of time—an acceptance that life is time-limited, framed by birth and death.

Patient and therapist select a primary focus for the fixed 12-session treatment that Mann calls the "central issue." The presenting complaint is connected to this underlying issue, with Mann maintaining that a preset, fixed time limit energizes both patient and therapist in a particularly unique way—most especially in helping to overcome resistance.

Working at Harvard University, Peter Sifneos (1972) describes his technique as "short-term anxiety, provoking psychotherapy." The therapist's role is strongly interpretive and confrontational, clearly guiding what takes place in the treatment room. Sifneos has a clear set of criteria for selecting patients appropriate for brief therapy. They must have a clear complaint, they should be "psychologically minded," and be strongly motivated for the work. The distinguishing characteristic of this approach is that the active stance of the therapist is in the service of keeping the tension level high throughout the treatment, constantly interpreting the patient's reactions in the transference. Following Freud's rule of abstinence (Freud 1919), where therapist withdrawal is linked to optimal frustration of the patient, Sifneos supports the view that anxiety facilitates the work of the analysis. He seems to be providing the patient with a new stress, namely the therapy itself, allowing the therapist the opportunity to see the patient's maladaptive patterns more quickly.

Short-term dynamic psychotherapy (STDP) is the name given his approach by Habib Davanloo of McGill University in Montreal. The essential elements (Davanloo 1992) of the treatment and the selection process involve: (1) establishing a central focus, (2) assessing the patient's capacity for responding to interpretations, and (3) assessing the patient's ego defense organization. Sessions involve the "triangle of persons": interaction with the therapist (the transference–countertransference relationship); then, interaction with significant others in the here and now, outside therapy (current life); finally, interaction with those from early life where roles and interactive patterns first developed (past life). Davanloo also works with the "triangle of feelings": the initial feeling is from a reaction to the escaping drives; next, the feelings related to covering and displacing secondary feelings acting as defense; and finally, the anxieties signaling the failure of defense.

COMPARING THE APPROACHES TO DOING BRIEF THERAPY

Can we determine which approach to brief treatment will best fit a particular patient who has a particular style and particular presenting symptoms and complaints? David Malan's emphasis on cognitive interpretations makes him a "nondirective, neutral teacher." The dramatic, explosive nature of hysterical patients responds well to Malan's intellectual, even-handed style.

Lewis Wolberg, strongly stressing an affective working alliance, highlights providing the patient with empathic support and a sense of security. His approach is best suited to those struggling with identity issues, as well as those passive-dependent patients who respond well to empathic responses.

Unlike Malan or Wolberg, Peter Sifneos is confrontational, provocative, and displays the widest range of affect in his work. Because of a tendency to harshness, those trained in Sifneos's technique must be vigilant not to feed sadistic inclinations, while at the same time avoiding a reaction-formation to excessive passivity. Patients struggling with oedipal issues, with containing aggressive drives, and with impulse control problems seem to best fit with Sifneos's more confrontive approach.

Because of James Mann's investment in structure and framework, patients with poor capacities for inner self-regulation do well with his technique. During the opening of treatment, patients with dependency traits initiate an idealized transference to the therapist as "parent-in-charge." Also, Mann's gentle organizing technique does not erupt major resistances in more infantile, passive patients.

Habib Davanloo does not fit neatly into any assessment system. He believes in the broadest range of acceptability of patients for brief therapy. He is known for the ability to mobilize affect in previously repressed patients, with particular suitability for patients with phobic and obsessive symptoms, as well as those whose primary defenses are intellectualization and isolation of affect. For Davanloo, neither the degree of mental illness nor the complexity of the focal problem determines the choice of treatment; they only affect the length of treatment. The same technique is used in all cases. Normal neurotics with an oedipal focus are treated in 5 to 10 sessions, and those with a focus involving loss in up to 15 sessions. Those believed to have a deeper pathology will take up to 40 sessions.

It has been held by some (Flegenheimer 1994, pp. 157–176) that matching the patient and therapist is more significant in brief therapy than long-term treatment since over the more extended therapy, with a relatively neutral stance by the therapist, the patient–therapist relationship will work through more and more transference issues, and will thus be more colored by reality. As Flegenheimer (1994) writes:

> In brief therapy it is necessary for the therapist to be active from the beginning. . . . This does not mean the abandonment of therapeutic neutrality or revealing the therapist's personal life. . . . However, it is not possible to be an active brief therapist and not reveal consider-

ably more personality traits and characteristics than in a more classical analytically oriented long-term therapy. Therefore, the personality of the therapist will become an important determinant of the formulation of the therapeutic alliance and the course of treatment. [p. 161]

PRESENT ISSUES IN BRIEF THERAPY

There are a number of issues raised by short-term and time-limited therapy, some real and some exaggerated. Modifications mentioned earlier: (a) the setting of a brief time limit; (b) the face-to-face nature of the contact; (c) the intense focus on a specific conflict; and (d) the more active stance of the therapist, all tend in varying degree to shift the nature of the therapeutic relationship. All of the brief therapists mentioned above introduced their theoretical explanations, metaphysical frameworks, and sets of practice techniques more or less independently of the others. Even among those who unquestionably support brief therapy there is little consensus as to which techniques are more effective than others or which patients would most benefit from a short course of therapy.

The charge among a significant segment of the psychoanalytic community is that brief therapy is superficial. This charge is clearly unwarranted. It is also claimed that its results, even when positive, are fleeting and reversible under subsequent stress. This seems no more true than with the longer-term psychoanalytic therapies. Finally, it is said that brief therapy's positive results are what Freud called "transference cures" and "flights into health." Again, the criticism is not supported by follow-up studies, and is made by those having a built-in bias in favor of long-term analytic therapy.

The major justifications for a brief dynamic psychotherapy are as follows:

It works as well as the longer variant, yet saves time, energy and money.

It fits certain situations better:

–Crisis intervention, particularly when the patient in crisis has a personality with strong structural features.

–Clear, solution-oriented, problem-solving situations, most commonly couple, marital, or family difficulties, or work and career problems.

It fits certain patients better:

—The modification to brief therapy is supported because of a patient's inherent ego defect, which makes it impossible to tolerate the long-term experience.

It is necessitated by external circumstances:

—The patient cannot afford the financial cost of long-term therapy. (Third-party payers will only provide coverage for short-term therapy.)

—Patient or therapist is constricted by time considerations.

COMMUNICATIVE PSYCHOANALYSIS AND BRIEF PSYCHOTHERAPY

Communicative psychoanalytic psychotherapy is adaptable to short-term psychotherapy, since it offers an interactional model (Langs 1975, 1976, 1979) to counteract, or at least minimize, the potentially harmful effects of a shortened and pressurized brief therapy experience. Communicatively trained therapists are cautioned to continually listen for unconscious reactions involving the conditions of therapy, which can be presented indirectly in the patient's narrative. The technique uses a stimulus–response paradigm to interpret the patient's inner and outer worlds in relation to the therapeutic experience. As explained by Grotstein (1984), it challenges practitioners to reexamine the meaning of therapy, the theories they embrace, their interventions, and their commitment to themselves, their patients, and the use of insurance procedures. Communicative therapy can be used in its original form as an analytic technique, or can be used to inform the therapist's listening powers in short-term therapy. The communicative approach provides us with tools for listening to the voice of the unconscious, and for hearing its echo in the patient–therapist interaction.

CONCLUSIONS

Short-term psychoanalytic psychotherapy involves a series of modifications, the most central of which is its brief, time-limited nature. Others include: (a) the face-to-face nature of the contact; (b) the strongly focused attention to specific conflicts; and (c) increased activity, consisting of frequent questions by the therapist, and directed guidance for the patient toward areas considered more important than others. It must be stressed that these modifications are not introduced by necessity, that is, in consideration of a patient's ego defect, forcing a shorter, time-limited treatment. The alterations are introduced a priori for external reasons in response to the financial and time pressures. Still (if we attend to the numerous reports of participating patients and therapists), brief therapy has been a powerful and effective modality.

The brief, time-limited form is not a substitute for longer-term psychoanalytic psychotherapy. Rather, it is another tool therapists can add to their toolbox. The two methods can enhance each other in intersecting ways. Psychotherapists can introduce strongly focused periods in longer-term treatment, while being more active in a non-adversarial, confrontational style. This offers us another effective tool in treating more severe pathologies. Conversely, brief treatment gains from applying psychoanalytic principles and techniques; in understanding unconscious communication in the bipersonal field; in listening, formulating, and intervening in a very focused manner; and in understanding the holding nature of a secure therapeutic frame. Here, knowledge from longer-term analytic therapy can illuminate the entire spectrum of brief, dynamic psychotherapy.

REFERENCES

Alexander, F., and French, T. (1946). *Psychoanalytic Therapy*. New York: Ronald Press.

Davanloo, H., ed. (1992). *Short-Term Dynamic Psychotherapy*. Northvale, NJ: Jason Aronson.

Eissler, K. R. (1953). The effect of the structure of the ego on psychoanalytic technique. *Journal of the American Psychoanalytic Association* 1:104–143.

Ferenczi, S. (1920). Further developments of an active therapy in psychoanalysis. In *Further Contributions to the Theory and Practice of Psycho-Analysis*. London: Hogarth, 1950.

Ferenczi, S., and Rank, O. (1924). *The Development of Psychoanalysis*. New York: Nervous and Mental Disease Publishing Co.

Flegenheimer, W. V. (1993). *Techniques of Brief Psychotherapy*. Northvale, NJ: Jason Aronson.

Freud, S. (1905). On psychotherapy. *Standard Edition* 7: 257–269.

—— (1919). Lines of advance in psycho-analytic therapy. *Standard Edition* 17: 157–168.
—— (1937). Analysis terminable and interminable. *Standard Edition* 23: 216–253.
Grotstein, J. (1984). The higher implications of Lang's contributions. In *Listening and Interpreting*, ed. J. Raney. New York: Jason Aronson.
Jones, E. (1955). *The Life and Work of Sigmund Freud, vol. 2.* New York: Basic Books.
Langs, R. (1973). *The Technique of Psychoanalytic Psychotherapy, vol. 1.* New York: Jason Aronson.
—— (1975). *Technique in Transition.* New York: Jason Aronson.
—— (1976). *The Therapeutic Interaction.* New York: Jason Aronson.
—— (1979). *The Supervisory Experience.* New York: Jason Aronson.
—— (1988). *A Primer of Psychotherapy.* New York: Gardner.
—— (1992a). The self-processing class and the psychotherapy situation: a comparative study. *American Journal of Psychotherapy* 1:75–90.
—— (1992b). *A Clinical Workbook for Psychotherapists.* New York: Karnac.
Mahler, M. (1969). *On Human Symbiosis and the Vicissitudes of Individuation.* New York: International Universities Press.
Malan, D. (1976). *The Frontier of Brief Psychotherapy.* New York: Plenum.
—— (1980). The most important development since the discovery of the unconscious. In *Short-Term Dynamic Psychotherapy*, ed. H. Davanloo, pp. 13–24. Northvale, NJ: Jason Aronson, 1992.
Mann, J., and Goldman, R. (1994). *A Casebook in Time-Limited Psychotherapy.* Northvale, NJ: Jason Aronson.
Rank, O. (1924). *The Trauma of Birth.* New York: Brunner, 1952.
Sifneos, P. E. (1972). *Short-Term Psychotherapy and Emotional Crisis.* Cambridge, MA: Harvard University Press.
Spitz, R. (1965). *The First Year of Life.* New York: International Universities Press.
Walter, B. (1940). *Theme and Variation.* New York: Knopf.
Wolberg, L. R., ed. (1965). *Short-Term Therapy.* New York: Thieme-Stratton.

❑ ❑ ❑

COGNITIVE-BEHAVIORAL TECHNIQUES

Crisis intervention, cognitive theory, and behavior management refer to systems that provide the basis for some of the more popular short-term modalities compatible with today's managed care environment. These brief descriptions are an attempt to capture the essence of these theories. In general, these short-term therapies share a six-step model, which includes:

1. Data collection/assessment
2. Definition of treatment goals and objectives

3. A treatment plan, including possible referral for adjunctive treatment
4. Implementation of techniques (interventions)
5. Evaluation
6. Follow-up

Although crisis theory (Golan 1986) has its roots in psychodynamic personality theory, particularly ego psychology, it also calls on concepts from stress, learning, systems, role, and other theories. Cognitive theory rejects the psychoanalytic concept of the unconscious as the primary driver in psychic life. For clinicians, the crisis approach offers a conceptual reference for brief-focused interventions in a wide range of pressure-filled situations. It is being offered as the treatment of choice in many settings. The use of crisis intervention depends on the clarification between acute, time-bounded crises and longer-term developmental and transitional stresses that might best be treated by other methods.

Crisis intervention recognizes that each individual is subjected to periods of internal and external stress that may disturb the equilibrium with his or her surrounding environment. These periods are usually triggered by some hazardous event—but may also build up under pressure over a long period of time. The person, in a state of tension and anxiety, calls on his or her usual problem-solving mechanisms to deal with the situation. He or she quickly discovers that they don't work. As the tension increases, he or she turns to emergency coping measures, which are also ineffective. When the problem cannot be resolved, avoided, or redefined, the tension peaks. At this vulnerable point, a precipitating factor can bring about a turning point and the individual may enter an active state of crisis marked by disorganization and disequilibrium. This is usually followed by a gradual reorganization until a new state of equilibrium develops.

As the crisis situation is developing, the person may see the stressful event primarily as a threat to his instinctual needs or his sense of autonomy or well-being; as a loss of a person, attribute, or capacity; or as a challenge to survival, mastery, or growth. Each of these elicits a characteristic emotional reaction that reflects the subjective meaning of the event to the individual. Threat elicits an increased level of anxiety. Loss brings about feelings of depression, deprivation, and mourning. Challenge stimulates a moderate increase in anxiety combined with a kindling of hope and expectation, which releases new energy for problem solving.

The duration of the crisis, dependent on many factors, is time-limited. A typical state of active disequilibrium usually lasts from four to six weeks. Each class of crisis situation appears to follow a specific sequence of stages in which the person's emotional and behavioral reactions can be anticipated. Fixation and disequilibrium at a certain point may provide a clue as to where a person is stuck and what lies behind his continuing inability to master the situation. During the unraveling of the crisis situation, the person appears to be particularly amenable to help. He or she is open to outside intervention and change, and a minimal but well-focused effort often has maximal effect. During the integration stage, new ego strengths and adaptive styles may evolve, enabling the person to cope more effectively with future problems. On the other hand, if help is not available at this point, maladaptive patterns will be adopted that may weaken the individual's ability to function adequately in the future.

One patterned approach to crisis intervention (Parad et al. 1976) is based on four essential steps:

1. Identification of the precipitating event and its meaning for the client.
2. Identification of the coping means used by the client.
3. The search for alternative ways of coping that might better fit the situation.
4. Review and support of the client's efforts to cope in new ways.

The implementation phase of crisis intervention deals with setting up and working out specific tasks. These are designed to solve specific problems in the client's current life situation, to modify previous inadequate ways of functioning, and to learn new coping patterns. Treatment is keyed to the achievement of limited goals. The techniques include reassurance, encouragement, advice, advocacy, and warning clients of the consequences of maladaptive resolutions of the problem. Important behavior concepts include guidance, role rehearsal, reshaping, modeling, teaching, coaching, prompting, and positive reinforcement.

Like crisis intervention, cognitive theory (Werner 1986) rejects the concept of the unconscious as the primary force in psychic life. Treatment focuses on the thoughts, emotions, expressed motives, and behavior of the client. Change consists of expanding or modifying individual consciousness until perception more nearly approximates reality. This is done by talking to the client and/or guiding the client into direct experiences that will alter his or her distorted thinking.

Cognitive theory is a general category including Alfred Adler's individual psychology, Albert Ellis's rational-emotive psychotherapy, William Glaser's reality therapy, and Harold Werner's rational casework, among others. The main points of the theory (Werner 1986) are:

1. Thinking determines behavior. Inappropriate behavior is caused by inaccurate perceptions.
2. Our basic patterns of behavior are influenced by our goals. We pick a lifestyle we think will help achieve our goals.
3. Our lives are not controlled by unconscious forces, yet we can be unaware of where our attitudes come from or the effect of our behavior on others.
4. Aggression is a reaction to feelings of threat or frustration, and not an instinct.
5. We are not inevitably controlled by instinctual drives.
6. Emotions can also be traced to thinking. There is no such thing as an unconscious emotion.
7. Motives, too, can't be unconscious. They are the result of thinking.
8. Everyone is inherently creative and has the resources of strength and courage to become everything they are capable of becoming.
9. Cognitive theory is socially oriented. Thinking is influenced by our society, environment, relationships and experiences.

Albert Ellis, the father of rational-emotive therapy, regarded man's emotional disturbances as largely the result of irrational beliefs. He professed that we can eliminate most of our emotional or mental unhappiness by learning to maximize rational and minimize irrational thinking. Irrational beliefs are transmitted by the culture, the family, or significant others. Some of the irrational beliefs postulated by Ellis (1962) that may lead to emotional disturbance include:

1. We must be loved and approved by everyone.
2. We must be perfect in everything we do.
3. Some people are bad and should be punished.
4. It's devastating when things aren't the way we want.
5. Happiness is externally caused.

6. We should dwell on bad things that might happen.
7. Difficult situations should be avoided.
8. We should depend on others.
9. Our past history determines our present behavior.
10. We should be very upset over other people's problems.
11. There is one right and perfect solution to all human problems.

Many psychotherapists are integrating some form of cognitive therapy into their practices. In response to the need for briefer and more focused therapy, Leahy (1996) describes specific procedures based on cognitive principles for the assessment and treatment of depression, anxiety, and marital conflicts. Safran and Segal (1996) integrate findings in the fields of cognitive psychology, infant development, and emotion theory as the new information relates to psychotherapy. Although cognitive theory can generate brief therapy, the principles are complex and require professional attention to new findings and integrations in the area.

Behavioral therapy (Thomlison 1986) refers to the systematic application of techniques intended to facilitate behavioral change. They are based principally but not exclusively on the conditioning theories of learning. The theory emerges from the work of Ivan Pavlov and B. F. Skinner. Pavlov's studies on the salivation reflex of dogs led to the process known as respondent conditioning. Skinner developed the foundation for contemporary behavioral therapy. At the heart of his theory is the concept of reinforcement. An individual's behavior can be increased in frequency of occurrence if such behavior is positively reinforced. In addition, the frequency of the behavior can be decreased by administering punishment or withholding reinforcement (a process called extinction).

The first step is to recognize that behavior in any situation does not stem from inner traits that are a concrete and unchangeable part of the personality. Behavior management focuses on specific behavior in specific situations. Whether we want to increase or decrease a behavior, it is the relationship of the behavior to the situation that must be analyzed and controlled.

Situations can be divided into three events: behavior, those events that come before it and those that come afterward. Psychologists call these associated events antecedents and consequences. The sequence is antecedent–behavior–consequence, A–B–C. That is the context in which to view human behavior.

An undesirable or problematic behavior is identified and labeled as a target behavior. Also identified are the antecedents and consequences, those environmental events that control or maintain the conditions for the problem behavior. The use of positive consequence to increase desirable behavior is the strength of the social learning approach to behavior therapy, and is not always easy to apply. Physical punishment is considered an unacceptable way of decreasing the frequency of an unwanted behavior.

Systematic desensitization procedures, used in the treatment of phobias and anxiety, lean heavily on Pavlovian principles, and have been greatly expanded by Joseph Wolpe (1990). His theory regards anxiety as an automatic response learned in a situation perceived by the individual as anxiety-provoking. Wolpe's desensitization requires that the individual learn relaxation techniques, including relaxation through imagery. While in a relaxed state, the patient is confronted with a hierarchy of anxiety-provoking situations, from the least anxiety-creating to the most. The procedure is repeated until the patient has successfully dealt with the entire hierarchy.

Cognitive-behavioral approaches share one common element: they attempt to help the patient regard his or her problem in a new way (Leahy 1996), through the processing of thoughts that are validated in actual behavioral assignments. All require the identification of negative self-statements, private thoughts, or self-talk that serve to inhibit performance. These irrational thoughts are cognitively restructured and the patient begins to identify positive, constructive self-statements. In each approach, alternate thought processes are substituted for the negative statements to provide a successful confrontation of the situation. The complexities of processes in cognitive therapy are gaining increased recognition (Safran and Segal 1996).

Although managed care has become a reality in today's marketplace, it would be foolhardy to adopt managed care as a solution to America's health problems. When evaluating the potentially positive and negative effects of managed care, psychotherapists work with the knowledge that therapy is most effective when it meets the needs of the patient above all (Barron and Sands 1996).

At best, therapy depends on the capacity of the clinician to understand the patient's dilemma and intervene in an appropriate manner in light of the circumstances surrounding the patient's life, including his or her financial condition. Hopefully, professional judgment will influence health care systems as well as psychotherapy.

III

Finding Solutions*

It was a bright cold day in April and the clocks were striking thirteen.
–George Orwell, 1984

This sense of identity provides the ability to experience one's self as something that has continuity and saneness, and to act accordingly.
– Erik Erikson, Childhood and Society

Part III offers possible solutions to the problems posed by managed care organizations. Although MCOs have threatened the professional identity of psychotherapists, there is still time to recover and reclaim our profession. However, in order to continue to preserve professional identity and integrity, as psychotherapists we need to examine ourselves as well as our practices. It is time for psychotherapists to ask ourselves, once again, some important questions. The first question is the one from our adolescence: Who am I? When we originally were exploring answers to this question, we developed some important ideals that have remained with us. We chose psychotherapy not from greed but from the desire to understand why people behave the way they do, from the genuine need to help others, and from the desire to grow through relationships with other people. Along the way to becoming professional psychotherapists, most of us were patients in psychotherapy, from which we emerged, hopefully, with a sense of being a person of value and a person capable of contribution and satisfaction.

The second question is one from our earlier adulthood: How do I see myself professionally? The work that a psychotherapist does is important and it is effective (Seligman 1995). Psychotherapists have an identity that includes a sharing of essential characteristics and goals with

*The information found here serves as a general resource guide for alternatives to managed care practice. Mention of an organization, site, school, or product is not necessarily an endorsement.

other people. Professional mental health clinicians all subscribe to a rigorous code of ethics. Managed mental health care organizations have challenged the importance and effectiveness of psychotherapy, the ability of psychotherapists to evaluate and treat our patients, and the ethics of the profession. Psychotherapists need to meet these challenges with informed responses, educational programs, and affirmation of our ethical commitments.

The third question is the question of today: What can I do to increase satisfaction and minimize anxiety and anger? First, remember the limitation of metaphors. Big Brother is not really here. Psychotherapists are not really helpless against the forces of MCOs. It might be useful in making decisions today to remember the hopes and plans that were active while in graduate school and in postgraduate training. There are paths to solutions that can be started right now.

Part III addresses some professional choices available to psychotherapists in this era of managed care. Chapters 10 and 11 present examples of areas and techniques that increase opportunities within managed care but can also provide foundations for psychotherapy practices outside of managed care. The specialized areas and techniques are called *coordinate choices* here because they represent points where the interest and abilities of the psychotherapist meet the requirements of most MCOs. Chapter 13 presents new directions for psychotherapists in three very different areas: computer possibilities for online psychotherapy issues, a proposed classification for anger disorders, and new perspectives on religion and spirituality. Chapter 13, Flight, presents the careers of several psychotherapists who chose to practice outside the managed care environments. Whether working within a managed mental health care organization or outside the system, psychotherapists still may elect to improve mental health care delivery. Chapter 14, Fight, presents the work of several groups of psychotherapists who created organizations to contest the injustices and inadequacies of MCOs.

10

Coordinate Solutions with Special People

There are psychotherapists who want to work with managed care because they believe that the managed care system is viable and acceptable, perhaps even preferable, to older approaches to mental health care delivery. For these psychotherapists, the first step is becoming a provider. Although becoming a provider may be difficult, at one point or another the MCOs will need new providers to replace those who leave. There are several ways for psychotherapists to increase their chances of becoming providers (see Part II). Probably the single most helpful step a psychotherapist can take to being accepted as an MCO provider is to have an area of specialty that suits the needs of the MCO to which the therapist is applying. MCOs appear to need psychotherapists with special training in many areas, including the treatment of people with alcohol and substance abuse problems, children and adolescents, elderly people, and victims of trauma. In addition, there is a renewal of interest in the psychotherapeutic treatment of patients with chronic illnesses such as asthma, cancer, diabetes, and coronary artery disease. The tragic spread of acquired immunodeficiency syndrome (AIDS) has created the need for psychotherapists trained to treat these patients and their families.

We call these *coordinate solutions* because they represent areas where the interests or specialties of psychotherapists meet the requirements of MCOs. The following is a sample of coordinate solutions.

TREATMENT OF PEOPLE WITH ALCOHOL AND SUBSTANCE ABUSE PROBLEMS

Alcohol and drugs permeate our society. Theories about the causes range from genetics to self-medication to learned helplessness. The economic, psychological, and social costs are high. Big Brother has been watching in the sickrooms and the bathrooms and has been looking over the attendance reports and the productivity charts. The actuaries in the system behind Big Brother are well aware of the expenses incurred by employers and insurance companies because of alcoholism and other addictions.

It has been estimated that 15.1 million Americans suffer from alcoholism or alcoholic dependence. Over 30 percent of Americans admit that they sometimes drink too much. Alcoholics tend to live 10 to 12 years fewer than nonalcoholics, suffering from a wide range of diseases that includes cirrhosis of the liver, heart disease, infectious disease, fetal alcohol syndrome, and, some believe, cancer (Kornblum and Julian 1995).

The use of other addictive substances also has dismal effects on society. Cocaine has been used by over 22 million Americans, with 1 million regular users. Heroin is used by 2 million Americans, with 1 million physically dependent addicts. The College on Problems of Drug Dependence (1994), a drug abuse research group, compiled the following estimates on the cost per patient of drug abuse in America:

Drug abuse treatment	\$3,000–\$8,000 per year
Incarceration	\$40,000–\$80,000 per year
Untreated (cost in crime)	\$50,000–\$100,000 per year
AIDS	\$100,000

Obviously, the need for alcohol and substance abuse counselors is great. In the past few years there have been many new programs established for education and training in this field. There are numerous opportunities for nonmanaged care psychotherapists as well as for psychotherapists working with MCOs.

The public awareness of the problems of alcohol and substance abuse and the concerns of business and industry have led to changes in legislative regulations with regard to the requirements for treating people with addiction problems. New government departments, regulations, and controls are emerging. Together with the intensification of awareness and with new regulations there is, of course, new confusion about which regulations apply to psychotherapists in private practice. Cheri Sciaca, a psychotherapist at the Counseling Service at Vassar College, has researched information on the regulation of alcohol and substance abuse counselors for the following summary of one state's attempt to organize regulations in the treatment of people with alcohol and substance abuse problems. Her article "Alcoholism and Substance Abuse Counselors in New York" follows.

❑ ❑ ❑

The regulation of alcoholism and substance abuse counselors is different in every state, often involving licensing, certification, or credentialing. In New York State alcoholism counselors are credentialed under the Mental Hygiene Law as Credentialed Alcoholic Counselors (CACs). Initially, CACs were considered separate from CSACs (Credentialed Substance Abuse Counselors). These two divisions were merged, coming under the Office of Alcoholism and Substance Abuse Services (OASAS) in Albany.

CACs can work in a variety of settings, including acute care and detoxification programs, inpatient psychiatric hospital and rehabilitation centers, outpatient rehabilitation programs, alcoholic clinics, drinking driver programs, and community residences in public, private and voluntary sector agencies. Some of the services they can provide include alcohol assessments, referrals, crisis interventions, consultation, education, and prevention. The Canon of Ethical Principles provides guidelines for the practice of alcoholism counseling and includes commitments to self evaluation, self improvement, and professional development as well as to refraining from the use of mind-altering substances when such use would result in personal or professional denigration or violation of law.

The theoretical basis for the CAC credentialing procedures derives from the position that addiction is a physical disease with psychological components that can only be arrested—not cured—by total abstinence from alcohol. The disease process model of addiction is seen as similar in many respects to coronary diseases or diabetes in the manifestation of both physiological and psychological determinants and treatment components. This view has been accepted by the American Medical Association and the American Psychiatric Association and is a departure from the previously held model of alcoholism as a moral failing. It is commonly held that the disease model of alcoholism has led to fewer signs of stigma attached to individuals seeking treatment for alcohol abuse or alcoholism.

There are other theories of chemical dependency, which are not necessarily inconsistent with a biologically based position. Examples of approaches to understanding alcohol and chemical dependency include the self-medication model, which proposes that the person is using substances to mask underlying difficulties, the learning model, which views chemical dependency as a learned behavior that needs to be altered, and the social model, which takes into account environmental factors and deficits. There is evidence that models of addiction that integrate components from a number of models and methods of treatment tend to be more effective than individual models of treatment.

Initially, individuals could follow either of two tracks to become counselors in the treatment of addictions. The first track was designed for people in recovery from states of addiction and the second track evolved for people with a formal graduate school education. It is interesting that most training programs and treatment facilities gave preference to people with addiction-recovery experiences over those with higher educations. This position has changed. The refined selection procedures include requirements for candidates to have formal education, but most programs also provide credits for personal experience.

While many states have requirements for certification similar to the requirements in New York state, the training and licensing requirements vary widely among the states. For example, Virginia offers two credentials: Certified Addictions Counselor (CAC) and Certified Substance Abuse Counselor (CSAC). Currently, there is a move to create a single category called Credentialed Alcoholism and Substance Abuse Counselor (CASAC). Educators and legislators on several state committees have been studying models of addiction and treatment based on recent research reports. The committees have developed rigorous standards for counselors providing addiction treatment services.

In New York State, a candidate for credentialing must demonstrate that he or she has attained the minimum qualifications and standards as stated in the Mental Hygiene Law. At present the requirements include 450 documented hours of relevant education and training completed within the past 10 years and a minimum of one year, or 1680 hours, of full-time work in providing services for people with addictions. Candidates also must complete a program of professional education and a training program that includes courses on counselor–client relationship, federal and state confidentiality laws, professional education and training in ethics, and a minimum of 9 hours of professional education and training in AIDS. A two-part examination for certification includes development of treatment plans as well as the traditional testing of academic knowledge. Every three years counselors must apply for re-credentialing, showing evidence of at least 60 hours of relevant continuing education.

❑ ❑ ❑

In an attempt to provide a uniform national credential for psychologists, the American Psychological Association (APA) offers a certificate of proficiency in the treatment of alcohol and other psychoactive substance use disorders. The APA office of professional psychology in Washington, D.C. provides information about the national certification program. Professional psychotherapists who are interested in treating people with addictions and who acquire the credentials necessary for certification will find opportunities for practicing in this field. Many MCOs readily approve many more sessions for the treatment of addiction disorders than for the treatment of other problems in mental health. For more information, see the Resource Guide in the back of the book or contact the APA certification program at:

APA College of Professional Psychology
750 First Street, N.E.
Washington, DC 20002-4242
(202) 336-6100

In the course of reviewing research in the field of chemical dependency, Brett N. Steenbarger, Ph.D. (1977) found certain conclusions that are important to psychotherapists interested in treating people with addiction disorders. For example, among 3000 alcoholics who completed treatment, there were reduced medical expenditures of from 23 to 55 percent. Other studies found that health care costs are twice as high in families of alcoholics as compared to families of nonalcoholics, and as many as 30 percent of hospitalized patients are addicted to alcohol.

Steenbarger also notes that the most successful interventions are ones that are supportive, build skills, and increase motivation. Following therapy, about one fourth of all addicted patients maintain their recovery for longer than six months. The remaining three-fourths of addicted patients show signs of relapse within three to six months after treatment. In view of the outcome process that so frequently includes episodes of relapse, psychotherapists need to consider plans that include the possibility of further treatment. It may be best to view psychotherapy for people with addictions as a series of time-limited treatment periods that take place intermittently for as long as necessary.

One of the problems in treating addictions is in setting goals that are too far-reaching for the addicted person causing her or him to feel discouraged and to lose the motivation to continue in therapy. Alan Marlatt, Ph.D. (1996) addressed several of these issues in his presentation of a cognitive behavior model of relapse that includes a harm reduction approach to addictive behaviors.

Robert E. Lichtman, Ph.D., C.A.C. (1996) refers to important distinctions among models of addiction treatment in his summary of alternative treatment and self help programs. Lichtman noted that, "While programs like Rational Recovery and Smart Recovery are generally abstinence based, harm reduction models such as Moderation Management and Moderate Drinking stress the cost/benefit analysis approach and consider abstinence as one choice among many" (p. 20).

The addiction model for understanding certain human behaviors has been extended beyond addictions to alcohol and chemical substances. Professional and popular literature reveal recent interest in behaviors referred to as various food addictions, sexual addiction, shopping addiction, and gambling addiction. With regard to gambling, APA Senior Congressional Fellow Michael R. Stevenson, Ph.D. (1996) notes that Senator Paul Simon has proposed legislation that would create a national committee to study gambling issues, including topics of problem gamblers and teenage gambling.

Psychotherapists exploring some of the behaviors other than alcoholism and substance abuse that are currently being labeled as addiction might find it helpful to consider established categories other than addictions when formulating diagnostic and treatment issues.

For example, *DSM-IV* (APA 1994) refers to gambling as an impulse disorder that may be associated with a substance disorder, but people with gambling disorders are included in a section along with the four other groups of people included as having impulse disorders not elsewhere categorized. Likewise, there is a substantial body of research with regard to eating disorders and sexual dysfunctions. Compulsive or impulsive shopping may accompany other symptoms that are indicative of a mood disorder or substance abuse disorder.

F. Michler Bishop, Ph.D., C.A.S. (1997) makes the case for considering multiple diagnoses when evaluating patients who demonstrate addictive behaviors. Claiming that two models makes work with addictions more effective, Bishop also suggests that the newer models of addiction such as Stages of Change and Harm Reduction also help prevent demoralization on the part of the client and on the part of the therapist. Diagnosis of multiple disorders may lead both to better care of patients and, with regard to MCOs, to certification of more sessions. Bishop suggests that psychotherapists would find it helpful to take continuing education courses and to study for the APA approved proficiency examination in alcohol and substance abuse.

ISSUES RELATED TO MEDICAL DISEASES

Disease management (DM) is a term that is fairly new in health care organizations. DM refers to a systems approach to treating medical illnesses. The theory underlying DM is that treating the patient as a whole person rather than treating outbreaks of illness will result in both better health outcome and long-term cost reduction. DM programs typically manage patients who suffer from high-cost conditions such as asthma, diabetes, and cancer. Programs are usually run by organizations that take care of the specific population, such as cancer patients or asthma patients, or organizations in partnership with MCOs. In the DM system, there are both primary care and support professionals who work in cooperative efforts. Support professionals include psychotherapists to whom patients are referred by case managers. Medical professionals treating particular DM populations may also refer patients to psychotherapists.

There has been increasing public recognition of the idea that many diseases have psychological implications. There are psychological issues related both to the course of a disease and psychological consequences of having a disease. Paul Ellwood, Jr. (1996), who is recognized as the father of current MCOs and a major contributor to health policy, says that companies want health plans to demonstrate quality in treating ailments that keep people out of work or make them unhappy and inefficient, such as depression, low back pain, and asthma. Ellwood, as usual, is pointing to the central issue. DM will continue to be an important area for MCOs because psychotherapy with patients who have mental health problems related to certain physical ailments results in increased efficiency at work. Psychotherapists have coordinate treatment possibilities with MCOs if they are interested in treating people with any of these ailments, or interest in the connection between mental health disorders and physical disorders, or in the treatment of families with a chronically ill family member.

In an early attempt to deal comprehensively with the major issues in the psychotherapy of cancer patients, Jane Goldberg (1981) clearly presents a range of views regarding the work that is being done in both understanding the treatment of cancer patients and understanding the social and psychological implications of having cancer. Despite Goldberg's excellent compilation, many of the problems that she discussed remain current and still represent areas that psychotherapists today need to confront. For example, psychotherapists are likely to be helpful to children with cancer and to their families, especially when the psychotherapists work with other specialists in the care of the cancer patients. As stated by Sharon B. Murphy (Eastman 1996), Chief of Hematology and Oncology at Northwestern University Medical Center in Chicago and Chair of the Pediatric Oncology Group, the new standards of care presented by the American Academy of Pediatrics reflect repeated studies showing that children with cancer do better when treated in a cooperative group setting. Murphy said, "If we don't put standards out there, we're going to have erosion of care. Fewer kids are going to be treated correctly, and more are going to die" (p. 39).

Murphy's warning is especially important in view of the reported rates of success with appropriate treatment of children with cancer. Although cancer is the chief cause of death by disease in children under the age of 15, and although the cancer rate apparently is increasing among children, the mortality rates for children with cancer have decreased 62 percent since 1960 (Eastman 1996). At the same time that studies show success with appropriate treatment, the number of cases involving inappropriate levels of care has geometrically expanded, according to G. A. Monaco, a lawyer and a founder of Candlelighter, a national support organization for parents of children with cancer and also an advisor to Children's Brain Tumor Foundation of Virginia, which advocates for survivors, families, and physicians. Monaco, however, believes that MCOs are educable, but only through a business perspective. Monaco recommends approaching MCOs from the point of view that it is a better idea to put money into appropriate care than into punitive damages (Erickson 1996).

On the side of the MCOs, there seem to be some changes in the treatment possibilities for children with cancer. In a new move for MCOs, the

Blue Cross/Blue Shield Association has announced the establishment of a pediatric cancer network that member companies can use for their subscribers. Blue Cross/Blue Shield President Pat Hays said, "One way managed care has gotten off track is that it has become a business arrangement instead of being quality-driven" (Eastman 1996, p. 31). Hays continued to explain that the new network is based on a consensus among the medical community about what works best for pediatric cancer. W. Archie Bleyer, Head of Pediatrics at MD Anderson Cancer Center in Houston said that the network will give immediate access to state-of-the-art care to children with cancer and that this immediacy will avoid potential problems in care caused by delay (Eastman 1996).

While the concern of Blue Cross/Blue Shield with appropriate medical care for children with physical disease is welcome, the medical personnel involved with the networks did not give sufficient attention to the emotional needs of children or their families. This omission occurred despite the fact that studies supporting the relationships among physical and mental well being are increasing.

Several leading experts in health psychology have discussed assessment and treatment of people with physical disorders. Gatchel and Blanchard (1993), for example, present discussions that illustrate the potential for psychotherapeutic intervention in such traditionally medical areas as irritable bowel syndrome, headache, asthma, dermatological disorders, rheumatoid arthritis, Raynaud's disease, and temporo-mandibular disorders. Blascovich and Katkin (1993) also inform psychotherapy specialists about the evidence linking psychological stress and disease. Both researchers and practitioners in health psychotherapy are involved with a range of issues related to psychological aspects of physical illnesses.

According to Gary R. Vanden Bos, Ph.D. (1995), APA Executive Director of Publications and Communications, medical specialists are increasingly recognizing the value of psychotherapy to the care of chronic illness in both childhood disorders and in the general population of people suffering with illnesses. Two recent books contribute to knowledge in this field: *Adaptation to Chronic Childhood Disorders* by Robert Thompson, Jr. and Kathryn Gustafson (1996) and *Managing Chronic Illness: A Biopsychosocial Perspective*, edited by Perry Nicassio and Timothy Smith (1996).

Recent studies of genetic components of emotional disorders promise to blur even further the distinctions between psychological and physical disorders. Based on research with identical and fraternal twins, Lykken and Tellegen (1996) concluded that genetics play a major role in the ability to be happy.

Two groups of researchers, one in Israel and another at the National Institute of Health in Bethesda, Maryland, reported detecting a partial genetic explanation for a personality trait called novelty seeking. In an interview for *The New York Times* (Angier 1996), Dr. Richard Ebstein of Jerusalem and Beersheva, Israel, said that these findings represent the first report of a link between a specific gene and normal behavior.

While novel-seeking behavior may be a component of normal behavior, it may also be a contributing factor in behavior of concern to professionals in the fields of disease management. Novelty seeking is a behavior that has been associated with addictive behaviors and other antisocial activities. As this time, there seems to be little practical advice that a psychotherapist can derive from these genetic findings, but the information can be helpful in developing new perspectives to normal and pathological behaviors. The work of Robert Plutchik, Ph.D. (1994) concerning emotions and biology may provide a basis for initial understanding of some of the recent genetic findings.

It is important for psychotherapists to consider their role on disease management teams. As new laws are passed to control MCO restrictions, it is likely that medical personnel will refer patients for the psychotherapy that will benefit them. Please note again that the correct completion of HCFA forms will help patients receive the psychotherapy services for which they are covered. In all likelihood, patients referred to psychotherapists will exhibit symptoms of anxiety, depression, compulsive behaviors, or other Axis I categories. As stated in Chapter 7, psychotherapists can list more than one Axis I category on OTRs, but on HCFA forms it is necessary to list each problem on a separate line. Thus, for a person who is suffering depression and anxiety related to, for example, a new job in an area far from his or her present home, and is also experiencing the medical diagnosis of dysthymic heartbeat, the psychotherapist would list at least three code numbers: 309.28 on line 1 for adjustment disorder with depression and anxiety; 316.00 on line 2 for psychological factors affecting a medical condition; 427.90 on line 3 for cardiac dysrhythmia. However, only 1 and 2 would appear in HCFA column E because the psychotherapist in this case is treating an adjustment disorder and other psychological factors related to the medical condition, but not the medical condition specifically. Psychotherapists who specialize in the treatment of people with medical disorders need to be familiar with both the multiaxial assessment methods of *DSM-IV* (1994) and with standard HCFA forms.

PSYCHOTHERAPY WITH OLDER ADULTS

No one disputes the fact that an aging brain affects an aging mind, but it is often difficult to separate the effects of genetically programmed aging of the brain and environmental influences. At times, evaluation is necessary to determine sources of distress in order to determine appropriate treatment. At other times, the goal of the psychotherapist is to help the patient clarify problems and goals. The interaction of physical disorders, stress-related disorders, and emotional reactions results in problems for older people.

Older adults frequently present their problems as difficulties with sleep or with eating and diet. They also express worries about learning and memory. While it is frequently necessary to work with the evaluations and manifestations of physical disorders, psychotherapists also can encourage and help motivate people to become active in mentally and physically stimulating activities that improve their well-being. With appropriate psychotherapy, older people can face their problems with creativity, compassion, growing understanding, and humor.

Older people most frequently need psychotherapeutic help with issues related to physical illness. For example, there are about 4 million people in the United States who have survived strokes, and one in four of these stroke survivors suffers from intense anxiety that frequently is undiagnosed by physicians or treated with the wrong medication (Astrom 1996). Of the 80 stroke patients who participated in the study, 31 percent showed symptoms of distress sufficient to diagnose generalized anxiety disorder (GAD) at three months after surgery, 24 percent at one year, and 19 percent at three years. About two-thirds of the stroke patients diagnosed with GAD also suffered from depression.

As more people survive strokes, there will be an even greater need for psychotherapists to treat patients who are excessively anxious or depressed or who otherwise express problems that indicate mental health issues. Treatment of survivors of any life-threatening illness requires expertise in the area. Although psychotherapeutic treatment of so many people, probably more than one-third of survivors of strokes, will be expensive, neglecting their treatment or providing wrong treatment is likely to result in even more expensive consequences.

Trends in mental health services for older adults have included over-reliance on inpatient treatment, inadequate integration of mental health services in nursing home organizations, and insufficient referrals from general medical providers. At present, many elderly people who suffer from mental health problems, such as depression or anxiety, turn to their physicians for help in understanding their symptoms. This is likely to change in the near future. Among the increasing population of older people, there is a growing number who are wise to their needs, capable of evaluating effective treatment and advocating appropriate treatment for themselves. The need for specially trained psychotherapists to work with the particular problems of elderly people is expected to grow.

In response to the needs of an ever-increasing older adult population, many hospital administrators plan to open geriatric treatment units and services. One of the advantages of hospital-based programs is the opportunity to provide comprehensive interdisciplinary assessment of cognitive, behavioral, psychological, social, and functional problems of older individuals. If the hospital programs are to succeed, the interdisciplinary teams will have to work closely with families and referring psychotherapists. Thus, the opportunity to work with this unique population will benefit from the interchange of referrals, information, and education between hospital staff and psychotherapists.

TREATMENT OF HIV/AIDS PATIENTS AND FAMILY

There are more than one million people with human immunodeficiency (HIV) infection living at this time in the United States. The mental health implications for people with HIV infection are enormous. Psychotherapists will continue to be needed to identify, assess, and manage the psychological problems experienced by HIV-infected patients, their spouses, partners, friends, and adolescents with HIV infection has profound impact on their lives, the lives of their families, and on the psychotherapists who treat them.

In addition to the one million people living with HIV/AIDS, there are about 300,000 people who have already died of AIDS-related illnesses. Barry Schoub (1994), director of the National Institute of Virology at the University of Witwatersrand, Johannesburg, South Africa, is convinced that these deaths represent only the beginning of the devastation that will result from the AIDS epidemic. Comparing AIDS to the Spanish influenza epidemic that killed more than 20 million people at the end of World War I, Schoub predicts that AIDS will be recorded as one of the worst illnesses to afflict humankind. Psychotherapists who specialize in treating people who are in states of loss, grief, and mourning are frequently welcomed by people who have lost a family member or friend to AIDS.

There have been several reports from institutes and hospitals where HIV/AIDS patients are treated. Gillian Walker (1991) presents case studies from the Ackerman Institute AIDS and Families Project to illustrate issues with families of drug-abusing and gay victims of AIDS, as well as with families with children who are born with AIDS and families with children with hemophilia. Walker also discusses the need to treat families in which one or more members test HIV-positive but do not show symptoms. Odets (1995) also presents material especially important for psychotherapists who see HIV-negative patients. Odets gives consideration to denial of the HIV-negative condition, identity issues, and survivor guilt and related family matters. Nancy Boyd-Franklin, Gloria Steiner and Mary Boland (1995) draw upon experiences at the National Pediatric HIV Resource Center, Children's Hospital of Newark, New Jersey, to address special issues, such as caring for the professional caregiver and examining multi-systems approaches to caring for afflicted families. In addition to concise discussions of the major psychological aspects of HIV and AIDS, Michael King (1993) provides an assessment of reports and studies from around the world. *Therapists on the Front Line* (Cadwell and colleagues 1994) contains a helpful annotation that includes references for specific treatment populations, impact on the therapist, and when the therapist is HIV infected.

The American Psychological Association (APA) participates in a range of activities in the fight against AIDS. Peter Freiberg (1996) describes the activities of the APA's office on AIDS, which ". . . establishes links between researchers, community-based organizations, and funding agencies; provides training and consultation for psychologists working with people affected by HIV/AIDS; . . ." (p. 34).

The National Library of Medicine in Bethesda has provided contracts to three libraries for the development of AIDS-related information. There are now resource centers at libraries in Riverside, California, in New York City at the New York Public Library, and at the Newburgh Free Library in Newburgh, New York. Rowena McDade, Project Coordinator for the HIV/AIDS Information Service of the Newburgh Free Library states that the resources of the library are available to all interested people (McDade 1996).

PSYCHOTHERAPY WITH CHILDREN

There is an increasing need for psychotherapists who work with children. Although the traditional methods of treating young children, notably child psychoanalysis and long-term play therapy, are based on principles that are not consistent with the requirements of MCOs, this important area of mental health treatment continues to develop in theory, education, and practice.

Most MCOs include provisions for the treatment of children but these provisions do not allow individual considerations any more than do the provisions for adults. MCOs generally suggest the use of medication for many childhood disorders. There is a frightening trend to overmedicate children (see Part I). At the same time, there is little doubt that some children respond well to medication. It is extremely difficult to convince most managed care organization case managers that individual children have individual needs. The process of securing the best treatment, even within the limits of managed care allowances, often requires that the psychotherapist spend considerable time and energy negotiating the appeal process for appropriate treatment.

Since the advent of managed care, there has been research and redesign in developing short-term therapies with children. Some short-term therapies, such as evaluations for medication and techniques for specific behavioral issues, may be effective. One of the more extreme of the current models is the 12-Hour Therapy with Children Program presented by Lawrence E. Shapiro (1996). Dr. Shapiro presents in four seminars a complete model for delivering therapy and counseling in 12 one-hour treatment protocols. More familiar types of short-term therapy for children include systems based on behavioral principles. The principles of behavioral therapy are based on research in the fields of classical and operant conditioning, social learning, and cognitive behavioral theories. There are considerable research findings to support the use of behavioral therapy with children (see Reisman and Ribordy 1993, for research summaries). Even in view of such findings, most clinicians feel more comfortable having a range of therapeutic treatments from which to draw the best interventions for each child.

It is indeed frustrating for psychotherapists to appeal to MCO case managers to approve treatment procedures. Nonetheless, child psychotherapists find many reasons to work with managed care. For one thing, once a psychotherapist is known to the MCOs as a provider who tries to treat each child in the most appropriate way, the case managers are likely to be more receptive to that provider's requests for sessions.

More relevant to the purpose of maintaining one's integrity, psychotherapists find that many of the children referred for therapy by MCOs or by primary providers are experiencing problems that can be treated with short-term therapy. Referrals frequently involve non-compliance with medications for such illnesses as diabetes, problems with sleeping or eating, anxieties, or even phobias regarding school. Very frequently a parent has asked for a consultation concerning a child who has developed problems following parental separation. In these cases, psychotherapists may ask to see one or both parents in order to help the parent to address the problem. Such solutions are appealing to psychotherapists who believe that most children feel uncomfortable about being in therapy and, as a result, do their best when they know that psychotherapy will be kept to as few sessions as possible. Of course, the shorter courses of therapy are preferred by the MCOs.

Behaviors that teachers or parents find extremely difficult to control are probably the most common reason for referring children to psychotherapists. Although some of these children will respond to the techniques of short-term therapy, many of the children demonstrate behaviors that are symptomatic of disorders requiring more extensive treatment. If, following a consultation and evaluation, a psychotherapist finds that a child's problems require longer treatment, the therapist will usually find it useful to discuss a treatment plan with the parents and, in so far as possible, with the child. The issues of length of treatment, type of treatment, and payment for treatment are important material for therapy. With regard to payment, the MCO case managers may agree to certify sessions for each of the people in the family who has a medically necessary condition. That is, the case managers may certify the maximum number of sessions available for the child's disorder, and also the maximum number that can be supported for the treatment of the mother's disorder that may be classified, for example, as an adjustment disorder, a generalized anxiety disorder, depression, or even an addiction disorder. In addition to approving sessions for the mother, case managers may approve sessions for the father who may be suffering from a disorder that contributes to the presenting problem of the child. Parents may suggest alternate payment arrangements in order to avoid further MCO involvement. Whatever financial arrangements are discussed, however, it is advisable to record the arrangements and to have all parties sign an agreement.

An extremely important area in child psychotherapy is the treatment of traumatized children. MCO administrators appreciate psychotherapists who evaluate and treat victims of trauma. Cynthia Monohon (1993) discusses the signs of psychological trauma that are usually first noted by a parent but may become obvious to teachers or physicians. Most children under the age of 11 are not likely to speak about their painful feelings. Children who are experiencing extreme distress are likely to show changes in behavior. Signs of trauma vary with the age of the child and with the type of trauma. The sources of childhood trauma include sexual molestation, physical violence, witnessing domestic violence or group violence, severe accidents, community catastrophes, and exposure to a terrifying individual experience. Events such as the loss of a sibling does not automatically involve trauma for a child. The experience of the death must be understood in order to know whether the child has experienced a traumatic event as well as a sorrowful one. Monohon lists some of the signs of trauma, including behavioral regression, unwanted images and thoughts, withdrawal and constriction, complaints of aches and pains, accident-proneness and recklessness, and anniversary reactions (Monohon, pp. 24–43). Sadly, sexually abused children sometimes show none of these indications of abuse. One of the few reliable signs of sexual abuse is sexualized behavior that is inappropriate for the age of the child.

In *Treating Traumatized Children*, Beverly James (1989) discusses clinical work with traumatized children. She develops four major areas for treatment: communication, sorting out, education, and perspective. Her methods seem appropriate for use with children who have managed care referrals.

Haim Ginott (1994) believes that prompt individual therapy is the preferred treatment choice for children exposed to traumatic events. For children with other types of disorders, Ginott often suggests group therapy because many of the problems of childhood are centered around social adjustments. Ginott lists descriptions of children considered suitable for treatment in groups, to include withdrawn children, immature children, children with phobic reactions, children with sexual identity issues, children who are overly obedient, orderly, and excessively generous, children with habit disorders, and certain children with conduct disorders. Psychotherapists with skills and interests in group therapy may find satisfaction in extending their practices to include the treatment of children.

PSYCHOTHERAPY WITH ADOLESCENTS

Although traditionally grouped with children, adolescents present separate sets of problems and behaviors. There is a need for specialists to treat adolescents in both individual psychotherapy and in group therapy. The treatment of adolescents offers the psychotherapist the opportunity to interact with a unique, lively, and exceptionally varied group of people. Adolescence is a time of intensity, idealism, and spontaneity that is frequently shared with enthusiasm. Many psychotherapists like to see adolescents because they bring freshness and spirit to sessions and an accessibility to treatment that is seen less frequently with older people. With the rapid changes of the adolescent years comes heightened potential for appropriate interventions and positive outcomes.

Psychotherapy with adolescents can be truly interactive. Psychotherapists are likely to experience the need to examine their own values as adolescent patients challenge value systems. As a therapist shows respect for the adolescent's rage against hypocrisy, both patient and therapist open possibilities for examining the meaning of honesty and commitment. On a most broad and hopeful level, it is worth considering that realistic support of adolescent idealism may lead to greater integrity in the next generation of adults.

Unfortunately, it has not been the search for the meaning of adolescent values that has brought recent attention to adolescence. Instead, increasing attention is focused on the problems demonstrated by adolescents. The reasons for this concern include the following:

1. Over 15 percent of our population is between the ages of 12 and 20. It has been generally estimated that at least 10 percent of these young people have mental health problems.
2. Adolescents have the highest arrest rate of any age group.
3. There is an increasing number of adolescents who consume alcohol and other drugs on a regular basis.

There are many sources available for exploring interest in adolescence. *American Psychologist* presented a special issue on the opportunities of adolescence in February, 1993. Miller (1986) provides an overview of important issues in the diagnosis and treatment of adolescence in his excellent book *Attack on the Self*. Novello (1993) brings several adolescent specialists together in *The Short Course in Adolescent Psychiatry*. Most training institutes recognize the growing need for specialists in this area.

PEOPLE SUFFERING WITH DEPRESSION

> *"Depression is a brutal disease. It flays you; it skins you alive. There is nothing to feel guilty about, nothing you can do except get help."*
> *–Rod Steiger, as told to M. Beck,* Newsweek, *May 20, 1996 (p. 26).*

Rod Steiger is one of many well-known people who have acknowledged the impact of depression on their own lives or the life of the person close to them. General Colin Powell urged people to get help with depression as he and his wife, Alma, appeared at a nationally televised press conference. General Powell casually said, "My wife has depression. It is very easily controlled with proper medication, just as my blood pressure is" (Beck 1996, p. 22). Author William Styron and newsman Mike Wallace also have discussed publicly their battles with depression (p. 20). These messages from prominent Americans are likely to have helped many people find the courage to seek therapy for depression.

In any given year about 8 percent of men and 13 percent of women in the United States suffer a major depressive episode (La Bruzza 1994), and that does not count the number of people who will show symptoms of a depressive disorder other than a major depressive disorder. Depressive Disorders and Bipolar Disorders are the two main groupings in the *DSM-IV* category of Mood Disorders. Mood disorders may be either primary or secondary to a medical condition or to the use of alcohol or an addictive substance. In addition there are two Adjustment Disorders with predominant symptoms of depression.

Depending on the type of depression and the individual circumstances, there are many ways to treat depression, including short-term treatment, long-term treatment, methods from almost every theoretical school of thought, and treatment in conjunction with medical professionals prescribing medication. Seligman (1993), who has been studying depression for decades, believes that of all the theories proposed for the treatment of depression there are only four therapies that work: two biological–medications and electro-convulsive shock treatment–and two psychological–

cognitive therapy (Beck 1976) and interpersonal therapy (Klerman et al. 1994). Further, Seligman believes that people with manic-depression who are in psychotherapy and are not being treated with lithium should leave that psychotherapy immediately.

Seligman probably knows as much, if not more, about depression as anyone in the world. In addition, he is a brilliant scholar who presents scientific evidence for his opinions, even in his works that are accessible to a general population as well as to psychotherapists (e.g., Seligman 1993). Nonetheless, there are people who do not agree with his conviction that there are only four ways to treat depression. Seligman's assertions about lithium may not be controversial among research scientists, but the use of lithium is controversial among two other populations. At least some clinicians remain uncomfortable with the diagnosis of bipolar disease or manic-depression with adolescent and young adult patients, for whom manic-mimicking, illegal drugs may be an unacknowledged factor contributing to their symptoms. The problem of diagnosis of bipolar disorder is especially relevant in clinic situations where people who have crashed after abusing cocaine may appear with symptoms of depression or drug-related psychosis.

The second group who might object to the use of lithium is the population of patients who are not likely to be represented in traditional medication trials: those patients, familiar to most clinicians, who refuse to take either any medication or specific medications such as lithium. Some clinicians find that treating these patients is still rewarding, and they will work with the individual patients to find sources of health and well-being other than medication. In fact, people with problems of depression who refuse medication may represent an appealing patient group for psychotherapists who want to be available to a non-MCO population as well as to patients with managed care plans.

11

Coordinate Solutions with Special Techniques

Just as there are problems that people experience that meet MCO requirements for approval of treatment, there are also treatment techniques that are especially appealing to MCOs. For example, many MCOs currently approve of group therapy as a treatment modality in certain situations, such as alcohol or depression. The psychotherapist who enjoys running groups, however, may find that some of the most rewarding group experiences, such as groups with socially inhibited adolescents or women entering the business world, are outside the managed care approval lists. In these situations, it is wise to look at the individual patient's diagnosis. The adolescent youngsters in the group for socially inhibited young people may also exhibit anxiety, depression, phobic fears, or obsessive disorders. Women entering the business world after years at home may also show intense anxiety, phobias, or the symptoms of adjustment or stress disorders. Psychotherapists are usually familiar with the need to consider several equally applicable diagnostic categories when assessing a person's behaviors and needs. It is neither unusual nor unprofessional to enter more than one diagnosis on Axis I of a multiaxial assessment (*DSM-IV* 1994). When completing forms for MCOs, it is important that the psychotherapist choose from among the equally applicable diagnoses, the ones that appear in the *ICD-9* Code Book (1996) to enter as the first diagnosis. It is important to remember that the diseases listed in the *ICD-9* Code Book are the ones that are considered medically necessary. It is also important that the psychotherapist is able to show the MCOs that the techniques used by the psychotherapist are addressed to the symptoms of the disease.

MCOs appreciate mental health providers who have special skills such as fluency in a second language or, of course, in the methods of short-term therapies. There are so many short-term therapies being developed for clinical practice today that the new therapies can be divided into two groups. There is an older group, related to traditional therapies, that is more easily accepted by most psychotherapists, and a newer group that includes some exceptionally creative and even exploratory approaches. Irving Weisberg discusses the more established short-term therapies in Chapter 9 of this book. This chapter will include several treatment modalities that are especially suitable for psychotherapists who are exploring new approaches.

The psychotherapeutic treatments presented in this chapter, with the exception of group therapy, are considered to be adjuncts or supplements to psychotherapy. Although MCOs generally encourage their use, they do not necessarily pay for sessions where the procedure code refers directly to these treatments. Keep things as simple as you can when working with MCOs. When practicing psychotherapy, bill for psychotherapy using the standard code number.

In contrast to most other psychotherapeutic treatment, group therapy has its own CPT code number which should be used for billing. While group therapy is an established mode of treatment, there are new ways to practice group therapy. Some of the innovations are especially relevant to short-term treatment. Henry Spitz, M.D. (1990) discusses the reasons for using group therapy in managed care situations and guides providers through managed care regulations regarding group psychotherapy.

PSYCHOPHARMACOLOGY

The pharmaceutical company Eli Lilly and Company estimates that more than 21 million people have received a prescription for Prozac since the drug was first introduced about five years ago. Sales of Prozac have totaled more than two billion dollars annually. The reported success of Prozac in eliminating a range of distressful symptoms has impressed many mental health workers, along with the knowledge that the ability to prescribe medication carries many benefits including financial remuneration. It was before the introduction of Prozac, however, that psychologists began to formally seek prescription privileges. An American Psychological Association Task Force was established in 1991 to study the question of prescription privileges for psychologists. The task force recognized the need for further education for psychologists interested in prescribing medication and made suggestions for substantial training. The Task Force report (1992) noted that competence would take at least two years of full-time training with additional supervised clinical experience in decision-making in prescribing medication. The report proposed course work and practical experience that would be necessary to qualify psychologists for the ability to independently prescribe psychopharmacological medication.

As an argument against psychologists' prescription privileges, it has been suggested that social workers and psychiatric nurses would seek privileges too. It might very well happen that social workers and psychiatric nurses, if they receive adequate training and experience, will seek some type of prescription privileges. Following the lead of nurse-practitioner privileges under certain circumstances, it might be a good idea to permit selected privileges to all those professional health practitioners who are educated and trained in accordance with credentialing requirements and law.

The purpose here is not to argue the qualifications for practicing psychopharmacology but rather to examine the position of being a psychoparmacologist in this era of managed care. When American Psychiatric Association President-elect, Harold Eist, M.D., addressed the American Psychological Association Midwinter Conference in 1996, he said that it was time for psychologists and psychiatrists to work together to oppose interference from MCOs. Eist was blunt in saying that it would not matter whether psychologists get prescription privileges because the profession of psychology is being destroyed by managed care. He asked that professional groups stop battling and start focusing on the most important issue facing mental health care professionals, that of treating the mentally ill without big business interference.

Although it is acknowledged that mental health practitioners have to decide in what way they will address the issues of managed care, they may still consider the practice of psychopharmacology as a way to work either within managed care or outside of it. There seems to be a need for trained and committed psychopharmacologists. DeLeon and Wiggins (1996) report that of 135.8 million prescriptions for psychotherapeutic agents written in 1991, only 17.3 percent of these were written by psychiatrists, that is, 82 percent of the psychotherapeutic medications prescribed that year were written by internists and family practitioners who are not required to obtain advanced training in the mental health field.

It seems reasonable to expect that opportunities for clinical practice will exist for mental health practitioners who have the training to prescribe medications within the laws of their states. It is also likely that despite the disagreements among psychologists concerning medication, the training and use of prescribing psychologists will continue. An independent study recently completed on behalf of the Department of Defense (DOD) found that the first three psychologists who graduated from the DOD Psychopharmacology projects found generally positive reactions to the training received and the services rendered by the new pharmapsychologists (Saemon 1996). Attitudes among mental health providers varied as expected, with most clinical psychologists, clinical social workers, and primary care physicians agreeing that prescription privileges for psychologists would improve the quality of care for patients and most psychiatrists disagreeing.

There are two findings that will have greater effect on securing privileges than any intellectual argument or philosophical debate. First, most beneficiaries found that training for psychologists for select prescribing privileges was a good idea. The second and more convincing finding is that pharmapsychologists are cost effective when compared with prescribing physicians.

Leaving aside the argument about who should have prescription privileges, we come to the question of whether the area of pharmacological treatment of mental health disorders is a good choice. Again, it is important to start with one's own interests, abilities, and commitments. Are you willing to work with a biological model? To what degree? According to David Antonuccio (1996), organized psychiatry seems to have abandoned psychotherapy, despite the observation that psychiatrists were pioneers among the advocates of psychotherapeutic treatments for depression and anxiety. Part of the reason for the emphasis on the use of drugs in treatment is due to the huge influence of effective marketing by pharmaceutical companies. A question to consider is: In what ways are the influences of the psychopharmacological industry similar to the influences of managed care?

A psychotherapist who is willing to explore the difficulties involved in being a psychopharmacologist will also find that there are many rewards in the practice of psychopharmacology. Psychotherapists in this area find that they can still practice psychotherapy as well as work with other psychotherapists. Within the laws governing practices among different professionals, psychotherapists also can design a practice in which they work with physicians and other professionals.

HYPNOSIS

Many therapists, seeking to enhance their skills in brief, solution-focused treatment, have turned to hypnosis. Hypnosis training provides a new tool for working with patients. It also provides the practitioner a new level of confidence in working with pain, both mental and physical. Some (but not all) MCOs look favorably on these skills, since hypnotherapy is both short-term and solution-focused. Although most MCOs cover relaxation techniques, not all of them recognize hypnosis as a treatment modality. When applying to become an MCO provider, psychotherapists with skills in relaxation techniques or hypnotherapy should definitely list the skills. However, when filling out an HCFA form (see Chapter 2), psychotherapists at present must use only psychotherapy codes that are listed in the *Current Procedural Terminology* (AMA 1996). For example, Medicare code descriptions that may be suitable for these skills include behavior modifying therapy (G0073), interactive psychotherapy (G0079), and medical hypnotherapy.

For people who have not been trained in hypnosis, hypnotherapy may connote secrecy and confusion. We are all familiar with, and perhaps confused by, the manipulations of stage hypnosis, which is a show business presentation designed to entertain, awe, or amuse an audience. In contrast, real hypnotherapy is a helpful technique that is relatively easy for professionals to learn. It is not one person controlling the other but a team approach, with therapist and patient working well together. Most people have probably experienced trance states, perhaps without even realizing it. Perhaps a person driving a car arrives at a destination without being aware of just how she or he got there; or someone may be watching a movie and loses the sense of being himself. It can be that simple but, at the same time, much more complex.

For simplicity in this discussion we will use the terms *conscious* and *unconscious*. The conscious mind represents a higher level of mental organization and perception while the unconscious mind includes the cognitions, perceptions, and emotions that occur outside of our awareness and motivate our behavior. The number of activities carried out by the unconscious mind is large.

Consider driving a car. One would assume that driving is a conscious, focused activity. In reality, experienced drivers do not concentrate on holding onto the steering wheel or stepping on the accelerator—they do it unconsciously. Walking, talking, suddenly remembering things, and creative thinking are all part of the same process. The unconscious mind motivates behavior like drinking, smoking, or overeating. Hypnosis can direct these activities to a more positive outcome.

The underlying assumptions of hypnotherapy (Havens and Walters 1989) are equally applicable to other treatment techniques. They include the following:

1. *Pain is the primary symptom.* Pain, emotional pain, and suffering motivate people to seek therapy.
2. *Our multiple minds must interact.* People have a conscious mind and an unconscious mind.
3. *Injured interactions cause pain.* An injured, inadequate, or inappropriate relationship between the conscious and unconscious minds can give rise to a variety of painful emotional, behavioral, and interpersonal problems or symptoms.
4. *Injuries elude examination.* Clients are generally unable or unwilling to admit, examine, or experience the source of their pain, or they may fear the perceived consequences of doing so. These attitudes make it difficult to identify or soothe the pain and may perpetuate the symptoms.
5. *Pain leads to the source.* Pain is the best guide. It automatically draws attention toward the source of the problem. The therapist must focus on the pain and help the patient do so as well.
6. *Awareness promotes healing.* People are inherently self-corrective and self-healing. Once the source of the pain is identified, patients will reflexively correct or eliminate that problem if they can.
7. *Assistance may be needed.* Not all patients can correct their problems without help. Some need to learn new skills before they can do so. It is best if this learning occurs at an unconscious level.

As may be obvious there are similarities between this general technique and brief focused therapy. However, many proponents of hypnotherapy hold that hypnotherapy addresses the unconscious to help the patient heal himself, while brief focused therapy is a cognitive technique that deals with the conscious mind.

Based on the above assumptions, hypnotherapy starts with a diagnostic trance, which sounds similar to the one-session therapy advocated by some behavioral short-term theorists. The diagnostic trance scenario follows three steps (Havens and Walters 1989):

1. The patient is asked to close his or her eyes and to relax while concentrating on the unpleasant sensations or feelings associated with the presenting problem.
2. The patient is asked to wait patiently and quietly while observing those unpleasant sensations, and to report whatever thoughts or images suddenly come to mind.

3. The patient is then asked to find a thought or image which removes or displaces his/her unpleasant feelings.

If the patient finds the key thought or image that relieves the uncomfortable feelings, then therapeutic change is a matter of practicing the new skill until it becomes habitual. If the patient fails to discover the key thought or image, suggested alternatives will be provided to his unconscious in direct hypnotherapy.

In this way, the patient is thus urged to find his or her own solution. The therapist's role is to give the patient the opportunity to engage in the unconscious self-healing process. However, the "mere identification of the problem . . . does not guarantee that the patient has the conscious/unconscious resources needed to resolve that problem" (Havens and Walters 1989, p. 20). Some need further suggestions of alternative solutions before they know what to do. Others may have difficulty in operationalizing their newfound solution.

Why is the participation of the unconscious mind essential to the process? Havens and Walters (1989) explain:

> The complexity and uniqueness of each person prevents us from knowing the best action another individual can or should take in any given situation. In fact, even the conscious mind of that person has such a limited and biased view of the situation that it may be unwise or inappropriate to leave such decisions to it. [p. 20]

There are two types of hypnotherapy: direct induction and indirect induction. In a typical direct induction, the patient may be asked to sit comfortably or lie down, close his or her eyes and relax, tuning into the sound of the therapist's voice. One method to induce a trance goes through the various parts of the body from head to toe. Another may focus on a special safe, comfortable place where the patient can relax completely. Hypnosis II, a technique developed by Dr. Alex Matos (1982), even incorporates external noise and distractions into the induction. One-word triggers are then used to induce a light trance and program behavioral suggestions.

Direct hypnosis focuses on the problem, such as pain, lack of confidence, phobias, smoking, weight control, and others. Once patients have left conscious awareness and slipped into a light trance, they usually experience a floating sensation, but sensations other than floating may occur and are similarly useful in continuing the process. The unconscious mind is then instructed to imagine itself as it would like to be. A smoker might see himself as a nonsmoker, an obese person as slimmer, a phobic person as walking down the street without fear. The patient is talked through the experience by the therapist. Once a patient unconsciously accepts that he can do something, he has a much better chance of actually doing it. A person who believes he or she is a nonsmoker is a nonsmoker. People who believe that they can control their eating can control their eating. The same frequently appears to be the case for people with phobias or people who lack confidence.

Performing a direct induction is simple. In comparison, Ericksonian hypnosis is much more creative and requires more time to learn. Ericksonians use indirect methods to induce a trance. Through pacing and storytelling, a patient can be induced into a light trance. The therapist then uses stories that are designed to change or reframe the patient's problem. One such story, aimed at removing invisible obstacles, uses an analogy of horses constrained by an electric fence (Havens and Walters 1989). Once any one of the horses experiences the electricity from the fence, the horses do not dare to challenge it again. The fence becomes an invisible boundary created by the mind of the horse, and is still effective even when the electricity subsequently has been turned off. But once another horse goes through the fence, the rest of the horses will follow.

The encoded message to patients is to test the boundaries of their conscious minds, just like the horses. Erickson employed paradoxical communication to bring about behavioral change with many patients. In couples therapy, for example, he encouraged a husband and wife to revert to a previous pattern of unwanted behavior. He then urged them to select out of that pattern "that which needs to be salvaged" (Haley 1985, p. 85). Having salvaged a part of the pattern, it was then easier to discard the old, unwanted behavior and to move on.

A major difference between Ericksonian techniques and psychoanalysis involves the processes of coding and decoding analytic material. In psychoanalysis, the therapist attempts to decode the hidden meaning in the patient's narratives. In Ericksonian hypnosis, the therapist encodes stories for the patient. Although the techniques of encoding and decoding are useful skills for a psychotherapist, they are not acceptable terms to MCOs. Because MCO personnel may not be familiar with certain techniques, they may associate them with long-term treatment. Consequently, it is probably best for psychotherapists to subsume such skills in another category of psychotherapy that is listed in the CPT.

There are many ways to use hypnotherapy skills with MCO-referred short-term patients at present. For example, hypnotherapy might be the treatment of choice for hospitalized patients who want to give up smoking during their time in the hospital. It is likely that there will be increased opportunities in managed care for psychotherapists whose skills and interests include the use of hypnotherapy techniques.

NEURO-LINGUISTIC PROGRAMMING

Another exciting technique is neuro-linguistic programming (NLP), developed by John Grinder and Richard Bandler at the University of California in 1972. According to O'Connor and Seymour (1990), Grinder and Bandler developed NLP through their studies of the functioning of people with exceptionally high achievements. It brought together concepts and techniques from the work of Fritz Perls, the originator of gestalt therapy; Virgina Satir, one of the earliest and most innovative of the family therapists; and Milton Erickson, who is recognized for his scholarly contributions to psychology as well as for his exploration of the uses of hypnosis. Grinder and Bandler combined various techniques of hypnosis into a model that can be used effectively as an aid to improving communication skills and promoting accelerated learning, personal change, and enhanced enjoyment of life.

NLP aims to give people more choices about what they do in life. The more choices, the greater the chance of success. O'Connor and Seymour (1990) put it succinctly: "If you always do what you've always done, you'll always get what you've always got. If what you are doing is not working, do something else" (p. 9).

Central to NLP are five *basic filters* or behavioral frames. They include:

- An orientation toward outcomes rather than problems
- How rather than why
- Feedback rather than failure
- Possibilities rather than necessities
- Curiosity and fascination rather than assumptions.

In NLP, changing a problem orientation into an outcome orientation is called a reframe. Learning the new frames starts with unlearning the old pattern entrenched in the unconscious, then relearning the new orientation until it becomes habitual.

The four stages of learning include:

1. Unconscious incompetence, in which you don't know that you don't know.
2. Conscious incompetence, in which you are aware that you don't know.
3. Conscious competence, in which you are learning but it demands your attention.
4. Unconscious competence, in which you do it naturally without prethought.

NLP urges an unlearning process (stages 4 to 2) and relearning (stages 2 to 4) with refined skills, more choices, and greater flexibility.

NLP is suitable for managed care practices because it is a short-term procedure. The techniques are useful for a range of symptoms and appear acceptable to most patients. The use of mnemonic devices is characteristic of NLP techniques; in fact, the NLP process is summarized by the acronym POSERS:

Positive: think of what you want rather than what you don't have.
Own part: think of what you can actively do to achieve your outcome.
Specific: imagine your outcome as specifically as you can.
  Step up: What will this outcome do for me? If not enough, go to a larger outcome.
  Step down: What prevents me from doing it? If impossible, go to a smaller outcome.
Evidence: How will I know I have what I want?
Resources: What resources do I have to get what I want? What other resources do I need?
Size: Is the outcome too big or too small for me?

NLP centers on communication and evaluating the effects of one person's communication on others. Noting that about 55 percent of communication involves body language, about 38 percent appears related to voice tonality, and only 5 percent is directly based on the words that are used, the proponents of NLP emphasize how much more there is to communication than the words that are spoken.

The teachers of NLP observe that feelings are frequently, at least in part, controlled by the people expressing the feeling. Grinder and Bandler elaborate upon the observation that "Emotions make excellent servants, but tyrannical masters" (O'Connor and Seymour 1990, p. 45). NLP includes behavioral techniques used in attempts to change inner realities, information from biological research, and sources from several other disciplines as part of several models. The field of NLP is promising for those psychotherapists who like to work with the interactions between biological and psychological behaviors.

EMDR

Eye Movement Desensitization and Reprocessing (EMDR) has been used for the reprocessing of painful memories with patients who are suffering from the effects of traumatic events. According to Francine Shapiro (1995), the originator of EMDR techniques and the recipient of the 1994 Distinguished Scientific Achievement in Psychology Award presented by the California Psychological Association, EMDR procedures are effective with many patient groups including phobia sufferers and people with dissociative disorders, as well as the people with whom EMDR was developed, most notably sexual abuse and crime victims. Dworkin and Cullen (1996) report that more than 14,000 worldwide clinicians have been trained in EMDR. Dworkin is currently working to win MCO approval of EMDR techniques. Despite some controversy, there is an increasing number of studies supporting the effectiveness of EMDR on alleviating the symptoms of post-traumatic stress disorder. EMDR is an eight-phase system that is used in conjunction with a comprehensive treatment program. Although eye movements assist in activating disturbing material and its processing, they are only one component of the treatment procedure. Proponents claim that EMDR unblocks the patient's natural information processing system. The theory here is that the patient's system had been blocked by trauma causing the same message of fear to occur repeatedly, just as if the traumatic event were happening again. EMDR stimulates the patient's natural healing processes to discard the fear and shame of traumatic events and resolve the emotional effects of the trauma.

Licensed mental health care professionals must be thoroughly trained in the methods before using EMDR because patients usually experience the same level of distress in treatment as they did in the original trauma. When EMDR is successful, it may accelerate the treatment of patients who experience severe and incapacitating forms of stress reactions.

GROUP THERAPY

The Dutch philosopher known as Benedict De Spinoza observed over three hundred years ago that human beings are social animals. Since that time researchers from a range of theoretical backgrounds have supported the same observation. Sociobiologist Edward O. Wilson (1975) noted that social vertebrates, the category of organisms that includes both human beings and primates, have the advantage of being able to modify their behavior "... according to observations of success or failure on the part of the group as a whole" (p. 382).

The development of group therapy as a treatment modality has a strong foundation in theoretical contributions and practical considerations. Abraham Maslow (1954, 1972) placed a human being's need to belong to a group right after the most basic needs of hunger, sleep, and safety. To one side of the theoretical and humanistic position of Maslow is the presentation of W. R. Bion (1974) of the way groups act, feel, and learn. Bion studied patterns of behavior fundamental to both psychoanalysis and group dynamics, bringing the application of psychoanalytic group work to groups in industry, the military, and the community.

Psychotherapy with groups of people has a long history. At present private psychotherapists conduct various types of group therapy with a wide range of patients. There are also professional psychotherapists who are consultants for self-help groups, for groups in industry, and for groups in schools. There are compelling reasons for treating adolescents in group therapy.

The success of group treatment for people with alcohol and other addiction problems has contributed to the development and growth of group therapy techniques. The list of areas in which group therapy is practiced is extensive. The following are examples of courses offered at one group therapy training program, The Center for the Advancement of Group Studies: forming and maintaining the group; working with transference and resistance in groups; using induced feelings; psychopathology in groups; and modern group methods in the health setting.

The Center offers two tracks, one for mental health professionals seeking training as group analysts, and one designed primarily for professional people in fields such as government and business in the fields of guidance, personnel, and teaching. It is based in New York City but also offers an off-site training program with training weekends in Portland, Oregon, and San Francisco. Group approaches for special populations, a division of the center, includes approaches used with special diagnostic groups such as people with AIDS, eating disorders, psychosomatic disorders, and addiction problems. Group therapy has been especially helpful for the victims and the perpetrators of sexual and physical abuse.

The American Group Psychotherapy Association (AGPA) was established in 1955 to promote group approaches to the delivery of human services. In 1995, at a conference of the Eastern Group Psychotherapy, a regional affiliate of the AGPA, there were several presentations aimed directly at the creation of short-term models that are compatible with managed care goals. For these models, instructors help group therapists learn specialized skills to guide their patients in selecting focal areas that are manageable within the given time frames and are applicable in a variety of inpatient and outpatient settings.

At the same time that certain group therapy specialists are developing models for short-term group psychotherapy to meet the demands of MCOs, other group psychotherapists are urging their colleagues to develop ways to stimulate a non-managed care practice. At one workshop, group specialist Stephanie Kravec, MSW, discussed realistic marketing, use of computers, direct mailings, and other activities that generate new referrals and consultation work. Kravec asked psychotherapists to bring ideas to a workshop where the participants would produce their own marketing material through a series of small group exercises.

Seminars usually reflect current themes as well as more traditional interests. At the Eastern Group Psythotherapy conference, there were many seminars that combined traditional methods with current concerns. Several seminars included work on dreams through group activities, an approach advocated by Jeremy Taylor (1992) in his popular book *Where People Fly and Water Runs Uphill*. Dr. Robert Langs uses dream fragments from group members to help them be in touch with their adaptive responses to emotionally-charged events. Langs developed a model for dream processing in groups in light of recent developments in the architecture and evolution of the mind.

James Sacks, Ph.D., Director of the Psychodrama Center of New York, noted that therapists who used psychodramatic methods have remained rather isolated from their analytically oriented colleagues. He invited group psychotherapists to learn various psychodramatic techniques, such as the double and role reversal, and to share their impressions of these techniques with other members of the group. Other topics of special interest included helping therapists work with groups of survivors of genocide and war traumas across generations, group therapy of dually diagnosed patients, and an experimental workshop focusing on prejudices as manifested in group process.

Psychotherapists enroll at group training institutes to learn about the forces that affect the behavior of individuals as they interact with other individuals in the family, school, corporation, religious institutes, and other groups. Psychotherapists who have training in group therapy are especially valuable to MCOs because payment for each individual in group treatment is less expensive, of course, than individual treatment. For the psychotherapist, group therapy is rewarding because it is helpful for certain people who do not respond as well in individual therapy as they do in group therapy. The growth of the field of group thrapy is testimony to the enrichment experienced by psychotherapists and their patients as they work on issues through group processes.

12

New Directions

COMPUTERS AND PSYCHOTHERAPY

The rising demand for psychotherapy and the increasing pressure to control the cost of treatment may meet in a technological solution, namely the use of computers in mental health care. Exploration of the use of computers in health care is a rapidly evolving and enlarging field. Most of these explorations have been addressed to problems in medical disorders but the potential for use of computers in psychological problems is also being explored.

Medical users of computers have focused on information acquisition and retrieval. Computerized acquisitions and retrieval of demographic and financial data is the most advanced area in the field and is now standard in most hospitals and medical practices.

The automated acquisition and remote display of laboratory data is perhaps the next most evolved area. Laboratory data systems have gone through several generations of evolution and are now commercially available from a variety of vendors. In the near future, electronic laboratory records are likely to replace manual recording of data and distribution of individual reports.

The electronic acquisition and recall of clinical material, such as patients' symptoms and physical signs, is in a much more primitive state. Clinical material does not use the neat mathematical language of financial and laboratory data and is therefore not easily recorded or assembled into searchable arrays. Progress, however, is being made and the pace of further progress is accelerating. At the Beth Israel Hospital in Boston, for example, the paper chart has been replaced by a completely computerized medical record. Progress in the field and the technical and ethical obstacles to progress have been the subject of a yearly series of conferences under the auspices of Harvard Medical School and the direction of Charles Safran, M.D. (1996).

The use of computers to aid the clinical decision process is the least advanced area in medical use of computers. Advanced methods for searching the scientific literature are already widely available but the integration of this wealth of data into the minute-to-minute care of patients is in its infancy. Standard textbooks and databases such as the Physician's Desk Reference are available on CD-ROM, as are searchable collections of journal articles such as *Silver Platter* and *UpToDate*. The world's journal literature can be searched on-line through such services as *BRS Colleague* or *Medline* and searches can be efficiently formatted off-line and run on-line through the National Library of Medicine's *Grateful Med*®. Searches of these resources produce large volumes of material more suitable for after-hours study than for contemporaneous patient care. *UpToDate*, a commercially produced medical literature review service is designed to quickly answer narrow diagnostic and therapeutic questions that might arise during individual patient encounters. It is updated quarterly, available on CD-ROM and may soon be available on the Internet. Such a resource could be accessed while working on the computerized medical record and provide answers to clinical questions at the time that decisions are being made. *Physician's Date Queries* (PDQ), available from the National Career Institute, provides disease-specific treatment overviews for cancer. These statements are updated monthly by an expert panel and are available on-line. Although PDQ statements are not as easily searchable as *UpToDate*, they could be accessed while working on the computerized medical record, during the decision-making process. The integration of knowledge-based clinical alerts (Rind 1994) and practical guidelines (Safran 1996) into use of the computerized medical record is just beginning. Integration of diagnostic and therapeutic algorithms is also being explored.

In psychological treatment, the use of computers is both less and more advanced than in medical treatment. Computerized access to information is available through many of the same resources as for medicine. *Grateful Med*® accesses many psychological journals. PsycINFO™ is provided by the American Psychological Association (1400 North Uhle Street, Arlington, VA 22201 800–336–4980) and includes all the material in Psychological Abstracts plus additional items, covering over 1000 journals and technical publications.

Less academically-oriented psychological information is also available on-line. The Internet has become a subculture where people talk, play, work, and seek information. Within this new subculture is available a variety of mental health experiences.

John Grohol, Psy.D., Clinical Product Manager at CMHC Systems, reports that Internet mental health sites offer different forums ranging from "virtual support groups" to information and referral sources. Various considerations for on-line therapy are still in initial stages. As webmaster for CMHC Systems Mental Health Net, Dr. Grohol has seen phenomenal growth in a very short period of time.

Mental Health Net began as a simple community service on the World Wide Web. Within the first four months on-line, it attracted 100,000 visitors with a total of one million accesses. After six months it had expanded to 2,000 pages of information amounting to 23 megabytes of information. Grohol estimates that there are 8,000 to 9,000 accesses every day. And the number is increasing each month. "Both professionals and nonprofessionals use Mental Health Net," he says. "The most popular pages are those on depression, personality disorder, panic attacks, and anxiety disorder."

Mental Health Net offers six major categories on its home page: Reading Room Professional Resources, Mental Health Administration, Self-Help Resources, Calendar, and Other Links. In addition, it has an on-line mental health magazine called *Perspectives* and a Quickfind search feature. Mental health on-line is only beginning. Mental Health Net can be accessed at http://www.cmhcsys.com/mhn.htm.

Although mental health literature access is well advanced, several other problems are more difficult in mental health cases than in general medicine. First, the conversion of relevant psychological history and symptoms into a universally acceptable data set is even more difficult than it is with medical signs and symptoms. Second, the absence of universally accepted treatment paradigms for most psychological disorders impedes progress. There are few, if any, equivalents in psychotherapy to the medical dictum "Treat all strep pharyngitis with penicillin G for 10 days except in penicillin-allergic patients." Lastly, problems of confidentiality are even more severe in psychological uses of the computer than in medical uses.

These obstacles notwithstanding, the use of a computer for psychological treatment has one large potential advantage, compared with its use in general medicine. That advantage is a consequence of the fact that both the material to be examined and the main treatment modality consist of language. Therefore, an independent skilled observer and technical therapist is not always essential in psychological assessment and treatment. A patient cannot easily examine his or her own eye or ear or replace his or her own hip, but patients can recall their experiences, assess their moods, and enter such material into computers themselves. Patients can also read or listen to computerized responses themselves, without a human interviewer or therapist as an intermediary. Accordingly, psychological uses of computers have advanced in ways that medical uses have not. These uses include history taking, testing, and treatment.

In the area of history taking and testing, computers have been found to be reliable instruments (Greist et al. 1973, Petrie and Abell 1994) and many users find the interaction with a computer comfortable and less threatening than interaction with a human interviewer (Koback et al. 1994, Slade et al. 1966).

Computerized psychological testing is also well advanced. *The Structured Clinical Interview for DSM-IV (SCID)* (First et al. 1995) was first developed for DSM-III in 1983 and has been adapted to computer administration in a version called *Mini-SCID* (First et al. 1995). Another computerized interview program, *The Symptom-Driven Diagnostic System for Primary Care (SDDS-PC)* (Broadhead et al. 1995), is available in three formats: clinical-administered, desktop computer-administered, and computer-assisted telephone administration (CATI).

Computerized Symptom rating scales, side effect monitoring scales and quality-of-life scales are also being developed. These subjects were recently reviewed by Koback (Koback et al. 1996).

The equivalence of computer-based and clinician administered testing is being evaluated. The American Psychological Association has published guidelines for the use of computerized tests (*American Psychological Association Guidelines for Computer-Based Tests and Interpretation*, Washington, 1986). Validating studies of multiple forms of tests such as the *SDDS-PC* mentioned above are being conducted as are patient variables that influence response to computerized tests (Spinhoven et al. 1993).

The use of computers in mental health is least advanced in the area of psychological treatment itself, but progress is being made, and the potential is great. On-line forums such as those available through Mental Health Net mentioned above provide a sort of anonymous self-help. Although each forum has a system operator (sysop) who monitors and maintains the forum, sysops do not interact with the group as therapists nor is there a science of treatment by this method. The popularity of such forums suggests that on-line group therapy may be fruitful area for development. Clinical research and the evolution of this method should be facilitated by the large volume of interactions, the anonymity of the participants which should encourage their willingness to be studied, and the ease with which 100% of the interaction can be captured in discrete units for clinical study.

Programs which mimic therapy are commercially available. *PC Therapist* (J. Weintraub, Thinking Software, Woodside, NY) is an artificial intelligence program that imitates human interviews. The program is entertaining and convincing but does not apply any of the science of psychology in formulating its responses.

Computerized therapy systems based in psychological theory are under development. These systems are not as glib and entertaining as the *PC Therapist* but suggest promising avenues for future research. For example, a psychotherapy system based on retrieval of stories of alcoholism and sexual abuse has been discussed (Smith et al. 1993). This system is intended as an aide to a human therapist. In contrast, a program intended to substitute completely for a human therapist is the BT STEPS program. This is a behavioral treatment for obsessive compulsive disorders in which patients interact with a computer by telephone to develop a treatment plan of exposure and ritual preventive (E & RP) sessions specific to their problem. Patients then access their own E &RP session by touch tone telephone. The system is designed to be used under the supervision of a physician or mental health professional and can be used with or without psychopharmaceutical treatment.

Exploration of computer-based therapy remains limited and preliminary but one can envision the convergence of these pathways into an interactive treatment module which is engaging, private, readily available, and adapted by accepted principles of psychological assessment and treatment to each individual user. Such a device might be used by a skilled clinician as an adjunct to clinical treatment and psychopharmacology and in some cases might stand alone.

PRACTICE POINTER: A BASIC MAP FOR PSYCHOLOGISTS TO THE INFORMATION SUPERHIGHWAY

The Internet's global network of computers houses virtually limitless sources of information. Practicing psychologists who have begun exploring the Internet may be wondering how to find useful professional information on this vast resource.

E-mail. This is the most common Internet application. Using Internet e-mail, a psychologist may consult with colleagues or other Internet users on-line. Some psychologists may be interested in subscribing to an e-mail list, an electronic topical discussion group. E-mail lists deliver messages to anyone who has subscribed, allowing the reader to respond easily to all other list members. Some e-mail lists are restricted (for example, licensed psychologists only); others are open to anyone interested. Psychology-related e-mail lists cover such topics as community psychology, research design, and psychology of women. APA hosts several e-mail lists. The "practice" list is for APA members only and is used for discussing practice issues. To subscribe, send the message "subscribe practice" to "majordomo@lists.apa.org" without using the quotation marks.

The "PsyUSA" list is one of many non-APA mental health lists which may also be of interest to some psychologists. In addition to comments from list subscribers, the moderator for this list compiles useful information posted on other lists. PsyUSA is restricted to licensed psychologists, clinical psychology researchers, and clinical and counseling psychology graduate students. Send the message "subscribe PsyUSA" to "listserv@juvm.stjohns.edu."

World Wide Web. This is the fastest growing section of the Internet. The Web organizes Internet information onto a series of interconnected "pages" that incorporate text, graphics, video, and sound. A "point and click" method moves users from page to page or computer to computer.

Software known as a "browser" is needed to explore the Web. Many on-line service providers have browsers built in to their communication programs, while others allow the user to pick a browser. The popular Netscape Navigator is among many browsers that may be purchased from computer equipment stores.

The Web address for PsychNet, APA's home page on the Web is "www.apa.org." APA's page includes many Practice Directorate documents as well as materials from other areas of the association. APA has also created the Consumer Help Center (helping.apa.org) in conjunction with the ongoing public education campaign, "Talk to Someone Who Can Help."

A comprehensive list of Internet resources for psychologists, including information on numerous e-mail lists, is available from Grohol's Mental Health Page (www.coil.com/~grohol) and Mental Health Net (www.cmhc.com). Other sites of potential interest include FreudNet (plaza.interport.net/nypsan), Behavior On-Line, a "gathering place" for professionals in the behavioral science and related fields (www.behavior.net)

and the Health Care Financing Administration (www.hcfa.gov). Several state and provincial psychological associations also have their own home pages. A list of these associations can be found on PsychNet (www.apa.org/pubinfo/refer.html) (Herndon 1996).

ANGRY PEOPLE

Psychotherapists have always focused on anxiety as a symptom and signal of inner conflict. *DSM-IV* contains twelve anxiety disorders. Traditional psychotherapists generally treat anxiety disorders by exploring the conflicts that are out of the awareness of the patient and that are assumed to lead to the anxiety. Psychotherapists from behavioral psychology backgrounds are using techniques of behavior modification, such as systematic desensitization (Wolpe 1990), to treat phobia disorders. Although the techniques for treating anxiety have varied among psychotherapists, anxiety remains the most central affect discussed in psychotherapy literature. The various anxiety disorders remain popular diagnoses in psychotherapy reports. Currently, case managers in MCOs frequently write "anxiety" as the reason for referral to psychotherapists. (Caution: the term "anxiety" is insufficient to warrant payment from MCOs. Clinicians need to state the *code number* of the specific anxiety disorder as listed in *DSM-IV* or *ICD* to qualify a patient's condition as medically necessary.)

As clinicians and researchers examined new ways to conceptualize and heal mental disorders, there was a change in focus from anxiety to depression. No single explanation accounts for the increased diagnoses of depression during approximately the last forty years. It may be that mental health professionals have become more aware of the symptoms of depression, there may have been an increase in the cases of depression, perhaps as a reflection of the changes in society, or the increased reports of depression may simply reflect the popularity of this diagnosis. At any rate, the studies of depression led to important distinctions among kinds of depression and to the development of different techniques for treating the categories of depression. *DSM-IV* (1994) lists eight disorders that include depression as the major affect.

Martin Seligman (1994), who has spent much of his professional life studying depression, anxiety, and anger, believes that uncontrolled anger ruins more lives than schizophrenia, alcohol, AIDS, and perhaps even depression. Seligman also notes that there is a second impact of anger that may be just as shattering—anger between parents is the most depressing ordinary event that children witness. The results of anger are severe and pervasive, yet there are no anger disorders listed in the standard diagnostic manuals.

While the study of anger is not new, there has not been sufficient clarity of focus. The emphasis on underlying issues with anger has been addressed by psychologists who are familiar with the eastern philosophy of Buddhism. At the Naropa Institute in Boulder, Colorado, Chogyam Trungpa Rinpoche (1983) explains, "Whenever there is aggression and disliking in any aspect in the environment as you are growing up, that is the ground of insanity, from the Buddhist point of view" (p. 2). He continues by pointing out that the purpose of aggression is to keep oneself intact. The aggressive person has refused to deal with anybody else at all, and, in fact, the aggressive person frequently wants to attack anybody who touches him or her.

Kassanove and Sukhodolsky (1995) consider Zen Buddhism in relation to social constructivism, which holds that human beings construct a private reality that imposes meaning on events. The authors note that meaning can develop during the perception of the events or later, based on memory of the events, and the imposed meaning or structure can come from social, cultural, or biological forces. In this sense both the rational-emotive therapy of Ellis (1994) and the cognitive therapy of Beck (Beck et al. 1976) are social constructive forms of intervention.

Albert Ellis (1995) has discussed for about the past two decades the disadvantages of making oneself angry, enraged, and vindictive. Along with a few others (e.g., Tavris 1983), Ellis has been calling for more attention to anger disorders, noting that these disorders are common, and require clear definition, specific diagnosis, and effective treatment.

Recent studies of cross-cultural differences in emotional experiences provide important information with regard to anger. Tanaka-Matsumi (1995) cautions psychotherapists to consider cultural factors when assessing anger-related problems. Noting cross-cultural differences, she urges psychotherapists to be aware of the antecedents of displays of anger that vary in acceptability in different cultures. After Tanaka-Matsumi reviews the cross-cultural literature regarding anger, she discusses various antecedents of displays of anger that vary in acceptability in different cultures. Méndez-Villarrubia (1994), in a discussion of issues in the assessment of Puerto Rican and other Hispanic clients, also cautions psychotherapists to consider how cultural differences affect the presentation of symptoms in the interpretation of the illness. Méndez-Villarrubia addresses specific categories used primarily by Spanish-speaking people from the Caribbean, including *ataques de nervios*, a set of behaviors that frequently have been interpreted as expressions of resistance and anger at an oppressive system, whether that system is in the family or in a social institution.

Several researchers have reported success in treating anger. For example, both Deffenbacher (1995) and Feindler (1995) present strategies that begin with relaxation training, move on to remediation of maladaptive thinking habits, and then go on to improvement of social skills. As Kassanove and Eckhardt (1995) note, Deffenbacher's work addressed distressed college students in a program that usually lasted for less than ten sessions. The short-term effectiveness of these psychotherapeutic strategies suggests that they might be useful in treating patients referred by MCOs.

There are several other promising systems to treat people who present with problems related to their anger including Erin (1994), Beck (1976), and Ellis (1994). Kassanove and Eckhardt (1995) reviewed the literature concerning anger and reported that they remain optimistic about advances in the understanding and treatment of anger disorders. After stating that there is a pressing need to address the epidemic levels of aggression and violence observed in communities around the world, Kassanove and Eckhardt conclude that the future holds promise for psychotherapists who work with patients who present with anger disorders.

Although *DSM-IV* does not list any anger disorders, there is one diagnosis that includes the occurrence of aggressive behaviors as the essential feature: Intermittent Explosive Disorder. In addition, the diagnosis of Impulse Control Disorder Not Otherwise Specified is a category for impulsive behaviors that do not fit into other impulse-loss categories such as Substance Abuse. Although aggression disorders are not listed in the main sections of the standard diagnostic manuals, the *DSM-IV* Glossary of Culture-Bound Syndromes contains several entries that include anger as a prominent feature of the disorder. For example, *amok*, originally reported in Malaysia and now reported among men in several parts of the world, describes a period of brooding followed by an outburst of violent, aggressive, or homicidal behaviors. The cause of the syndromes *bilis* and *colera* are considered to be strongly experienced anger or rage. *Boufee delirante*, observed in West Africa and Haiti, refers to an outburst of aggressive behaviors and confusion. A Korean syndrome called *hwa-byung* is literally translated into English as "anger syndrome."

If a psychotherapist wants to work with an MCO with regard to the treatment of a patient with an anger disorder, it would be wise to see if a particular patient's symptoms meet the criteria for Intermittent Explosive Disorder or Impulse Control Disorder Not Otherwise Specified. Some of the culture-bound syndromes may also meet the criteria for a *DSM-IV* category, as, for example, *boufee delirante* may appear to be a Brief Psychotic Disorder.

For psychotherapists or researchers who want to measure the effects of treatment on states of anger, either for personal interest or for MCO reports, there are reliable anger scales. For example, Charles Spielberger (Spielberger and Sydeman 1994) developed sets of scales for the measurement of several affective traits and states. There are several tests that include measurements of anger in brief personality inventories for adults as well as adolescent patients.

PEOPLE WITH RELIGIOUS BELIEFS

Until recently, traditional psychoanalysts and psychoanalytic psychotherapists generally have not been hospitable to religious beliefs. There have been, of course, exceptions along the lines following such early theoreticians as William James (1902) and, in some ways, C. G. Jung (1938). But, for the most part, psychotherapists have avoided religious issues, a position that can be traced to the first psychoanalytic psychotherapist, Sigmund Freud. Freud had personal difficulties with religion. On the one hand, he upheld family values and traditional moral commitments in so devoted a manner that even the current advocates of traditional values would view his behavior as exemplary. On the other hand, Freud (1927) described religion as an illusion; an obsession; an irrational, infantile expression of conflict; and a symptom of other maladaptive attempts to resolve various conflicts.

It appears that many psychotherapists have followed Freud's contemptuous hand. As Strean (1994) points out, the majority of clinicians who have written on religion have referred to religious faith in extremely negative terms. Strean relates that the eminent psychoanalyst Jacob Arlow (1994) implored psychoanalysts to treat expressions of religious convictions in the same neutral way they respond to other clinical information.

While psychotherapy programs in the past have largely ignored the principles of organized religions, the leaders of organized religions have studied the theories and outcomes of psychotherapy for techniques that might be applied to help the religious population. In fact, as documented by Clebsch and Jaekle (1994), pastoral counseling has a long history in Christianity. Clebsch and Jaekle state that their study of the development of the western religious personality includes the

> . . . emphasis on the pastoral and other healing arts, which will still flourish today in the traditional patterns and at the same time are assuming novel and variegated forms. There remain recent (and by now conservative) patterns based on psychoanalysis and client-centered therapy. There are recovered forms such as meditation, body movement, and breath control, and there are really novel types such as love massage, bioenergetics, transactional analysis, existential analysis, and primal therapy. Pastoral or religious cure of souls today involves all these techniques and more.

Religions in addition to mainstream Christianity also have included openness to the techniques of psychoanalysis and psychotherapy. Feigue Cieplinski (1993), who is both a psychoanalyst and a religious school educator, draws upon child psychoanalytic principles in addressing the identity issues of Jewish young people. Cieplinski's discussion of identity is especially valuable for psychotherapists interested in understanding the need for persistent self examination within a system and within a group of people with shared characteristics. She notes the complexities of identity that include the process of integrating into our personalities the models we imitate, the cultures in which we live, and the teachings we assimilate.

Following injunctions as old as the ancient Talmud, the Association of Orthodox Jewish Scientists (AOJS) (Schwartz 1996) has supported training seminars for psychotherapists committed to observance of religious principles. The AOJS (1996) has produced a series of taped seminars concerning treatment issues including the following topics: children of divorce in the Orthodox community; issues in the treatment of single people; treating the Orthodox couple regarding fertility issues; clinical issues with bereaved parents; and managed care and Orthodox mental health professionals.

Traditional institutes of religious training frequently include courses in psychotherapy. The orientation of the Blanton-Peale Graduate Institute is psychoanalytic; its affiliation is with the Andover Newton Theological Seminary, New York Theological Seminary, Union Theological Seminary and Fordham University. The Blanton-Peale Institute offers courses in drive theory, self psychology, ego psychology, and object relations in an intense and extensive learning experience, but it also provides the opportunity to integrate the religious journey of the student into the psychotherapeutic work.

Although many religious training programs included courses in psychotherapy, many people looked in directions other than religion for answers to problems in life. As science in general and psychology in particular grew more powerful and more popular, many people turned away from the organized religion of their parents. The pursuit of science provided intellectual adventure and varied opportunities, yet scientists had intentionally avoided the more vague areas of human experiences such as values and identity. While science had been developing approaches to study subjective and ill-defined human needs, major religions were reorganizing to absorb some secular themes. The process for each area is, of necessity, slow and people are by nature impatient for answers and in need of guidance. Many people experienced profound emptiness. To their credit, psychoanalytic theoreticians observed the experiences that many people were having and they did attempt to address the problem through various approaches and orientations. Many people rejected the religious identities of the past but could not yet integrate a new identity through their scientific studies. At about this time several psychotherapists wrote books that reached both the psychotherapeutic community and the self searching population at large. *The Road Less Traveled* by M. Scott Peck, has been a consistent best seller since 1979 when it was published with the subtitle *A New Psychology of Love, Traditional Values and Spiritual Growth.* Dr. Peck's book is aimed at people who are suffering through problems and who respond to directives similar to those provided by religion. In much the same way as other popular psychotherapy books of this era, the book contains references to religions other than the ones with which most of his readers were familiar. For example, Peck starts his discussion of problems and pain with a reference to the first of the truths taught by the Buddha which is "life is suffering" (p. 16). For many readers the reference to Buddhist philosophy is more appealing than, say, the common refrain of older Jews that "life is hard," or of traditional

Christian teaching that "Christ suffered for your sins," even though these initial comments all serve to elicit similar thoughts about human pain.

For many people who rejected their own religions but failed to find solace in science, there is now a growing body of studies that scientifically study spiritual activities. For example, Elizabeth Targ (Wallis 1996), clinical director of psychosocial oncology research at California Pacific Medical Center in San Francisco recruited 20 faith healers to pray for severely ill AIDS patients. One of the healers reported that she draws on Christian, Buddhist, and Native American traditions (*Time*, June 24, 1996, p. 59). In another study of the treatment of AIDS patients, D. W. Sherman (1996) is enabling nurses to overcome their fears of caring for AIDS patients.

The adult children of people who endeavored to "trust in God" now flock to Tibetan sages and shamans of exotic cultures. The works of Deepak Chopra (1996), a writer who synthesizes Indian philosophy and Western medicine, have reached millions of people. Brian Weiss (1988) teaches past-life therapy to mental health professionals (Omega, Summer 1996, p. 40).

Rebecca Clay (1996), reporting that religious institutions play a central role in African-American life, points to the counseling role of the clergy in the three main African-American religious groupings that include Protestantism, Catholicism, and the Nation of Islam. Winston Gooden, Ph.D. (Clay 1996), an associate pastor at the First African Methodist Episcopal Zion Church and an associate professor at Fuller Theological Seminary's Graduate School of Psychology in Pasadena, California, describes African-American religious organizations as a refuge from racism, and a place for celebrating survival. The religious institution, Dr. Gooden says, presents a communal ritual space in which people can experience their own sense of being special, and feeling more important and more powerful than they feel in the wider society. Dr. Gooden sees religious participation as "a wonderful preventive force in terms of mental health" (Clay, p. 46).

At this point in history, people appear to be returning from their spiritual quests with a new understanding of themselves and others and with values and an approach to life that bring them satisfaction. Nonetheless, for many people the search for answers in exotic places and systems has not provided the balanced perspectives, creativity, and comfort for which they longed. They did bring back from other cultures helpful and productive ideas and techniques that for several years have been incorporated into psychotherapy. For example, many psychotherapists have incorporated techniques of meditation into their practices.

Those who went from our society to others also brought back a new awareness of spiritual needs and feelings. The new awareness has changed the attitudes of many people in the healing professions. The quest for spiritual comfort seemed different to many people than the quest for religious comfort. Spirituality became a respected aspect of psychotherapy for many participants in treatment.

One of the benefits of the acceptance of the search for spirituality values has been the increased tolerance shown by scientific investigators and clinicians for religious people. Rebecca Clay (1996) quotes Harold Keonig, director of The Program on Religion, Aging and Health at Duke University: "We see people who are distressed, people who are turning to religion for comfort. We see their behavior as something associated with psychiatric illness, when they're really just grabbing at something to give them comfort. We're misinterpreting what's going on" (Clay, p. 48).

It may be that psychotherapy has integrated as much spirituality and as many techniques of the healing arts of other societies as it can absorb at the present time. The traditional religions practiced in the west are responding to the new age approaches to healing mind and soul. At a week-long retreat at the Omega Institute, courses in Sufi Retreat and Tibetan Buddhism are complemented with a course on Jewish Mystical Tradition and on Soul Making in the Christian Mystical Tradition.

Just as the leaders of traditional religions are reaching out to retrieve the wandering members of their flocks, members of the psychotherapy communities are reaching out to incorporate areas that were formerly neglected. For example, Shafranske (1996), in *Religion and the Clinical Practice of Psychology*, brings together an overview of opinions regarding the relevance of religious issues in psychotherapy today.

Psychotherapists, then, may consider working with populations of people who were previously underserved. Psychotherapists can find courses, texts, and other materials to help them to treat these populations. For example, Herbert Strean (1995) provides guidance for psychotherapists, with or without religious convictions, in the treatment of Orthodox Jews. As mentioned previously, the AOJS has materials and other sources for Orthodox Jewish psychotherapists working with people who have specific problems. The Blanton-Peale Institute in New York is associated with several Christian seminaries but maintains a nondenominational commitment and a cross cultural faculty and student body. Several traditional psychoanalytic institutes, including the Post-Graduate Center for Mental Health in New York City, have begun to offer programs in pastoral counseling. Universities such as Harvard in Boston and Johns Hopkins in Baltimore are continuing to hold seminars for the purpose of studying the needs that draw people to spirituality and the results of spiritual beliefs on individuals and groups.

13

Flight

Flight addresses the many psychotherapists who, for one reason or another need to develop practices outside of MCOs. There are two types of psychotherapists in this category: those who have problems getting on—or remaining on—the lists of MCOs, and those who choose to work outside of managed care for personal reasons. Psychotherapists in either of these positions might consider a specialty that is needed by people who are willing to pay for their own treatment. This chapter presents solutions that psychotherapists have used to explore new ideas or expand their areas of interest. It starts with the example of two people who learned new techniques to establish a practice based on their interest in helping children to express anger, and continues with examples of other people who have succeeded in non-MCO areas.

THE CHILL STORY

In 1984 Alan Schneider moved from Manhattan, where he had both a full-time position at the Veteran's Administration Hospital as a psychiatric social worker and a private psychotherapy practice, to a rural area in upstate New York. The dramatic change in locations was accompanied by a similarly dramatic change in the nature of his work. Trained in psychoanalysis at National Psychological Association for Psychoanalysis (NPAP) while completing his coursework in family and community education at Columbia University, Schneider was used to a formal, structured approach to his work. However, his desire to relocate to the country began a series of events that was to take him in a new and unanticipated direction.

During the first few years he was in a rural environment, Schneider was able to complete his dissertation, begin a small practice, and start a family with his wife, Deidre Laikin, an established novelist and also a former elementary school teacher. As the years passed, Schneider's practice grew steadily. Although he often found himself involved in crisis intervention, supportive therapy, and advocacy for children rather than in strict psychoanalysis or even psychoanalytical psychotherapy, he liked the people with whom he worked and he liked the seclusion and serenity of his work.

In the late 1980s, the local economy began to falter and there was a marked drop-off in full-fee patients. Occasionally, Dr. Schneider waited for insurance payments and carried a "balance due" for several months. By the early 1990s, as economic conditions in this rural area worsened, more and more patients requested reduced fees. At about this time, several MCO representatives began to visit his office and urged him to join as a provider. Dr. Schneider resisted. He knew there would be difficulty finding reliable office workers who would understand the need for strict confidentiality in psychotherapeutic work, and he was well aware of the increased paperwork burden such an affiliation would require. In addition, his frequent conversations with physicians on the West Coast, where managed care had long been an unpleasant fact of life, made him wary of joining. But his potential client base was increasingly affiliated with local MCOs.

Alan Schneider and Deidre Laiken (1980, 1995) had written two books on emotion. Dr. Schneider had helped build his practice through public speaking and being a host on radio shows. Now confronted with the demands of managed care, Dr. Schneider wondered if he could find another way. He knew affiliating himself would mean the end of his independence as a private practitioner. The reimbursement provided by the MCO was considerably less than his normal full fee. This would mean he would be working longer hours yet receiving less financial compensation. In addition, he would be supervised by employees of the MCO, a situation bound to leave him frequently feeling frustrated, helpless, and angry.

Dr. Schneider began to see an alternative. Even this small town, surrounded by dairy farms and cornfields, was not immune to the national epidemic of school violence and teen suicide. The local superintendent of schools requested that he speak to the faculty on student anger and the prevention of violence. The talk was a success. Within a few months the superintendent asked Dr. Schneider to provide instruction to teachers in conflict prevention. The CHILL program was born.

Together with his wife, Schneider created a program that promised to "Change Hostility Into Listening and Learning." What began as a seed of an idea rapidly grew into a healthy and challenging business. Alan and

Deidre created a unique seminar business that used all their past experience in psychotherapy and education. Under their direction, CHILL became a therapy group for stressed-out staff and a learning experience for new teachers, and it provided everyone from students to cafeteria workers to secretarial staff with a way to handle potentially dangerous impulses. Alan and Deidre considered CHILL a logical expansion of an idea they had nurtured for many years: emotional education.

In 1994, the CHILL program received a Federal Violence in the Schools Grant, an innovation in the school grant program, and a grant from the local Community Action Alliance. Alan and Deidre conducted seminars with parents, students, teachers, and community leaders on topics from neuro-linguistic programming to "SuperLearning" to hypnosis. Although by that time the MCOs had a firm grip on virtually all businesses in the area, Dr. Schneider maintained his practice without becoming a provider. He saw CHILL, public speaking, hypnosis, and consulting work at first as welcome adjuncts to a traditional psychotherapy practice. As he gained skills in treating children diagnosed with learning disabilities and attention deficit disorder, his practice changed and became completely outside the influence of Big Brother.

Most recently, Alan Schneider and Deidre Laiken developed a line of tapes (1995b) and books explaining CHILL techniques and philosophy. When Dr. Schneider looked clearly at the direction to which managed care was pointing for mental health professionals in his community, he chose an alternate route. He has created a new area in which to apply the skills and interests of a psychotherapist.

ART THERAPY

Judith Duboff is a registered art therapist (ATR). The art therapy profession has a national accrediting board, which is going through the steps to receive state licensing for art therapists. So far, this has been accomplished only in New Mexico. Until the rest of the states provide the opportunity for licensing, art therapy remains outside the managed care network in those states.

Being denied insurance reimbursement has motivated Ms. Duboff to create therapeutic settings that are appealing to people who enjoy privacy and creativity. Ms. Duboff holds classes (or groups) for parents and children, for mothers and adolescent daughters, and for women trying to make changes in their lives. Art therapy is an especially appropriate treatment for children who are reluctant to talk. The following case studies describe important treatment communications in art therapy, the first with a child and the second with a family.

> A suicidal, sexually abused girl painted three flowers in a bouquet with a red bow in her first art therapy sessions. As treatment progressed and she dealt with the shame and anger that were the results of having been raped repeatedly by her stepfather, she drew many flowers being trampled and apparently ignored signs that said, "Don't step on the flowers." A turning point came in treatment after she drew a horse being forced to take a carriage over a bumpy road. Although the horse said, "No, I will not," it was forced to continue anyway. She was able to understand the parallel to her experiences of being raped, and no longer blamed herself. She then painted a girl watering wilted flowers in a garden. At the end she drew growing flowers that were not being damaged.

> A 5-year-old girl was withdrawn and shy at school. Her initial artwork showed her father and sister on both sides of the paper and a clay cow. In the first family art therapy session the father painted the 3-year-old sister as a grown woman until his wife said "That must be me; she's grown up," and then he added a smaller figure representing the child. The other girl was not even in the picture. The therapist alternated individual sessions for the girl and family sessions. The mother was very infantile and helpless in the beginning. Her self-esteem and her creativity seemed to grow hand in hand. At one point she made dolls that sold at fairs. As she became a more effective mother, the father and she renewed their relationship and developed a proper hierarchy in the family. Both girls received appropriate nurturing. The 5-year-old became more at ease and outgoing at school. One of the last clay pieces she made was two adjoining caves (that looked exactly like two breasts) with one girl in each of them.

These descriptions of the activities in art therapy illustrate the observation, made throughout history, that art transforms the person creating the art as well as those to whom art communicates. Art therapy is a therapeutic modality that allows an opportunity for a person or a family to give form to imagination in artistic expression and create new channels of understanding, communication, and healing.

It is an alternative approach in many ways. The art therapist's office is filled with drawing materials, paint, clay, and a large work table. The process of art-making, which is a central aspect of art therapy, provides an alternative means of conscious awareness that is expressed symbolically and then is seen and understood in the safety of the therapeutic alliance with the art therapist.

PSYCHOANALYSIS

The practice of psychoanalysis is intellectually stimulating and personally satisfying. Many young professionals have pursued the goal of becoming a psychoanalyst with years of postgraduate psychoanalytic education and training.

Although the practice of psychoanalysis seems to be flourishing, there are, at the same time, many warnings to young professionals that psychoanalysis cannot continue to exist. Of course, the cry of the death of psychoanalysis has been around since it was first presented, but the intensity of the rumors of its death has become more pronounced in this day of MCOs. While the demise of psychoanalysis is unfounded, the observation is accurate that psychoanalysis, unless it is considerably modified, is outside the realm of managed care. Psychoanalysis depends on privacy, trust, and the ability to unfold at a rate that meets the needs of the patient. Even the opening phase of psychoanalysis proceeds at a pace determined by the needs of the individual patient. A recent meeting of the Institute for Psychoanalytic Training and Research (March 15–17, 1996) in New York City focused on the opening phase of psychoanalysis as a process that creates a particular therapeutic alliance. It is in this secure environment that the patient finds the courage to expand the capacity for self-reflection. Self-reflection is a concept that is not likely to be part of the lexicon of a managed care organization. Nor is the concept of truth, which is an integral component of psychoanalysis. Bail (1981) said, "While direct access to the truth is available, it would seem, to poets and mystics only, those less fortunate have finally been able, in this century, to take advantage of the most remarkable heuristic device of modern times: psychoanalysis" (p. 63).

In an address called "A Winnecottian Analyst Meets Managed Care" at a conference of The Psychoanalytic Society of the Postdoctoral Program at New York University, Leanne Domash (1994) stated, "Winnicott's attitude of deep waiting, of suspending understanding, clashes so starkly with utilitarian managed care principles as to send the analysts into an existential panic" (p. 1). The panic that Dr. Domash is experiencing can be averted if psychoanalysis is practiced outside of managed care.

The observation that managed care is inconsistent with the professional principles of psychoanalysis is appearing with increasing frequency. In a letter to *The New York Times*, Ernest Brod (1996), Vice President of the Society of Modern Psychoanalysts, presents the position of the Society's advisory that "confidentiality, standards of care, and appropriate treatment modalities cannot be achieved within managed care. In order to remain true to their professional principles, practitioners of psychoanalysis must not participate in managed care networks" (p. 12). Brod warns that until MCOs recognize the need for trust and privacy inside the office of the therapist, increasing numbers of psychotherapists and patients will bar the door against the intrusion of another entity in the room.

Nina Thomas (personal communication, July 1995) seems to be in agreement with the position stated by Brod. Thomas, a former president of the New Jersey Psychological Association, is currently the chairperson of the National Mental Health Forum, an organization with the goal of educating consumers to the necessity for long-term treatment in psychoanalysis. The philosophy of the Forum is based on the need for psychoanalysts to separate themselves from reliance on reimbursement by insurance companies. The Forum advocates a formula by which psychoanalysts would provide a scale of fees in order to include people who would not otherwise be able to participate in therapy several times a week.

Although there is agreement that the current crisis in mental health care makes it necessary for psychoanalysts to reexamine their ideology and commitments, there is also agreement that psychoanalysis is far from dead. In fact, the reexamination of psychoanalysis appears to be revitalizing the practice and the communication among psychoanalysts. Once it is accepted that psychoanalysis is surviving and, in fact, gaining new adherents, the next step is to examine the direction that it will take.

How does a person go from wanting to be in private practice to actually being engaged in a psychoanalytic or psychodynamically oriented private practice? Most graduates of medical programs, doctoral programs, or masters degree programs in social work or nursing who are interested in psychoanalysis plan to participate in an established program in a major city. In many of the institutes for psychoanalysis, there is access to patients and supervision, with referrals provided to trained candidates and graduates. The American Psychological Association's Division for the Study and Practice of Psychoanalysis and Psychoanalytic Therapy, Division 39, has announced that plans are under way for the development of an outreach program, with the goal of extending programs to outlying areas that do not have the abundance of analytic resources that are found in the larger metropolitan areas. *The National Directory of Psychotherapy Training Institutes* (Baum and Pounds 1993) provides information about free-standing, independent institutes that offer training in psychoanalysis and psychotherapy.

Allan Schore, Ph.D. (1996), of the Department of Psychiatry and Biobehavioral Sciences, University of California School of Medicine, presented recent studies from a spectrum of disciplines which provide more detailed information regarding early socioemotional development. Schore finds that current research provides data to update Freud's structural theory and generally supports the tenets of psychoanalysis. Working toward a multilevel perspective, Schore integrates new insights about human interactions from developmental and clinical psychoanalysis, current ideas about the origins of social functioning from the developmental sciences, recent reports on emotional phenomena from the behavioral sciences, and the latest research on limbic structures from the brain sciences. In order to generate an overarching model of emotional development, Schore's model and the supporting studies are relevant to psychoanalysis and encouraging to psychoanalysts.

Schore is predicting that psychoanalysts will incorporate awareness of the biological functions underlying psychological interactions and will include, as a long term goal of treatment, inducing literal structural alterations in the patient's right hemispheric orbito frontal affect regulating systems. Schore believes that the alterations produce a representation of the positive functions of the analyst, thereby contributing to a self system that is more tolerant of intensity of affects and more adaptive to intrapsychic and interpersonal functioning.

In contrast to Schore's interpretations, Alan Stone, M.D. (1995), Professor of Law and Psychiatry on the faculty of Law and Medicine at Harvard University, finds that recent research in areas such as memory has cast doubt on the usefulness of psychoanalytic techniques. Stone, however, has not yet given up on psychoanalysis. He believes that psychoanalysis remains the best way to explore the mysteries of one's self, but that it is not an adequate form of treatment for most of the problems presented by people seeking psychotherapy. In his own practice Stone says he focuses primarily on problem solving and on helping patients find new ways of interacting with the important people in their lives. In addition to new techniques, Stone welcomes psychopharmacology as a way to relieve human suffering. In response to the question, "Where will psychoanalysis survive?" Stone said

> Freud's famous conclusion was that when our patients' neuroses are cured by psychoanalysis, they have to deal with ordinary human suffering on their own. Perhaps it will be no further offense to Freud for me to suggest quite the opposite. When a patient's symptoms are treated, he may then need a psychoanalyst to help him deal with his ordinary human suffering. That is the therapeutic domain in which the art of psychoanalysis will survive. [p. 11]

Psychoanalysis is changing in response to cultural influences as well as to biological research. The important psychoanalytic goal of helping patients achieve independence is under scrutiny as analysts from non-European orientations bring different meaning to the concept of independence. In a traditional sense, the goal is to become more internally independent which might—or might not—lead to the ability to enjoy the interdependence of family life and community interactions. In a more current psychoanalytic exploration, the acceptance of family or group interdependence as a variant of a healthy, satisfying, and adaptive way of life is leading to reconsideration of the inner structures that contribute to the ability to enjoy life.

Working with people from different backgrounds and experiences from the traditional psychoanalytic patients has changed aspects of psychoanalysis in direct ways. For example, there have been in the past very few reports of psychoanalysis with poor people. Now, as psychoanalytically trained clinicians attempt to treat poor people in clinics, the psychoanalytic tenets of privacy and anonymity are not applicable, leading some psychoanalysts to create new ways to practice.

Not only are psychoanalysts treating patients of different economic and cultural backgrounds, but patients are coming to psychoanalysts who are themselves from different cultures. In addition, people who were trained during the last three decades are now the leaders in psychoanalysis. In many ways, these people are injecting into the psychoanalytic process the cultural values that sprang from recent societal changes such as feminism and egalitarianism, thus changing the function of the field.

According to Tori De Angelis's (1996) report in the *APA Monitor*, psychoanalysts are creatively meeting modern challenges while retaining their original focus on deep meanings and inner structures. They are meeting new challenges by examining basic tenets of psychoanalysis in light of the knowledge derived from cultural considerations. De Angelis (1996) quotes psychoanalyst Rose Marie Perez Foster, Ph.D.: "We're beginning to ask, do our assumptions about human nature and human development apply to all people, or just to a small group of Europeans on whom the theory was originally based?" (p. 43). Perez Foster is editor with Michael Moskowitz, Ph.D. and Rafael Javier, Ph.D. (1996) of *Reaching Across the Boundaries of Culture and Class: Widening the Scope of Psychotherapy*.

PSYCHOTHERAPY SKILLS IN LEGAL AREAS

There are several areas that involve the exploration of new roles, adapting skills into different types of practice. To illustrate, consider forensics. Forensics is a specialty outside of managed care that redirects skills into a different type of work. Areas such as divorce mediation, custody evaluation, and work for the courts all benefit from the mental health professional's training, but are not actually psychotherapy.

A psychotherapist who is trained in family therapy will find his or her training useful in the field of divorce mediation, but divorce mediation is often more specific in its goals. Sylvan Schaffer (1995), who provides legal counsel at the New York State Psychological Association and who is both a psychologist and an attorney, warns that divorce mediation involves areas, such as taxes, investments, and real estate, in which psychologists are not usually professionally trained. Schaffer also discusses the need for psychologists to be aware of the rules affecting privilege and confidentiality as they apply to the mediation process. With awareness of the special legal issues, psychotherapists may want to consider this challenging and rewarding professional field.

Like divorce mediation, child custody evaluations require specific training in legal considerations and procedures relevant to doing child custody evaluations or family treatment and in psychological testing. Further training is necessary to do custody evaluations. In addition to training, specialists in the area suggest finding an experienced supervisor and consulting with an attorney if there are any legal questions (e.g. Ochrach 1996).

There are other areas of court-related activities that may interest psychologists. For example, the American Board of Vocational Experts (ABVE) lists activities that are relevant to the occupational functioning of people who have had their functioning altered by physical, mental, emotional, or social impacts on their lives. The psychological factors underlying such situations are important elements in testifying with regard to an individual's ability to perform work. Members of the ABVE have academic preparation in the areas of rehabilitation, psychology, and counseling. ABVE holds conferences for mental health professionals who are interested in being vocational experts (ABVE 1996).

Forensics can include custody and competency evaluations, the growing areas of divorce mediation, and other types of mediation as well. Psychotherapists, however, need to remember that there are many issues to consider in dealing with forensics. Schaffer's (1995) article on consent agreements in forensic assessments provides an outline of areas for consideration by mental health professionals.

THE COMMUNICATIVE EXPERIENCE

On a late October Sunday in 1994, an overflow crowd of psychotherapists jammed into a picturesque church hall in Stockbridge, Massachusetts, to mark the seventy-fifth anniversary of the venerable Austen Riggs Center, a small, private, not-for-profit open psychiatric facility. Since 1919, the Center has offered a haven for the emotionally ill that is dedicated to intensive psychodynamic psychotherapy, both short- and long-term, in an open setting. Riggs clearly was in trouble. The onslaught of managed care had cut deeply into the institution's traditional cash flow, placing the Riggs programs in jeopardy. The crisis cast a pall over the international scientific symposium entitled "The Inner World in the Outer World."

Sixteen months later Riggs is back on its feet, thanks primarily to the efforts of Edward Shapiro, Medical Director and CEO. What accounted for the transformation? Does it provide any insights into the problems of dealing with managed care? The answers were provided by Dr. Shapiro at a 1996 meeting of the Freudian Society in New York City. And they did not include transforming Riggs into a center for short-term behavioral modification.

Using the treatment of personality disorders as a "lens," Shapiro (1996) assessed the impact of managed care on the establishment of a reliable framework for dynamic treatment. Managed care had disrupted the treatment "frame" (Baranger and Baranger 1966, Langs 1976, Milner 1957), causing a reconsideration of the relationship between interpretation and management in the therapeutic setting. In theory, once patient and therapist agree on a framework, interpretation can become the principal treatment technique. However, Shapiro noted, with the increased presence of the third-party payer, establishment of the frame was disrupted by difficulties in negotiating payment, frequency of appointments, and duration of treatment. The pressures created by a form of business and behavioral management that is concerned with resources and symptoms seriously alter the way patients can engage in deepening therapeutic work. "To maintain our integrity and keep our therapeutic enterprise grounded in reality, we were forced to reexamine the basics of our treatment setting in this new context," he added.

The concept of the frame is not new to psychotherapy and has been detailed by others over the past 40 years (Baranger and Baranger 1966, Langs 1973, 1976, Milner 1957, Raney 1982). The frame has footholds in external reality and the analytic dyad. It is a boundary (Milner 1957) that ". . . marks off an area within which what is perceived is taken symbolically, while what is outside the frame is taken literally" (p. 158).

Langs (1982) stresses that the "ground rules (frame) are clearly among the most essential determinants of the modes of relatedness, cure, and interaction between the patient and therapist, and influence the entire unfolding of the therapeutic experience" (p. 69). "The honesty, integrity, and insightfulness of the therapist and of the therapeutic experience depends on the therapist's actual management of this dimension of the therapeutic relationship" (p. 490).

In order for therapy to take place, it is up to the therapist to provide a safe, predictable therapeutic space. With this kind of security, a patient can risk opening up his inner world. A "misalliance" (Langs 1978) occurs when that arena is invaded by managed care. Under the pressure of managed care, many therapists have lost their ability to manage the framework of dynamic psychotherapy. Financial and treatment parameters are now being managed by a third party that has been incorporated into the treatment room. Insurance in the treatment room (Langs 1973, Raney 1972) is a powerful force of resistance.

The way the psychotherapist manages the issues of frame management and interpretation (Langs 1976) is a reflection of how he manages between his inner and outer worlds and is an indication to the patient of the therapist's character. It is at this boundary that the patient and therapist meet to engage in interpretive treatment. "There can be no interpretation without competent management, no useful management without interpretation," Dr. Shapiro (1996) says. A secure framework represents a negotiated reality that incorporates the limitations of resources represented by third-party managers. By incorporating this limitation into the framework, the therapist can help the patient understand his or her transference meaning and the effect on his or her past or present behavior.

At Austen Riggs, Shapiro reported that therapists were faced with incorporating into the treatment the external limitations of the therapy, the meaning of them, and how that meaning has governed the patient's past and present behavior. The staff developed a management structure that brought together the insurance companies, the patients, and the clinicians. Shapiro showed, for example, how one patient finally realized that he was using the hospital setting as an overprotective mother. When the patient came to this realization, he broke out of the insurance dependency and got a job to support his own therapy. The repetition of the family dynamics was reduced and treatment advanced to a new level. Shapiro urges therapists to get out of the "rescue business" and return to their craft, which is interpretation. Fighting with insurance companies is not a therapeutic activity for the patient, the therapist, or the case manager.

A secure therapeutic setting has a central, significant impact on the patient's motivation for change. The ideal frame calls for total privacy to allow patients to talk about their deepest secrets and be held in an empathic environment that is predictable and consistent.

In most first sessions, patients are introduced to the limitations created by inviting managed care into the treatment room. The issues of confidentiality and privacy are interpreted not only as an issue between the patient and the insurance company, but also as an issue between the therapist, patient, and insurance company. Money is a reality, interpreted in relation to what is going on in the session and in relation to the therapist as well as the patient and his problems. Instead of blaming the insurance company, patients and therapists are encouraged to look at their contributions to the situation.

> One case example involves a 48-year-old woman with a dependent personality disorder who was referred for treatment by an EAP. She lived in

the downstairs apartment of her mother's house with an abusive boyfriend who controlled everything she thought and did. With the constant interference and unsolicited advice of her boyfriend, the patient found it difficult, if not impossible, to make everyday decisions. The therapist interpreted to her the repetition in the therapeutic frame of her relationship with her boyfriend. The patient was inviting the insurance company to make decisions about the treatment, which could be regarded as similar to the relationship with her boyfriend. The patient, saddled with financial problems, required more intensive treatment than allowed by the EAP. Both the patient and the therapist were interacting in a two-family treatment environment with the EAP acting the part of the intrusive boyfriend.

The interpretation led her to take her first steps toward independence. By the end of the sixth session, the patient had ended her relationship with the boyfriend and forced him out of the house. She also evicted the EAP and took on a second job to help pay for private therapy at a reduced fee.

The communicative approach is a set of techniques that attempts to empower the patient as well as the therapist. Insurance and managed care companies have transformed the profession, as well as therapists and patients. Subscribers who expect mental health coverage receive restricted behavioral training to cope with their problems. Some managed care patients find this educational process helpful and many of them believe that it is the nature of psychotherapy. For many, new problems mean a return to treatment in search of new solutions. This is education, not psychotherapy. However, for the more serious, understructured patients who require long-term treatment, managed care as it appears today cannot address these problems appropriately. It simply cannot afford to deal with issues of pathology or quality of life, nor should we expect that it will.

Insurance coverage for mental health services does not require a complicated and unwieldy bureaucracy. A simplified schema for insurance coverage might include:

An insurance policy to cover a fixed number of sessions per year. Such a policy might provide 6, 13, or 26 sessions, and be priced accordingly.

A standard fee will be authorized for psychiatrists, psychologists, and clinical social workers. Without a cadre of paid case managers, the insurance company will be more cost-effective. It need only track how many of the authorized sessions a subscriber has used. Co-payment will be negotiated between patient and provider.

The subscriber can use his or her sessions with any accredited therapist of his or her choice. When the sessions run out, there is an option for paying the therapist privately or waiting for the next annual allotment of sessions.

Billing should not require disclosure of a diagnosis. Instead, bills sent to insurance companies should include the name and address of the patient, the dates of the office visits, and the amount due. Confidentiality can further be secured by using numbers rather than names, thus keeping unnecessary data from all administrative personnel.

Such a plan would eliminate outside interference in treatment, reduce the inordinate paperwork created by outpatient treatment reports, restore some confidentiality to the treatment room, and simplify the overburdened billing process. It would also bring a new level of honesty back to mental health care.

14

Fight

Many psychotherapists have chosen to oppose MCOs on the basis of principles that they are determined to advocate. These psychotherapists have reached out to other professionals, politicians, and mental health consumers to form various organizations. Some organizations, like the American Mental Health Alliance, provide professional services in a nonmanaged care system based on professional ethics. Others, like the National Coalition for Mental Health Professionals and Consumers, are advocacy groups working for change. Some groups are local or regional, others national. They are all part of a powerful movement to challenge the present health care system. Chapter 14 introduces psychotherapists to a sample of fight solutions, presenting the ideologies and experiences of these movements in the words of their own members.

HOW CLINICIANS CAN FIGHT BACK AGAINST MANAGED CARE

Sheila Peck, a marketing and advertising consultant in Island Park, New York, has a special interest in helping psychotherapists to resist managed care techniques. When she learned that we were including ways to confront MCOs in this book, she volunteered to write the following essay, addressed especially to new clinicians.

❑ ❑ ❑

I'm traveling to a conference about managed care on a train from New York to Chicago. Here, there is no insurance—no phones, no computers, no faxes. This is part of what I like about traveling by train. For a few hours I'm insulated from the mundane, able to forget everything for a short while.

In the dining car, as is the way with Amtrak, they seat me with two other passengers and we chat, getting acquainted. After the usual hellos and comments about how much fun it is to ride by train, we trade destinations.

Jill is going to visit her family in Cleveland. Jim is a teacher from Michigan who, as a hobby, travels the country by train whenever he is on vacation. I'm headed for a managed care conference in the heartland. Suddenly, over Amtrak's lovely dinner, Jill catches her breath.

"I'm an office manager for an orthopedist," she announces. "I hate managed care."

Jim, concerned that his evening conversation is taking a negative turn, asks cautiously, "Are you both on the same side?" He doesn't want controversy in the dining car.

"Yes!" we nod emphatically.

"Good," he sighs, relieved. Then he draws himself up proudly and divulges, "Well, you might not like it but I don't have to worry about managed care. I only pay five dollars a visit."

Jill and I glance at one another.

"Then you have managed care," I tell him.

"What do you mean?" he inquires testily, pulling out his insurance card. He displays it on the table.

"Do you have to use specific doctors in a network?" I ask patiently.

"Well—yes," he acknowledges. "What is managed care anyway?" he asks, puzzled.

Jill and I eagerly tell him.

Jim listens silently. When we finish there is a long pause before he speaks. "Is there anything I can do about it?" he asks us in a very small voice.

There it is. The peace of Amtrak has been invaded by managed care after all. With the knowledge that it follows us wherever we go, I finally decide to sit down and spend some of these hours zipping through America writing about managed care.

I dedicate this discussion to the beleaguered New York orthopedic office manager and the Michigan teacher, Jill and Jim. Here are some things they—and you—can do to fight back. And it will be a fight. The advent of managed care has generated a crisis for all of us: clinician, consumer, and society in general.

How to Handle the Crisis Within Yourself

The Chinese pictogram delineating the word "crisis" consists of two symbols: one represents "danger" and the other "opportunity." Because our first reaction is often panic, many clinicians have been addressing the danger while we have often overlooked the opportunity.

"Opportunity for what?" you may ask, thinking only about the problems managed care has caused for our patients and ourselves. There is an opportunity for changing, learning, and growing. After all, isn't this what our profession is all about?

However, before you accept the managed care chance for change, ask and answer several questions:

1. Is this fight worth it to me?
2. Can I deal with the possibility of getting thrown off a panel?
3. Can I imagine being relieved if this happens?
4. Am I willing to take the necessary time to stage a real fight?

If you answer "yes," you're ready to do battle.

Remember, this "crisis" may be a real opportunity for you. Think about the ways in which you may adapt.

For instance, you may decide to develop a managed-care-free practice and learn more about marketing and public relations. Or you may enhance your advocacy skills as you learn to play managed care's game and fight for your clients. You can become a better diagnostician—a positive change that the demands of managed care have helped me achieve.

If you are a newer clinician you have, by necessity, become expert at practice building without managed care, because you probably have not been accepted on many panels. If you are a veteran, you may experience the relief and freedom that can ensue when you are terminated from a panel or decide voluntarily to leave. When this happened to me recently, both the patient and I found it liberating.

In speaking about managed care to clinicians in a variety of venues, I have found that the primary symptom of the crisis is a lack of hope. Psychotherapists ask the same rhetorical question over and over again: They make the rules and what can I do about it?

This discussion is intended to help you regain hope, to change the internal defeat engendered by managed care into energy that will empower you. Just look at how much you can do.

In order to have time for this fight, given the demands of managed care paperwork and telephone calls, make sure you set aside the equivalent of one session per week to use for the battle. In addition, you might add a second "session" to complete the necessary marketing or learning skills to build an increasingly larger part of your practice without managed care.

Managed care often effectively devalues our work and, as a result, lowers self-esteem. After all, it's only "talking," right? One meaningful way to fight back is to realize that the managed care organization is trying to make money. That's all—the bottom line. Most MCOs do not care about effective treatment. This point has nothing to do with the importance of our work. If you think about your pro bono patients, current or past, you'll realize that the quality of your work is unrelated to the amount you're getting paid. If you are good at what you do, no managed care organization can take that away from you, no matter how many sessions they may deny.

How to Explain the Ground Rules to Your Patients

Because the initial meeting is such an important part of forming the therapeutic bond, I generally explain the ground rules in the first session so that the patient understands the external factors of managed care and the limitations imposed by lack of confidentiality. Most of them do not realize the limitations created by managed care because they have been educated about the supposed inviolability of the patient–therapist relationship. If you do work with managed care, be careful about what you put into the Outpatient Treatment Report. Remember, this may be with your client *for life*.

In a speech given at "Preserving Psychotherapy," a November, 1995, conference co-sponsored by the National Coalition of Mental Health Professionals and Consumers, Inc. and the Georgia Mental Health Coalition, John Chiaramonte, L.C.S.W., an expert on vendorship and managed care, reminded listeners that the battle is about "advocating for quality care for psychiatric patients, maintaining your integrity as a mental health provider . . . and participating in advancing the evolution from a system which can abuse patients to one which protects consumers. Be clear that above all else, this [fight] is a consumer protection movement." Help your patient to be a good consumer and self-advocate. Include in the treatment process these external managed care factors since it is a reality of their treatment.

How to Fight with Managed Care

If you choose to fight with managed care it may be hazardous to your practice's health. So follow these instructions with discretion. When you call MCOs make sure you get the name of the person with whom you are speaking. Write it down in your records. In the past you would only be given first names: "This is Terri," or "This is Joe." Now they will supply surnames but not necessarily first names which can be a problem if you hear "This is Mr. Smith," or "Mrs. Jones speaking." In a sense, you are on firmer ground than they are. You know that you're working for the well-being of your patients. The managed care organization is working for the well-being of themselves.

If you are calling because you have been denied treatment that you believe is necessary, there are some actions you might take. Request the grounds for refusal. If you are told that treatment is "not medically necessary," ask what it means. Ask for a letter rejecting the request for treatment. Remember that many utilization reviewers are not clinicians so they know only managed care language. If you were working with a patient who came from a different culture (and managed care is a very different culture) you would have to speak in a different manner to be understood. Therefore, use managed care organization-speak in an attempt to get what you need for your patient. Keep in mind that some gatekeepers are limited by company policy as to what they can do. You can always request a review or to speak to a supervisor. Frequently, the utilization reviewers operate from canned speeches.

One way to help establish "medical necessity" when you render an Outpatient Treatment Report, is to keep Axis III of *DSM-IV* in mind. Axis III is the part where you include physical illnesses or problems. If this fits, you can link the physiological difficulty to the treatment you are offering for emotional problems, thus forging a more solid link to "medical necessity."

How Else Can You Fight?

Be aware that these suggestions are hazardous to your managed care practice. Some of them are to be used only when all else has failed and when appropriate. Use your own judgment as an advocate for your consumer/patients.

1. Ask the utilization reviewer how the managed care organization would handle the situation if this patient were suicidal or had a breakdown. How would the company feel if the patient wrote a suicide note naming the managed care organization responsible for the situation?
2. Point out to the managed care organization that longer-term therapy might actually be cheaper. Make a cost-comparison analysis, though don't expect logic to prevail.
3. Find out from the patient's insurance booklet the maximum allocation of sessions and ask for it up front where appropriate. Point out that this might be more cost-effective.
4. If you know that the managed care organization continually allows fewer sessions than advertised, consider a nuisance truth-in-advertising suit.
5. Contact your Better Business Bureau.
6. Tell your State Insurance Commission. This little-used tactic often gets results, particularly in connection with HMOs.

If They Won't Accept You on a Panel

Wait for the law to change. Remember that no matter what legislation your state might pass, if the client's company is self-insured, it is still covered by ERISA, a federal law that supersedes state regulations. However, ERISA regulations will be modified in the near future.

1. Emphasize your specialties or your particular niche.
2. Ask the MCO representative how to keep your application with them. Providers do leave MCOs for many reasons. There will be vacancies.
3. Concentrate on building a practice without managed care.

Building Your Practice without Managed Care

Keep in mind that it isn't as hard to build a practice without managed care as you may think. For one thing, there's a large self-pay market out there. For instance, many people, even if they have insurance, are reluctant to use it given the way in which the safeguarding of confidentiality is overlooked. Other potential self-payers have exhausted their benefits or may not possess any insurance. Some clinicians make financial payment plans in advance with clients based on patient ability to pay. Remember to take into account the amount of time you will not be devoting to paperwork and telephone-waiting if your client is self-pay. According to some recent calculations, about half the money we receive from managed care goes to pay for time spent in nontherapy functions, so that even a cut of 50 percent for private pay patients may not be an actual loss. You must figure this out for yourself.

There are many marketing skills either to learn or to hire someone to do for you. For those who are public relations savvy, you can find numerous no- or low-cost ways to publicize your practice. Be on the lookout for seminars on this topic presented by your professional societies. Many of them are helping their members in this fashion.

Here are some practice-building ideas:

1. Hire a practice consultant.
2. Develop a marketing plan for yourself.
3. Find your own niche, which utilizes your particular skills and let people know about it.
4. Talk to your colleagues about niche marketing. Let them know about who you are and how you practice, emphasizing that your skills may serve as a useful adjunct to their practice. This means finding a tiny piece of the psychotherapy market and adopting it as your niche. It doesn't mean you can't have a general practice, only that you are announcing that this particular molecule is yours. Theoretically, the more you refine your niche, the more unique you are.

For example, I have a background in marketing. The niche I chose when managed care began to eat away at my autonomy and my ability to provide effective treatment for my clients was developing a practice consultant service for my colleagues. Without the advent of managed care it is doubtful I would have moved in this direction. For me, the managed care crisis has presented a real opportunity: I can use the skills of my prior career and still continue to see some clients.

Even More Ways to Fight Back

1. Some clinicians form group practices or guilds which concentrate on the self-pay market. There is much strength and hope to be gained from affiliating with colleagues.
2. Form a clinicians support group to share managed care "horror stories" and work out a strategy of response. As a function of this group you could develop practice marketing ideas to share with each other. Each of you will have his or her own talents, concepts, and experiences to contribute. In addition, your group can collect data for later presentation to press and legislators.
3. I strongly recommend that every clinician and consumer join the National Coalition of Mental Health Professionals and Consumers, Inc., a national grass-roots organization that devotes itself entirely to fighting managed care.
4. Inform your local newspapers and other media about what's going on. More and more national media outlets have been writing about the abuses of managed care and HMOs. Get involved. Write an effective press release. Media is most interested in how managed care affects patients and consumers, so avoid presenting it from a "poor therapist" point of view.
5. Advocate within your professional organizations—insist that they take an anti-managed care stand. Because some clinicians accept the industry and don't want to risk being ousted from panels, our organizational leaders sometimes try to please all members and thus avoid speaking up officially on the topic.
6. Don't leave out the legislative system. Keep in touch constantly with your senators and representatives on local, state, and national levels, asking critical questions vis-à-vis managed care and HMOs.

There are many laws regulating managed care that keep coming up in legislatures all over the country. Find out what *yours* are. Make sure you have an adequate understanding of what each bill says and support the appropriate legislation. Write letters, send e-mail, and sign petitions. Check your professional organizations and see what legislation they are supporting. Let your legislators know how you feel as a professional and as a voter. And keep telling them about it.

John Chiaramonte said in Atlanta, "In order to get politicians to pass laws to protect consumers, it is necessary that they [and we] be thoroughly informed of the problems that exist. To this end it is necessary to get consumers, the press, and advocating organizations involved in continually feeding materials to the legislators. It is essential that we clinicians survive long enough . . . to accomplish this."

Changes are already happening around us. They will continue only if we all fight back. Your world, your practice, and your patients will all go on with or without managed care. Empower yourself and your patients. And to Jill and Jim, those managed care strangers-on-a-train, I hope this discussion can help you, too.

❑ ❑ ❑

NATIONAL COALITION FOR MENTAL HEALTH PROFESSIONALS AND CONSUMERS

Leading the grassroots fight is the National Coalition of Mental Health Professionals and Consumers (NCMHPC) with headquarters on Long Island, New York. Associated with the national group are 15 state coalitions from Maine to Florida and Delaware to California. The major goals of the Coalition are:

- to expose the problems and abuses of managed care and managed competition
- to work toward regulating the industry
- to work toward replacing managed care and managed competition with a pro-patient medical and mental health care system.

Karen Shore, NCMHP President, describes the purpose of the organization:

> Treatment decisions have been taken out of the hands of the psychotherapists and put into the hands of gatekeepers employed by corporations. Humanistic values are being undermined by managed care, which is a concept born out of the idea of reducing costs through competition. Its aim is to industrialize health care. . . . [Under MCO control] . . . we must stand by and watch good treatment be destroyed for profit and see graduate schools cease teaching intensive therapy because they must make their graduates "marketable" to managed-care companies. . . . It is frightening to find ourselves too afraid to protest, and it is profoundly demoralizing to know that we and our patients are merely properties on this industry's mammoth game of Monopoly. What will America do when being a health care professional is no longer tolerable to intelligent, ethical, caring people?
>
> The goals of the organization are the preservation of personal privacy, protection of the integrity and quality of psychotherapy through public and professional education, and legal and legislative actions. The Coalition has been successful in bringing the critical issues to the attention of the public. They are organizing lawsuits against managed care companies and they lobby national and state lawmakers on the need for reform. Every Coalition member receives a lobbying kit as well as periodic bulletins to alert them of important developments in the field. In addition to an annual conference, the Coalition also organizes conferences and political protest campaigns.

"Our wonderful profession, based on empathy, concern, and a love of education and training, is being sacrificed to corporate profits," writes Karen Shore (1995b). "I urge you to join the Resistance."

AMERICAN MENTAL HEALTH ALLIANCE

The American Mental Health Alliance, Inc. (AMHA) is a Massachusetts-based interdisciplinary organization of licensed mental health professionals that makes and manages contracts for mental health and substance abuse treatment services. These contracts are offered directly to businesses, municipalities, government agencies, and other organizations. AMHA is organized as a worker cooperative organization, with policies shaped by its more than seven hundred members. Member-professionals have invested money in AMHA, but earn money only by providing service to clients, not by dividing profits.

The AMHA effort, guided by sound clinical practice, offers an alternative to the current movement to industrialize mental health care for profit. The founders of AMHA believe it is crucial to preserve choice of practitioner and treatment modality, facilitate access to services for patients, preserve the basic rights of patients, including privacy and confidentiality, preserve the curative therapeutic relationship between patient and therapist, and encourage professionals to work in a way that is ethically responsible and consistent with their training. Because AMHA members believe that profit motives often create a conflict between shareholder interests and patient needs, any AMHA surpluses are used to maintain needed reserves, enhance services, and contribute to prevention.

The basic belief of AMHA is that its members, acting in professional collaboration, can provide mental health and substance abuse treatment with true excellence. AMHA principles include protection of an ethical psychotherapy practice, emphasizing the primary responsibility of the therapist to the patient rather than to a third party. AMHA holds that the best treatment decisions are made by an empowered patient–professional dyad. AMHA members handle quality assurance collaboratively and effectively, with no micromanagement of professionals. AMHA has, in addition, made a commitment to doing first-rate research on mental health treatment.

AMHA recognizes the need to develop a national presence in order to make national contracts with multistate companies. At the same time, however, research shows that corporate clients tend to be more satisfied with the performance of locally based health care groups than with those based elsewhere. Thus, it is reasonable to plan autonomous AMHA groups in each state or region, and to link these in a federation that assists its members in organizing and operating. Presently, there are AMHAs in 17 states.

NATIONAL COALITION FOR PATIENTS' RIGHTS

The National Coalition for Patients' Rights is a non-profit organization comprised of medical professionals and concerned citizens dedicated to restoring confidentiality to health care. They work to pass true confidentiality legislation, prevent infringements on privacy, and raise public awareness through advocacy and public education.

The privacy of medical records is being compromised by existing law and societal trends. It is legal for doctors to disclose sensitive information about their patients. This may become mandatory if certain legislation passes. At the same time, many managed care companies and hospitals now computerize patient records and are forming electronic networks to share information.

National Coalition for Patients' Rights is dedicated to strengthening confidentiality in the doctor/patient relationship by:

1. Strictly limiting the amount of clinical information required by insurers for processing claims or determining the need for services.
2. Providing a mechanism for confidential, independent clinical review if insurers dispute treatment necessity.
3. Requiring informed consent from patients for any information to be entered into or accessed from a computer network.
4. Protecting consumers and providers from penalties such as denial of health benefits or imposed fines, for refusing to disclose more extensive data than would be legally required, or for declining to computerize medical information.

CONFIDENTIAL COUNSELING OPTIONS (CCO)

Confidential Counseling Options provides an alternative to selecting a mental health professional from the employment-related plan. HMOs, PPOs, and an increasing number of other types of insurance plans create a situation where mental health decisions are often made by personnel who have no knowledge of therapy or of the client. Through CCO, mental health care is self-directed and private. The duration and frequency of treatment are determined between the client and the therapist. CCO also offers an alternative to the trial-and-error method of choosing a therapist from the telephone directory. An appropriate match between a therapist and client is vital. Consequently, CCO offers access to a network of qualified, independent, and experienced professionals.

CONNECTICUT PSYCHOTHERAPISTS' GUILD

The Connecticut Psychotherapists' Guild is a network of independent psychotherapists concerned about loss of privacy, limitation of treatment choices, and other impacts of managed care on mental health care. They offer consumers detailed information about these impacts and promote alternatives to managed care psychotherapy.

The Guild is organized as a general partnership by the five founding members. In addition, over seventy independent psychotherapists have joined the Guild. A directory is published offering information about Guild values and structure, psychotherapy, controversies surrounding managed care, how to arrange for psychotherapy, and a list of Guild therapists, including their qualifications and special interests. Its goal is to help people make the best decision about their therapy.

BOULDER PSYCHOTHERAPISTS' GUILD, INC.

At the Boulder Psychotherapists' Guild, members have analyzed the managed care crisis and have come to four conclusions:

1. Quality psychotherapy, which holds the client's interests paramount, is often compromised by managed care and the insurance industry's interest in short-term cost reduction.
2. The crisis is likely to get worse for at least a couple of years before it gets better.
3. Economic and political factors guarantee that managed care will continue to be a powerful force in mental health care.
4. One of our best strategies for preserving quality psychotherapy is to increase the pool of self-paying clients.

The Boulder Psychotherapist's Guild is a marketing and referral network for independent, licensed psychotherapists. The network offers professional marketing services in order to promote the profession and inform clients about their options.

THE LEGAL CENTER FOR PATIENT PROTECTION

On the side of quality psychotherapy, professionals in the mental health community have joined with attorneys to establish The Legal Center for Patient Protection in Washington, D.C. Believing that litigation is the major weapon that will make managed care companies accountable for their practices, the organizers of the center have been filing lawsuits against several MCOs on behalf of patients and clinicians. Thus far, legal suits have helped to overcome an ERISA problem and have brought attention to numerous cases of denied benefits. It is hoped that the exposure of MCO abuses will lead to changes that permit psychotherapists to protect their patients and to practice with integrity.

15

Psychotherapy in the 21st Century

The future looks promising for psychotherapists both within health care programs and in private practice. The Bureau of Labor Statistics and the National Research Council (Murray 1996) project growth in demand for psychologists through the coming decade especially in therapy services for children. The Bureau of Labor Statistics placed social work among the top fifteen fields expected to show growth. Researchers at the department of social medicine at Harvard Medical School report increased needs for psychiatrists on an international level (Baldwin 1995). Psychiatric nurses are extending psychotherapy into new areas in hospital based practices (Sherman 1996). Managed care businesses are also establishing overseas branches, even in countries that have nationalized health care. The managed care firm, Value Behavioral Health, as one example, has been developing health care services for companies in Brazil and Spain, and is likely to expand its operations to other countries.

Bridget Murray (1996) notes future trends in psychotherapy in her summary of data related to jobs in the field. Murray acknowledges that the MCOs have affected psychotherapy by limiting sessions and that they are likely to cut mental health contracts even further. On the other hand, managed care is evolving and may become more hospitable toward psychologists. Murray includes the predictions of Ronald Fox, Ph.D., APA's 1994 president and a business consultant in Chapel Hill, North Carolina. Fox (Murray 1996) says that collaboration between psychologists and other health care providers is likely to increase because psychotherapy "lowers health care costs by driving down visits to the family doctor" (p. 52). Physicians will increasingly consult with mental health professionals about the treatment of patients with diabetes, asthma, heart conditions, and other illnesses that require patients to change eating, exercising, and other lifestyle behaviors. Issues related to controlling physical well being, such as weight control and involvement in health maintenance activities, are major growth areas for psychotherapists.

APA Research Director Jessica Kohout, Ph.D. (Murray 1996) observes that the growing ethnic minority populations will need psychotherapists to develop treatment for illnesses, such as cancer and panic disorders, that are culturally sensitive. Psychotherapists will be treating a growing number of elderly people who need help for depression anxieties related to physical disorders and numerous other conditions that emerge in an aging population.

Businesses will call upon psychotherapists to work with problems that impede employee work performance, including alcohol and substance abuse, interpersonal conflicts, and workplace violence. Psychologists who traditionally trained in testing and evaluation will find that this old specialty is reborn in measuring outcomes of various programs and in matching people with jobs, psychotherapy, and training programs. Other areas such as forensics, learning differences, and stress management will be growth areas for psychotherapists.

Kohout points out that increasing numbers of recent graduates in the mental health field are finding work with large health maintenance organizations. At the same time, many psychotherapists are treating patients who want to work on their problems without interference from managed care regulations. Psychoanalysts and psychoanalytic psychotherapists are changing to meet the needs of their patients from different cultures and classes. Psychoanalysis is also changing through considerations of the contributions of theoreticians and clinicians in developing areas such as attachment theory and psychoneurology.

The various disciplines are providing contributions to new psychotherapists and to the growth of traditional psychotherapies. Louis Ormont, Ph.D. (1993), who has taught group therapy methods at several graduate schools and training centers, says that modern group therapy takes shape and form from creative practitioners in every discipline. Stanley Meyers, Ph.D. (1997), Director of Training at the Center for Advancement of Group Studies in New York, predicts even greater growth in the practice of group therapy. Meyers notes that psychotherapists today have the opportunity to offer a range of psychoeducational group activities that have the impact of improving the lives of the participants, although the conditions addressed do not necessarily meet the criteria of MCOs. These workshops are time limited and include themes such as learning to enjoy music and coping with blocks to creativity. These theme-centered workshops serve the purpose of helping people to be comfortable with the group experience and they also open the door to further exploration for people who have been afraid to get the help that they need.

Some psychotherapists will learn to be business managers. They will participate in networking and in marketing their practices. There are others who will develop their practices in fields outside of managed care. It appears that many psychotherapists are choosing to participate in professional groups that demand change in the health care system and that offer alternative plans. Although psychotherapists will need to acknowledge and sometimes adapt to the changing situation for psychotherapy, opportunities will increase for them as they are called upon to address problems ranging from alcoholism and reckless driving to schizophrenia, AIDS, and trauma. Frank De Piano, Ph.D. (Murray 1996), dean of psychological studies at Nova Southeastern University in Fort Lauderdale, Florida, observes that as long as there are problems, there will be no shortage of jobs for psychotherapists.

The managed care industry will change considerably, but it will not disappear. The court system will provide limitations on many of the MCO practices that have frustrated and angered psychotherapists. MCOs will no longer be able to deny that they are making medical decisions by their refusal to provide payment for conditions they decide are not medically necessary. The MCOs are practicing medicine without the license to do so, and that will have to change.

On the other hand, some of the MCOs will continue to grow through mergers and other business techniques. They will, at least for a time, open areas in psychotherapy. As noted previously, MCOs are moving overseas and will need health care procedures for their new branches. MCOs will join together to lobby in Washington and they will develop defense teams and will open new areas as they continue to find ways to expand.

MCO leaders have identified managed care programs for workers' compensation as a major growth area. This is an area where psychotherapists can find opportunities. Over 20 states have passed legislation allowing companies to add managed care to their workers' compensation programs. Mental health care providers in workers' compensation programs will provide assessment, treatment, early intervention, EAP services, case management, and disability management services.

Programs that offer alternative systems to MCOs will also grow. InterStudy, the research organization that includes Paul Ellwood, Jr., will continue to study new plans sponsored by large practices, physician-hospital organizations, and integrated delivery systems.

In the 1960s, Dr. Ellwood promoted health care organizations. His vision of an egalitarian system to provide health care to all in an efficient structure failed to live up to its promise. In the 1990s, Dr. Ellwood contributed to proposals for a managed care system that was designed to promote efficient health care. The variations of managed care business have not worked, either. The National Coalition of Mental Health Professionals and Consumers, under the original leadership of Karen Shore and Joyce Edward, developed ideas for a system of managed cooperation. Perhaps in the next decade Dr. Ellwood will integrate the coalition's plan into his proposals in order to produce a new vision for mental health care delivery.

Computers will continue to bring both benefits and problems to the practice of psychotherapy. There will be increasing opportunities to use computers for keeping records, writing reports and other works, communicating with each other, finding information (including referral information), and exploring innovative ideas. Computers will offer numerous ways to conduct psychotherapy research and even, perhaps, to treat problems with some types of psychotherapy, especially in the area of cognitive behavioral programs.

16

Conclusion

The area of computer use in psychotherapy brings the discussion back to the warnings of *1984*. As the world becomes more and more computer literate, it becomes more difficult to maintain privacy. Are we heading for the day when every therapist's office has a computer screen with a managed care officer overseeing employee psychotherapy sessions? If the therapist's intervention is not in conformance with the established formulary, will the therapy be immediately terminated?

Although the future for psychotherapy does hold promise, there also will be new challenges to professional autonomy by each health care system that comes along. The challenges can be met if psychotherapists are willing to be aware of what is happening them and also willing to participate in taking control of their lives.

Managed care systems will change through legislated controls in some ways that will improve the situation for psychotherapists and through expansion, mergers, and industrial techniques, in ways that will compound difficulties and cause frustration.

Psychotherapists will need to advocate for themselves and for their patients. Psychotherapists, most importantly, will need to be aware of the challenges to their identity and their autonomy. First, psychotherapists need to be aware of the ways in which certain organizations work to achieve their purposes. Orwell certainly intended to warn people of the possible threats to freedom. The threat to freedom to control one's life is especially important for psychotherapists because psychotherapy aims at increasing an individual's freedom to make choices. Within limits, of course, psychotherapist and patient work toward being able to control their lives. It is important to be aware of the ways in which independence is challenged and freedom eroded. It is in the sense of being aware of what is happening to one's self and one's society that Orwell's *1984* provides a warning. As long ago as 1958, David Rapaport (1967) summarized the ways in which the organizations of *1984* challenged the individual's ability to control his or her own life:

> In the world of *Nineteen Eighty-Four*, the individual is robbed of his privacy—the environment invades it. Whenever the individual is alone he is watched through "telescreens"; whenever he is not driven by his work, he is driven by the "telescreen," which constantly bombards him with information and with instructions which he must obey. The language is so simplified that it can convey only factual information and orders; it carries no implications, connotations, allusions, or individual expression. Memory is undermined. When the political alliances of the state change, the books and newspaper files are destroyed and replaced by a revised version which fits the new circumstances. Finally, the fear of unknown but horrible punishment is kept constant. The lack of unobserved privacy coupled with the steady shower of information and orders, the lack of personal expression, the changing records which attack even the continuity vouchsafed by memory, and the mortal fear of punishment, are the means by which the world of *Nineteen Eighty-Four* robs the individual ego of its autonomy and turns the person into an automaton at the command of the environment. [p. 730]

Rapaport not only summed up the dangers of becoming automatons, he pointed to the solution. Human beings need to be involved with others, caring for each other, enlivened by love and participation in our lives and in the issues of our society. Former APA president Frank Farley, Ph.D. (1996) agrees with Rapaport that human beings protect their autonomy through love and involvement. Noting that the public agenda is dominated as much by love and sex as any other agenda, Farley urges psychotherapists to attend to these items. Farley is concerned with the lack of sufficient progress in ethnic and gender issues, but he is optimistic: "Children are more precious. Marriage is more for love. The heralded worldwide economic depression of the 1980s didn't materialize. Our psychological treatments are getting more effective. We're unraveling mysteries of the brain" (p. 775).

Ronald Fox, Ph.D. (1996), a senior partner in Norton, Fox, and Associates, a national consulting firm, calls upon psychotherapists to refute the claims of managed care and insurance industry officials that undermine the profession. The need for psychotherapy service is enormous. Fox says that mental disorders are more prevalent than ever, with about 48 percent of the population indicating a lifetime history of at least one emotional disorder. Of the population of 200 million people about 96 million will suffer an emotional disorder, but almost 60 million will receive no treatment. These numbers are in contrast to the claims made by representatives of MCOs whose profits increase as access to care decreases.

Bryant Welch, J.D., Ph.D. (1996) believes that managed care is terminally ill. He attributes the imminent demise to growing public protests that expose abuses in the system: the erosion of ERISA protection of MCOs from legal liability and the recognition by the courts of illegal MCO practices. Welch and his fellow lawyers are now able to file suits on the bases of malpractice, bad faith insurance denial, tortuous interference with doctor–patient relationships, breach of contract, and other causes of action.

The contributions of Dr. Welch and other lawyers to justice in health care are likely to have enormous impact on MCOs, but as even Welch acknowledges, managed care will not go quietly into the night. More likely, the legal actions will result in the death of certain MCO practices. With parts missing, some MCOs might actually dissolve, but it is likely that the system itself will evolve into another form of managed care.

During this upcoming time period when mental health care systems are coming apart and reforming into other systems, psychotherapists will have the opportunity to advocate for themselves and their patients. The best way to protect the profession is to join both professional organizations and interdisciplinary groups devoted to protecting the integrity and quality of mental health care. It is essential to be alert to the period of time when the managed care industry prepares to start its major changes. During that time, psychotherapists will decide whether they will survive managed care in the 21st century. If this book has only one purpose, it is to help psychotherapists put their skills to work to protect their professional integrity and personal satisfaction. Whether managed care dissolves under the new regulations or evolves into new forms, psychotherapists can survive. However, if therapists want to survive as autonomous professionals, there are specific areas that have to be addressed. Psychotherapists need to join their colleagues in educating the public about what psychotherapy can offer, in acting to preserve privacy and confidentiality, in developing and supporting principals for mental health care delivery systems, and in effecting legislation that protects mental health professionals and their patients. Through these means, psychotherapists will continue to practice our honorable and effective profession.

REFERENCES

Abrom, E. M. (1993). *The Freedom of the Self.* New York: Plenum Press.

Alderman, E., and Kennedy, C. (1995). *The Right to Privacy.* New York: Knopf.

Alpert, B. (1996). Wellcare management group: conflicting accounts. *Barron's*, March 18, p. 19.

AMBHA data documents growth of managed care (1996). *Mental Health Report*, April 6, p. 60.

American Board of Vocational Experts (1996). Fall Conference. Glenview, IL.

American Heritage Dictionary (1995). *The People's Chronology: Microsoft Bookshelf '95* [Computer program]. Microsoft Corporation.

American Medical Association (1996). *Current Procedural Terminology* (*CPT*). Chicago.

American Psychological Association (1992a). Ethical principles of psychologists and code of conduct. *American Psychologist* 47:1597–1611.

—— (1992b). Report of the ad hoc Task Force on Psychopharmacology of the American Psychological Association. Washington, DC: American Psychological Association.

—— (1992c). *PsychINFO Psychological Abstracts Information Services Users Reference Manual.* Washington, DC: American Psychological Association.

Anderson, F. (1996). The ethical basis of clinical confidentiality. British Medical Association Report. The Electronic Privacy Information Center [WWW document]. URL *http://www.epic.org/*, January 12.

Angier, N. (1996). Variant gene tied to a love of new thrills. *The New York Times*, January 2, p. A1, B11.

Anonymous (1995). The horrors of HMOs. Psych Central [WWW document]. URL: *http://www.coil.com/~grohol/*

Anthony, J. (1993). Who's reading your medical records? *American Health*, November, pp. 56–58.

Antonucci, D. (1996). Separating good marketing from good science. *The National Psychologist 5*, September, pp. 14–15.

Appelbaum, P. S. (1993). Legal, liability and managed care. *American Psychologist* 48 (3):251–257.

Appleby, E., Jr. (1995). Managed care extra: Who profits? Mental Health Net [WWW document]. URL *http:www.cmhcsys/mhn.htm.*

Asher, J., and Weeks, M. (1996). Scientists close in on multiple gene sites for manic depressive illness [WWW document]. URL *http://www.nimh.nih.gov/*, April 1.

Astrom, M. (1996). Generalized anxiety disorder in stroke patients. *Stroke* 27:270–275.

Austin, C. D. (1993). Case management: a systems perspective. *Journal of Contemporary Human Services* 74:451–459.

Bacha, S. M. (1995). Medicaid managed care: A looming boon or bust? *National Psychologist*, May/June, pp. 16–17.

Baek, S. (1994). The confidentiality conundrum. *Managed Healthcare*, April, pp. 52–53.

Bail, B. (1981). To practice one's art. In *Do I Dare Disturb the Universe: A Memorial to W. R. Bion*, ed. J. S. Grotstein. London: Karnac.

Baker, R. (1996). Harry! Louise! You lied. *The New York Times*, June 1, p. 19.

Baldwin, J. (1995). Our global village: report puts mental health on the international agenda. *Psychiatric Times 12*, August, p. 1, 21.

Baranger, M., and Baranger, W. (1981). Insight in the analytic situation. In *Classics in psychoanalytic technique*, ed. R. Langs, pp. 383–390. New York: Jason Aronson.

Barasch, R. (1996). Beware: stepped up fraud investigations include mental health providers. *National Psychologist*, March/April, p. 11.

Barr, S. (1993). Patient databases have placed privacy on its death bed. *The Washington Post*, available at America Online: keyword: Magazine Stand.

Barron, J. W., and Sands, H., eds. (1996). *Impact of Managed Care on Psychodynamic Treatment*. Madison, CT: International Universities Press.

Baum, L. A., and Pounds, B. G., eds. (1994). *The National Directory of Psychotherapy Training Institutes*. New York: Brunner/Mazel.

Beck, A. F. (1976). *Cognitive Therapy and the Emotional Disorders*. New York: International Universities Press.

Beck, A., Rush, J., Shaw, B., and Emery, G. (1979). *Cognitive Treatment of Depression*. New York: Guilford.

Beck, M. (1996). Follow the money. *Newsweek*, May 20, pp. 26–28.

Belar, C., and Deardorff, W. (1995). *Clinical Health Psychology: A Practitioner's Guidebook*. Washington, DC: American Psychological Association.

Bennahum, D. (1995). Docs for docs. Wired [WWW document]. URL: *http://www.hotwired.com/wired/*, March 31.

Bennett, M. J. (1988). The greening of the HMO: implications for prepaid psychiatry. *American Journal of Psychiatry* 145 (12):1544–1549.

Berkowitz, A. (1996). Our genes, ourselves? *Bioscience* 46 (1):42–52.

Berman, P. C. (1996). Judges balk when MCOs favor own financial health over patient well-being. *National Psychologist*, January/February, pp. 10–11.

Bias from gene tests feared (1995). *Newsday*, September 30, p. A4.

Biddle, N., Miller, S., Beals, C. K., and Hager, M. (1996). *Newsweek*, May, pp. 20–23.

Bion, W. R. (1959/1974). *Experiences in Groups*. New York: Ballantine Books, Inc.

Blanck, G., and Blanck, R. (1992). *American Object Relations*. Cape Cod Conference. Eastham, MA: New England Educational Institute.

Blascovich, J., and Katkin, E. (1993). *Cardiovascular Reactivity to Psychological Stress and Disease*. Washington, DC: American Psychological Association.

Blazer, D. (1994). *Intervention Strategies for Emotional Problems in Later Life*. Northvale, NJ: Jason Aronson.

Blue Cross and Blue Shield Association (1996). Who*Where*What*Key Competitors*How much [WWW document]. URL *http://pathfinder.com*.

Bollas, C., and Sundelson, D. (1995). *The New Informants: The Betrayal of Confidentiality in Psychoanalysis and Psychotherapy*. Northvale, NJ: Jason Aronson.

Bonstedt, T. (1992). Managing psychiatric exclusions. In *Managed Mental Health Care*, ed. J. Feldman and R. Fitzpatrick, pp. 69–82. Washington, DC: American Psychiatric Press.

Bowermaster, D. (1996). A last try at health reform. *U.S. News and World Report*, May 6, pp. 68–69.

Bowman, A. C. (1994). Integrated marketing. *Target Marketing Strategies for Managed Care Payers* (Conference proceedings). Health Care and Insurance Institute, Division of Institute for International Research, New York.

Bowman, L. (1993). The paperless future of health care. Mercury Center [WWW document]. URL *http://www.sjmercury.com/main.htm.*

Boyd-Franklin, N., Steiner, G. L., and Boland, M. C. (1995). *Children, Families and HIV/AIDS.* New York: The Guilford Press.

——, eds. (1995). *Treatment of HIV/AIDS Patients and Families.* New York: Guilford.

Breckenridge, C. (1995). President's Report. *National Federation of Societies for Clinical Social Work, Inc. Progress Report*, December, p. 3.

Broadhead, W. E., Leon, A., Weissman, M. M. et al. (1995). Development and validation of the SDDS-PC screen for multiple mental disorders in primary care. *Archives of Family Medicine, 4*, pp. 211–219.

Brod, E. (1996). Psychotherapist has duty to maintain privacy [Letter to the editor]. *The New York Times*, May 26, section 4, p. 12.

Browning, C. H., and Browning, B. J. (1993). *How to Partner with Managed Care.* Los Alamitos, CA: Duncliff's International.

Bunis, D. (1996). Do insurers care enough? *Newsday*, April 8, p. A4, A21.

Cadwell, S. A., Burnam, R. A., Jr., and Forstein, M. (1994). *Therapists on the Front Line.* Washington, DC: American Psychiatric Press.

Chiaramonte, J. (1995). New markets opened to clinical social workers. *The Clinician*, Fall, pp. 6–7.

Chipman, A. (1995). Meeting managed care: an identity and value crisis for therapists. *American Journal of Psychotherapy* 49 (4):558–567.

Chogyam Trungpa, Rinpoche (1983). Creating an environment of sanity. *Naropa Institute Journal of Psychology* 2:1–10.

Chopra, D. (1996). Journey to the boundless. Workshop presented at the Omega Institute for Holistic Studies, Chair, G. Kaufman, May. New York: Rhinebeck.

Church, G. J. (1994). Health care: Oh Noooo! Time Domestic Online [WWW document]. URL *http://pathfinder.com*, March 14.

Cieplinski, F. (1993). *Jewish Identity Through Literature.* New York: Jay Street Publishers.

Clay, R. (1996). Religion is the backbone of black life. *APA Monitor*, August, p. 46.

—— (1996). Psychologists may be less cynical of religion. *APA Monitor*, August, p. 48.

Clebsch, W. A., and Jaekle, C. (1995). *Pastoral Care in Historical Perspective.* Northvale, NJ: Jason Aronson.

Cohen, R. (1996). God, help me. *New Yorker*, June 3, p. 94.

College on Problems of Drug Dependence (1994). Drug abuse research and the health of the nation [WWW document]. URL: *http://freenet.vcu.edu/health/vatc/fact1.txt.*

Colwell, C. (1996). Computerizing your practice. *Nassau Newsnotes*, June, pp. 5, 11, 13.

Commission for Case Manager Certification (1996). *CCM Certification Guide.* Rolling Meadows, IL: Commission for Case Management Certification.

Computers and your health care records (1994). *Consumer's Research*, April, pp. 33–36.

Cooke, R. (1995). Tracing roots: genetic link to breast cancer for Jews. *Newsday*, August 30, p. A7.

Court: Benefits deceit merits trial (1996). *Newsday*, March 30, pp. 49, 51.

Cox, F., and Cox, L. (1996). *A Conscious Life*. Berkeley: Conari Press.

Culture and ideas (1996). *U.S. News & World Report*, September 2, p. 14.

Daly, R. (1996a). *The demise of ethics in the era of managed care: A phenomenological analysis of the impact of managed care of the psychoanalytic space*. Paper presented at a meeting of the Alumni Association of the Psychoanalytic Center for Communicative Psychoanalysis, New York, NY, May.

—— (1996b). Personal communication, March 16.

Davidson, T., and Davidson J. R. (1995). Cost-containment, computers and confidentiality. *Clinical Social Work Journal* 23 (4):453–463.

DeAngelis, T. (1996). Psychoanalysis adapts to the 1990s. *The American Psychological Association Monitor*, September, pp. 1, 43.

Deffenbacher, J. (1995). Ideal treatment package for adults with anger disorders. In *Anger Disorders*, ed. H. Kassanove, pp. 151–171. Washington, DC: Taylor & Francis.

DeLeon, P. H. (1995). Proceedings of the American Psychological Association Incorporated, for the year 1995. *American Psychologist* 50:633–682.

DeLeon, P. H., and Wiggins, J. G., Jr. (1996). Prescription privileges for psychologists. *American Psychologist* 51(3):225–229. *(SCID-I/P, Version 2.0.)* New York: New York State Psychiatric Institute.

DelPizzo, L. (1996). Personal communication, June 3.

Denkers, G., and Clifford, R. (1994). *A Survey of Psychologists' Experiences with Managed Care: Consumer issues*. San Mateo, CA: San Francisco Bay Area Psychologists Task Force on Managed Care.

Dentzer, S. (1996). Shedding light on managed care. *U.S. News & World Report*, May 6, p. 70.

deShazer, S. (1991). *Putting Differences to Work*. New York: Norton.

deShazer, S., and Berg, I. K. (1988). *Investigating Solutions in Brief Therapy*. New York: Norton.

De Zulueta, F. (1994). *From Pain to Violence*. Northvale, NJ: Jason Aronson.

Diagnostic and Statistical Manual of Mental Disorders (1994). 4th ed. Washington, DC: American Psychiatric Association.

Does therapy help? (1995). *Consumer Reports*, November, pp. 734–739.

Dolnick, E. (1996). Death by HMO. *Glamour*, February, pp. 161, 208–210.

Domash, L. (1994). *A Winnocottian Analyst Meets Managed Care*. Paper presented at the Seventh Biennial Conference of the Psychoanalytic Society of the Postdoctoral Programs, Inc. on the Changing Cultural Contexts of Psychoanalysis, New York, NY, March 5.

Dreyfuss, R., and Stone, P. H. (1996). MediKill. *Mother Jones*, January/February, pp. 22–27, 77–81.

Dworkin, M., and Cullen, M. (1996). Eye movement desensitization and reprocessing and EAP. *EAPA Exchange*, July/August, pp. 18–19.

Eastman, P. (1996). "Blues" pioneer new managed care pediatric network. *Oncology Times*, June, p. 1, 34–37.

Eaton, L. (1996). Aetna to buy U.S. Healthcare in big move to managed care. *The New York Times*, April 2, pp. A1, D8.

Ellis, A. (1995). Forward. H. Kassanove (Ed.). *Anger Disorders*. Washington, DC: Taylor and Francis.

Ellis, A. E. (1994). *Reason and Emotion in Psychotherapy. Revised and updated.* New York: Carol Publishing.

Ellwood, P., Jr. (1996). How doctors can regain control of health care. *Medical Economics*, May 13, pp. 178–192.

Elmer-Dewitt, P. (1996). The genetic revolution. *Time* 143:46–52.

EPIC (1995). Principles for federal privacy protection of medical records. The Electronic Privacy Information Center [WWW document]. URL *http://www.epic.org/*.

—— (1996a). Medical privacy public opinion polls. The Electronic Privacy Information Center [WWW document]. URL *http://www.epic.org/*.

—— (1996b). Who owns personal information? Anatomy of a privacy case. The Electronic Privacy Information Center [WWW document]. URL *http://www.epic.org/*.

—— (1996c). Threats to medical record privacy. The Electronic Privacy Information Center [WWW document]. URL *http://www.epic.org/*.

Erikson, E. H. (1950). *Childhood and Society*. New York: W. W. Norton.

Erikson, J. (1996). Increasing focus on families and physicians struggling against HMO cost-containment. *Oncology Times XVIII*, June, pp. 1, 34–40.

Facts about ERISA (1995). *National Psychologist*, January/February, p. 15.

Farley, F. (1996). From the heart. *American Psychologist 51*, August, pp. 772–776.

Feindler, E. L. (1995). Ideal treatment package for children and adolescents with anger disorders. In *Anger Disorders*, ed. H. Kassanove, pp. 173–174. Washington, DC: Taylor & Francis.

First, M. B., Gibbon, M., Williams, J. B., and Spitzer, R. L. (1995). *MiniSCID, Version 2.* North Tonawanda: NYMHS.

First, M. B., Spitzer, R. L., Williams, J. B., and Gibbon, M. (1995). *Structured Clinical Interview for DSM-IV Axis I Disorders–Patient Edition (SCID-I/P, Version 2.0.)* New York: New York State Psychiatric Institute.

Fisher, L. M. (1996). Don't call it Healthscape, and it's not a Web site. *The New York Times*, June 18, p. A1.

Flower, J. (1994a). The other revolution in health care, Part 1. Wired [WWW document]. URL: *http://www.hotwired.com/wired/*, April 18.

—— (1994b). The other revolution in health care, Part 2. Wired [WWW document]. URL: *http://www.hotwired.com/wired/*, April 18.

Flynn, L. M. (1995). The impact of managed care. NAMI [WWW document] URL *http://www.cais.com/vikings/nami/index/html*, April 18.

Former first ladies pitch for reform as national poll shows backing for mental health (1994). *National Psychologist*, May/June, p. 4.

Forslund, D., and Kilman, D. (1996). The virtual patient record: A key to distributed health care and telemedicine [WWW document]. URL *http://www.acl.lanl.gov/telemedicine/virtual.html*, February 29.

Fox, R. E. (1996). Charlatism, scientism, and psychology's social contract. *American Psychologist 51*, August, pp. 777–784.

—— (1994). Managed care: APA's president looks for productive approaches. *Psychotherapy Finances*, June, p. 1.

Frank, R. (1993). Health-care reform: an introduction. *American Psychologist* 48: 258–260.

Freiberg, P. (1996). APA supports a range of efforts to address HIV/AIDS. *American Psychological Association Monitor*, June, p. 34.

Freud, S. (1927). *The Future of an Illusion*. New York: Norton.

Freudenheim, M. (1994). Insurance companies expect battle over health care to shift to the states. *The New York Times*, October 23, p. A22.

—— (1996a). Managed care empires in the making. *The New York Times*, April 2, pp. C1, D1.

—— (1996b). H.M.O.'s cope with a backlash on cost cutting. *The New York Times*, May 19, pp. A1, A22.

Friedman, W. H. (1994). *How To Do Groups*. Northvale, NJ: Jason Aronson.

Fromm, E. (1961). Afterword to G. Orwell's (1949/1981) *1984*. New York: Penguin Books, pp. 257–267.

Gallagher, M., and Seltz, C. (1996). New study highlights five-year trends in benefits. Hewitt Associates LLC [WWW document]. URL *http://www.hewittassoc.com*, March 11.

Gallinari, K. L. (1995). Voices: Viewpoint: Relieving insurance pain for patients and courts. *The New York Times*, November 5, p. 11.

Gallo, N. (1994). Safeguarding your medical records. *Better Homes and Gardens* 72 (9):42–46.

Garfinkel, S. (1995). Separating Equifax from fiction, Part 1 & 2. Wired [WWW document]. URL: *http://www.hotwired.com/wired/*.

Garfinkel, Wild, and Travis, P. C. (1996). Personal communication, October 25.

Garrett, L. (1996). Dose of reality: drugs expensive. *Newsday*, June 15, p. A7.

Gatchel, R., and Blanchard, E. (1993). *Psychophysiological Disorders: Research and Clinical Applications*. Washington, DC: American Psychological Association.

Gatz, M., and Smyer, M. A. (1992). The mental health system in older adults in the 1990s. *American Psychologist* 47:741–751.

Geier, T. (1996). Culture and ideas. *U.S. News & World Report 121*, September 2, p. 14.

Ginott, H. G. (1961). *Group Psychotherapy with Children*. Northvale, NJ: Jason Aronson.

Glazer, D. (1994a). U.S. Healthcare profits. *NYSPA Newsgram* 2:4.

—— (1994b). VBH drops providers. *NYSPA Newsgram* 2:2.

Golan, N. (1986). Crisis theory. In *Social Work Treatment: Interlocking Theoretical Approaches*, ed. F. J. Turner, pp. 296–340. New York: Free Press.

Goldberg, C. (1991). *Understanding Shame*. Northvale, NJ: Jason Aronson.

—— (1996). Tort reform: A need or hoax? Long Island Commercial Review. The Electric Library [On-line service]. URL: *http://www.elibrary.com/*.

Goldberg, J., ed. (1981). *Psychotherapeutic Treatment of Cancer Patients*. New York: Free Press.

Goleman, D. (1993). What you reveal to a psychotherapist may go further. *The New York Times*, April 14, p. C12.

Goodman, M., Brown, J., and Dietz, P. (1992). *Managing Managed Care: A Mental Health Practitioner's Survival Guide*. Washington, DC: American Psychiatric Press.

Gorman, C. (1995). The doctor's crystal ball. *Time*, April 10, pp. 60–63.

—— (1996). Big brother wants you healthy. *Time*, May 6, p. 60.

Gray, G. V., and Glazer, W. M. (1995). Defining medical necessity in mental health. *Behavioral Health Management* 15(1):28–30.

Gray, P. (1996). Gagging the doctors. *Time*, January 8, p. 50.

Greenhouse, L. (1996). Justices uphold patient privacy with therapist. *The New York Times*, June 14, pp. A1, A25.

Griest, J. (1990). Treatment of obsessive compulsive disorder: psychotherapies, drugs, and other somatic treatment. *Journal of Clinical Psychiatry* 51:44–50.

Greist, J. H., Gustafson, D. H., Stauss, F. F., et al (1973). A computer interview for suicide risk prediction. *American Journal of Psychiatry* 30:1327–1332.

Grohol, J. M. (1995). Why managed care hurts you. Psych Central [WWW document]. URL: *http://www.coil.com/~grohol/*

Gruntal & Co. (1996). Healthcare and medical service growth trust. Hewlett, NY: Gruntal & Co. (Advertising brochure).

Haley, J., ed. (1985). *Conversations with Milton H. Erickson, M.D., Volume II, Changing Couples.* New York: Triangle Press.

Hamilton, J. (1995). Medicine's new weapon: Data. Business Week [WWW document]. URL: *http://www.businessweek.com/bwol.htm,* March 16.

Hammonds, K. (1996). The patient is stable—for now. *Business Week* [WWW document]. URL: *http://www.businessweek.com/bwol.htm,* January 8.

Havens, R. A., and Walters, C. (1989). *Hypnotherapy Scripts: A Neo-Ericksonian Approach to Persuasive Healing.* New York: Brunner/Mazel.

HB 2147 (1995). Medical records—access by patient [WWW document]. URL *http://www.state.va.us/dlas/ses19951/subjects/sbj032.htm,* July 1.

Health care privacy protection act (1996). NFSCSW [WWW document]. URL *http://www.webcom.com/nfscsw/.*

Health Care Reform Newsletter (1995). [WWW document]. URL *http://www.physics.fsu.edu/~/wv/lwv-tlh/HealthCare/2nd/.*

Health Care Systems Committee (1996a). "Gag Clauses" banned. NFSCSW [WWW document]. URL *http://www.webcom.com/nfscsw/.*

—— (1996b). Analyst predicts HMO winners. NFSCSW [WWW document]. URL *http://www.webcom.com/nfscsw/.*

Herndon, P., ed. (1996). Practice Pointer: A basic map for psychologists to the information superhighway. *Practitioner Update of the APA Practice Directorate* 4, October, p. 3.

Hillowe, B. (1996). Personal communication, April 19.

Himelstein, L. (1994). Attack of the cyber snoopers. *Business Week*, available at America Online: keyword: Magazine Stand.

How will the new parity law affect psychologists? (1997). *New York State Psychologist*, December, p. 10.

Howard, K., Kopta, S. M., Krause, M. S., and Orlinsky, D. E. (1986). The dose–effect relationship in psychotherapy. *American Psychologist* 41(2):159–164.

Howry, M. (1995). Tort reform: Is the system broken?: Who wins with reform? Proponents say it's the taxpayers, foes say it's insurers (Fourth in a four-part series). The Columbus Daily Reporter [WWW document]. URL *http://sddt.com/~columbus/Files2/tort.html,* December 29.

Hoyt, M. F. (1994). *Constructive Therapies.* New York: Guilford.

—— (1995). *Brief Therapy and Managed Care: Readings for Contemporary Practice.* San Francisco: Jossey-Bass.

Hullett, J. (1996). Personal communication, February 14.

Hymowitz, C. (1995). High anxiety: In the name of Freud, why are psychiatrists complaining so much? *The Wall Street Journal*, December 21, pp. 1, A6.

IBM Healthcare (1995). Finding fraud [WWW document]. URL *http://www.solutions.ibm.com/healthcare/*.

Iglehart, J. (1966). Managed care and mental health. *Health Policy Report* 334(2):131–136.

IN Jersey (1996). America '96: Hopes and Fears [WWW document]. URL *http://www.njw.injersey.com/*.

Interdisciplinary Committee for "Consumers Right to Know" Mental Health Legislation (1995). *Overview of "Consumer's Right to Know Legislation."* (Available from Ivan J. Miller, Ph.D., 350 Broadway, Suite 210, Boulder, Colorado 80303.)

International Classification of Diseases, 9th revision, Clinical Modification (ICD-9-CM), (1989). U.S. Department of Health and Human Services, HCFA, DHHS. Publication No., (PH.S) 89-1260.

Jackim, L. W. (1993). *A Legal Primer for Psychotherapists and Counselors*. Providence, RI: Manisses Communications Group, Inc.

James, B. (1989). *Treating Traumatized Children: New Insights, Creative Interventions*. Lexington, Massachusetts: Lexington Books.

James, W. (1902). *The Varieties of Religious Experience*. New York: Macmillan.

—— (1931). The importance of individuals. In *The will to believe and other essays in popular philosophy*, pp. 255–262. New York: Longmans, Green. (Original work published 1890.)

Jannes, J. J. (1996). *Short-Term, Problem-Focused Therapy*. Presentation before the Child and Family Consultation Group in New York, NY, April.

Johnson, K. (1996). In New York, Aetna will be understudy. *New York Times*, April 2, p. D8.

Jung, C. G. (1938/1967). *Collected Works*. Princeton, NJ: Princeton University Press.

—— (1956). *Symbols of Transformation*. New York: Pantheon.

Juster, I. (1966). What is "medical necessity"? *Coalition Report*, March/April, p. 9.

Kahr, B. (1996). *Breaches of confidentiality in the history of psycho-analysis*. Unpublished manuscript.

Kalous, T. D. (1996). Managed care is here to stay [Letter to the editor]. *APA Monitor*, February, p. 3.

Kassanove, H., and Eckhardt, C. (1995). An anger model and a look to the future. In *Anger Disorders*, ed. H. Kassanove, pp. 197–203. Washington, DC: Taylor & Francis.

Kassanove, H., and Sukhodolsky, D. G. (1995). Anger disorders: Basic science and practice issues. In *Anger Disorders*, ed. H. Kassanove, pp. 1–26. Washington, DC: Taylor & Francis.

Kiesler, C. A. (1992). U.S. mental health policy. *American Psychologist* 47:1077–1082.

Kilborn, P. T. (1996). Tucson H.M.O.'s may offer model for medicare's future. *The New York Times*, March 26, pp. A1, B11.

King, M. B. (1993). *AIDS, HIV and Mental Health*. Cambridge, England: Cambridge University Press.

Klerman, G. L., Weissman, M. M., Rounsaville, B. J., and Chevron, E. S. (1994). *Interpersonal Psychotherapy of Depression*. Northvale, NJ: Jason Aronson.

Kliman, A. S. (1986). *Crisis: Psychological First Aid*. Northvale, NJ: Jason Aronson.

Kluge, E. (1994). Health information, privacy, confidentiality and ethics. *International Journal of Bio-Medical Computing* 35(1):23–27.

Koback, K. A., Greist, J. H., and Jefferson, J. W. (1996). Clinical computing for physicians and patients. *Psychiatric Clinics of North America: Annual of Drug Therapy* 3:1–12.

Koback, K. A., Reynolds, W. M., and Greist, J. H. (1994). Computerized and clinician assessment with depression and anxiety: respondent evaluation and satisfaction. *Journal of Personality Assessment* 63:173–180.

Kolata, G. (1995). When patients' records are commodities for sale. *The New York Times*, November 15, p. A1.

Kolmansberger, K. (1996). Personal communication, January 3.

Koop, C. E. (1996). Manage with care. *Time* 148 (Special Issue), p. 69.

Kornblum, W., and Julian, J. (1995). *Social Problems*, 8th ed. Englewood Cliffs, NJ: Prentice-Hall.

Kroft, S. (1996). Do You Really Want to Know? (H. A. Radcliffe, Producer). *60 Minutes*. New York: Columbia Broadcasting Service.

Kronish, E., ed. (1994). Four approaches to psychoanalytic treatment today. *Issues in Psychoanalytic Psychology* 16(2). New York: Washington Square Institute.

LaBruzza, A. (1994). *Using DSM-IV*. Northvale, NJ: Jason Aronson.

Landers, S. (1996). Billing: The ethical, legal price tags. *NASW News*, March, pp. 3–4.

Langs, R. (1973). *The Technique of Psychoanalytic Psychotherapy*. New York: Jason Aronson.

—— (1976). *The Bipersonal Field*. New York: Jason Aronson.

—— (1978). *Technique in Transition*. New York: Jason Aronson.

—— (1979). *The Supervisory Experience*. New York: Jason Aronson.

—— (1982). *Psychotherapy: A Basic Text*. New York: Jason Aronson.

—— (1988). *A Primer of Psychotherapy*. New York: Gardner.

Lardiere, M. (1996). Personal communication, April 25.

Lazo, S. (1995). New drugs, Medco right Rx for Merck: payout rises for 20th year in a row. *Barron's*, July 31, p. N40.

Leahy, R. (1996). *Cognitive Therapy: Basic Principles and Applications*. Northvale, NJ: Jason Aronson.

Lewin, T. (1996). Questions of privacy roil arena of psychotherapy. *The New York Times*, May 22, A1, D20.

Lewis, N. (1996). Two marines who refused to comply with genetic-testing order. *The New York Times*, April 13, p. 7.

Lewyn, M. (1994). You can run, but it's rough to hide from marketers. Business Week [WWW document]. URL: *http://www.businessweek.com/bwol.htm*, December 10.

Lichtman, R. M. (1996). Division on addicts. *New York State Psychological Association Notebook*, p. 20.

Littlejohn, S. (1995). HCLA joins Gingrich in seeking stronger legal reform. The Health Care Liability Alliance [WWW document]. URL *http://www.wp.com/hcla/hclanews.htm*, June 21.

Lonky, N. M. (1995). Future possibilities in the managed care marketplace. Mental Health Net [WWW document]. URL *http://www.cmhcsys.com/mhn.htm*, December 18.

Lowman, R. L., and Resnick, R. J., eds. (1994). *The Mental Health Professional's Guide to Managed Care*. Washington, DC: American Psychological Association.

Lykken, D., and Tellegen, A. (1996). Is happiness inherited? *APA Monitor*, August, pp. 51–53.

Magnusson, P. (1996). Even Clinton is embracing medical savings accounts. *Business Week* [On-line], Available Dec. 19: *http://www.businessweek.com/*.

Maier, T. (1996). Doctors lose suit on Aetna Managed Care. *Newsday*, May 30, p. 8.

Marlatt, A. (1996). *Relapse prevention and harm reduction*. Presentation at New York State Psychological Association on Addicts Program, October.

Maslow, A. H. (1970). *Motivation and Personality* (2nd ed.). New York: Harper and Row.

Matos, A. (1982). *The Big Apple Diet*. Millbrae, CA: Celestial Arts.

Matus, H. (1996). Current healthcare issues. Paper presented at the meeting of the Center for the Communicative Psychoanalysis and Psychotherapy at the Bleuler Psychotherapy Center, Forest Hills, NY, January.

May, T. (1995). Tort reform: Is the system broken?: Medical aspect of reform effort pits physicians against lawyers (Third in a four-part series). The Columbus Daily Reporter [WWW document]. URL *http://sddt.com/~columbus/Files2/tort.html*, December 28.

McBride, S. (1996). Referral penalty on physicians to be limited. *The Wall Street Journal*, March 27, p. B6.

McCall, T. B. (1996). Some HMOs are bad news. *Redbook*, August, pp. 47–48.

McDade, R. (1996). Resources available from the HIV/AIDS Information Service. *Brochure at the Newburgh Free Library*, Newburgh, NY.

Medical Records Institute (1995a). Information about the Medical Records Institute [WWW document]. URL *http://www.medrecinst.com*.

—— (1995b). What is an electronic patient record? [WWW document]. URL *http://www.medrecinst.com*.

The Medicare News Brief (1996). *MNB*, December, pp. 1–8.

Meehan, B. (1996). From comfort to chaos. In *Impact of Managed Care on Psychodynamic Treatment*, ed. J. W. Barron and H. Sands, p. 73. Madison, CT: International Universities Press.

Meeks, B. N. (1994). Privacy is my life. Wired [WWW document]. URL: *http://www.hotwired.com/wired/*.

Mendez-Villarrubia, J. M. (1994). A. La Bruzza with J. M. Mendez-Villarrubia. *Using DSM-IV*. Northvale, NJ: Jason Aronson.

Merit Behavioral Care Corporation (1996). Fact Sheet, September, p. 2.

Meyers, S. (1997). Personal communication, Jan. 5.

Microsoft Corporation (1994a). Medicine, 1954. *The People's Chronology: Microsoft Bookshelf '95* [Computer program].

—— (1994b). Medicine, 1964. *The People's Chronology: Microsoft Bookshelf '95* [Computer program].

—— (1994c). Medicine, 1988. *The People's Chronology: Microsoft Bookshelf '95* [Computer program].

Miller, D. (1986). *Attack on the Self*. Northvale, NJ: Jason Aronson.

Miller, I. (1994). *What Managed Care is Doing to Outpatient Mental Health: A Look Behind the Veil of Secrecy*. Boulder, CO: Boulder Psychotherapists' Press.

—— (1995). *Managed Care is Harmful to Outpatient Mental Health Services: A Call for Accountability*. Boulder, CO: Boulder Psychotherapists' Press.

Milner, M. (1957). *On Not Being Able to Paint*. New York: International Universities Press.

Mitchell, A. (1996). Despite his reversals, Clinton stays centered. *The New York Times*. July 28, p. 1, 28.

Monohon, C. (1993). *Children and Trauma: A Parent's Guide to Helping Children Heal*. New York: Lexington Books, Maxwell Macmillan.

Morin, S., chair (1995). Five Year Report of the Policy and Planning Board, 1994. *American Psychologist* 50:620–632.

Moritsugu, K. (1996). Gene discrimination bills pass. *Newsday*, June 20, p. A19.

Murray, B. (1996). Students' future is rosier than they think. *APA Monitor*, September, p. 52.

Nadler, E. R. (1995). *Behavioral health measurements on outcomes and accountability*. Paper presented at the OPS/Behavioral HealthCare of New York Seminar, Kingston, NY, June 27.

—— (1996). *A proposal for the provision of demand management services*. Unpublished manuscript.

Nagel, D. (1995). Medical privacy? Technology is eroding confidentiality. *Newsday*, October 27, p. A7.

—— (1996). Personal communication, June 8.

Nagel, D. M., and Breitenstein, A. G. (1996). The end of personal medical privacy [Letter to the editor]. *Wall Street Journal*, June 7, p. A13.

NASW News (1996a). Managed care study reports therapy lead. 41(5):1.

—— (1996b). Nicole Brown disclosures draw discipline. 41(5):6.

—— (1996c). Supreme Court upholds social work privilege. 41(8):1.

National advocate's report (1996). NFSCSW national advocate's legislative updates and alerts [WWW document]. URL *http://www.webcom.com/nfscsw/lobby/updates.htm.*

Nau, D. (1996). Managed care utilization review. Mental Health Net [WWW document]. URL *http://www.cmhcsys.com/mhn.htm.*

NewsPage (1996a). HMO enrollment picking up speed; Medicare and Medicaid patients ensure that growth will continue [On-line service]. URL *http://www.newspage.com/*, March 27.

—— (1996b). Mercator Genetics establishes international clinical collaborations in Finland, Denmark, and Isreal [On-line service]. URL *http://www.newspage.com/*, April 22.

—— (1996c). Neurocrine Biosciences forms Canadian research and development company [On-line service]. URL *http://www.newspage.com/*, April 22.

—— (1996d). New Jersey psychologists file precedent-setting lawsuit against managed care company [On-line service]. URL *http://www.newspage.com/*, April 22.

—— (1996e). Blue Cross of California/CaliforniaCare Health Plans offers electronic claims program to all Prudent Buyer Plan Providers [On-line service]. URL *http://www.newspage.com/*, April 25.

—— (1996f). Electronic filing of claims opens new vistas for fraud [On-line service]. URL *http://www.newspage.com/*, April 27.

—— (1996g). Web-enrolled group LTC produces sign-ups of 20% [On-linc service]. URL *http://www.newspage.com/*, April 27.

—— (1996h). AHCPR unveils new inpatient data product [On-line service]. URL *http://www.newspage.com/*, April 29.

—— (1996i). Millions of Americans report health care problems [On-line service]. URL *http://www.newspage.com/*, May 5.

—— (1996j). Managed care discontent growing/cost reduction successful but consumers now press to retain wide access to care [On-line service]. URL *http://www.newspage.com/*, May 7.

—— (1996k). Work begins to standardize clinical charts on computer [On-line service]. URL *http://www.newspage.com/*, May 8.

—— (1996l). U.S. health official puts schizophrenia costs at $65 billion; new medications may offer cost savings [On-line service]. URL *http://www.newspage.com/*, May 9.

—— (1996m). Traditional health insurers losing ground [On-line service]. URL *http://www.newspage.com/*, May 10.

—— (1996n). Court denies Louisiana right to set ERISA plan's network rules [On-line service]. URL *http://www.newspage.com/*, May 18.

—— (1996o). South Dakota hikes insurance rates of state workers who smoke [On-line service]. URL *http://www.newspage.com/*, May 18.

—— (1996p). Mental health fight escalates/employers challenging benefit parity program [On-line service]. URL *http://www.newspage.com/*, May 2.

—— (1996q). Managed care executives and consumers speak out in national survey [On-line service]. URL *http://www.newspage.com/*, May 28.

—— (1996r). Psychologist admits to $3.5 million fraud [On-line service]. URL *http://www.newspage.com/*, May 28.

—— (1996s). New Jersey psychologists file precedent-setting lawsuit against managed care company [On-line service]. URL *http://www.newspage.com/*, May 29.

—— (1996t). Federal court rebuffs anti-managed care lawsuit against Aetna Health Plans [On-line service]. URL *http://www.newspage.com/*, May 30.

—— (1996u). Gag clauses irresponsible myth, HMO physician asserts [On-line service]. URL *http://www.newspage.com/*, May 30.

—— (1996v). Coalition says business study of mental illness parity is "full of errors and fatally flawed" [On-line service]. URL *http://www.newspage.com/*, May 31.

—— (1996w). New cost study casts doubt on employer numbers in health care reform debate; estimated one percent of private insurance costs result from severe mental illness [On-line service]. URL *http://www.newspage.com/*, May31.

—— (1996x). New study underscores costs and loss of choice under mental health "parity" mandate [On-line service]. URL *http://www.newspage.com/*, May 31.

—— (1996y). NMHA/Business community study slants impact of parity amendment [On-line service]. URL *http://www.newspage.com/*, May 31.

—— (1996z). Insurers argue DNA has role in setting rates [On-line service]. URL *http://www.newspage.com/*, June 3.

—— (1996aa). City of Hope researcher identifies genes associated with Tourette's Syndrome, attention deficit disorder, conduct disorer [On-line service]. URL *http://www.newspage.com/*, June 3.

—— (1996bb). Statement by Tipper Gore on Mental Health Legislation [On-line service]. URL *http://www.newspage.com/*, June 5.

—— (1996cc). Medicaid directors turn to managed care to cut costs, survey reports [On-line service]. URL *http://www.newspage.com/*, June 11.

—— (1996dd). N.J. seeks to limit use of genetic testing. [On-line service]. URL *http://www.newspage.com/*, June 19.

Nicassio, P., and Smith, T., eds. (1996). *Managing Chronic Illness: A Biopsychosocial Perspective.* Washington, DC: American Psychological Association.

Niedzielski, J. (1996). Managed care organizations keep spawning more MCOs. *National Underwriter Life & Health Financial Services,* April 29, p. 7.

Norman, K. C., and Moynihan, J. J. (1994). An electronic network strategy for managed care. *Managed Care Quarterly* 2(1):54–61.

Novello, J. (1993). *The Short Course in Adolescent Psychiatry.* Northvale, NJ: Jason Aronson.

Ochroch, R. (1996). Child custody evaluations. *NYSPA Notebook* 8 (3):1, 32.

O'Connor, J., and Seymour, J. (1990). *Introducing NLP: Psychological Skills for Understanding and Influencing People.* San Francisco, CA: Aquarian Press.

Odets, W. (1995). *In the Shadow of the Epidemic.* Durham, NC: Duke University Press.

Office staff update (1996). *Independent Health,* Summer, p. 11.

Office staff update: We made Newsweek (1996). *Independent Health,* Summer, p. 1.

Ormont, L. (1992). *The Group Therapy Experience.* New York: St. Martin's Press.

O'Rourke, P. J. (1995). *Age and Guile Beat Youth, Innocence, and a Bad Haircut.* New York: The Atlantic Monthly Press.

Orwell, G. (1949). *1984.* New York: Penguin Books, 1981.

Parad, H. J., Selby, L., and Quinlin, J. (1976). Crisis intervention with families and groups. In *Theories of Social Work with Groups,* ed. R. W. Roberts and H. Northen, pp. 304–330. New York: Columbia University Press.

Pear, R. (1994a). States again try health changes as congress fails. *The New York Times,* September 16, p. A1.

—— (1994b). States seek a voice in company health plans. *The New York Times,* December 1, p. A28.

—— (1994c). State regulators seek power over self-insured employers. *The New York Times,* September 20, p. A7.

—— (1996). Doctors may get leeway to rival large companies. *The New York Times,* April 8, pp. B1, B9.

Peck, S. (1996). Personal communication, April 6.

Perez Foster, R., Moskowitz, M., and Javier, R. (1996). *Reaching Across the Boundaries of Culture and Class: Widening the Scope of Psychotherapy.* Northvale, NJ: Jason Aronson.

Petrie, K., and Abel, W. (1994). Responses of parasuicidal patients to computerized interviews. *Computers in Human Behavior* 10:415–418.

Phillips, D. G. (1995). Professional standards and managed care. *National Federation of Societies for Clinical Social Work, Inc. Progress Report,* December, p. 11.

Plutchik, R. (1994). *The Psychology and Biology of Emotions.* New York: HarperCollins.

Policy post (1996). New electronic health information post privacy risks. Center for democracy and technology [WWW document]. URL *http://www.cdt.org/privacy/health/.*

Pollack, E. J. (1995). Managed care's focus on psychiatric drugs alarms many doctors. *The Wall Street Journal,* December 1, pp. A1, A11.

Polonsky, I. (1995). Fifteen ways to increase referrals from managed care organizations. *NYSPA Notebook* 7 (3):8.

—— (1996a). *Therapy and Treatment Questionnaires.* Oakland, CA: Professional Health Plan.

—— (1996b). They used the wrong map, but it led them in the right direction. *National Psychologist*, January/February, p. 6.

Pope, K. S., and Vetter, V. A. (1992). Ethical dilemmas encountered by members of the American Psychological Association: a national survey. *American Psychologist* 47(3): 397–411.

Pope, K. S., Tabachnik, B. G., and Keith-Spiegal, P. (1987). Ethics of practice. The beliefs and behaviors of psychologists as therapists. *American Psychologist* 42:993–1006.

Privacy Rights Clearinghouse Fact Sheet #8 (1994). [WWW document]. URL: *http://www.acusd.cdu/~prc/.*

PRNewswire (1995). Minnesota takes the lead on agreement to protect 41 million Americans [WWW document]. URL: *http://www.acusd.cdu/~prc/.*

Protos, J. (1996). Ten things your HMO won't tell you. *Smart Money*, March, pp. 134–144.

Psychologists marketing practices, survey shows. (1996). *National Psychologist*, March/April, p. 2.

Psychotechnology Online (1996). Welcome [WWW document]. URL *http://www.psychotechnology.com/.*

Publication Manual of the American Psychological Association, 4th ed. (1994). Washington, DC: American Psychological Association.

Radcliffe, H., producer (1996). *Do you really want to know?* (television). New York: *CBS News 60 Minutes.*

Raney, J. O. (1982). The payments of fees for psychotherapy. *Journal of Psychoanalytic Psychotherapy* 9:147–181.

—— (1984). *Listening and Interpreting. The Challenge of the Work of Robert Lands.* New York: Jason Aronson.

Rapaport, D. (1967). The theory ego autonomy. In *The Collected Papers of David Rapaport*, ed. M. Giel (pp. 722–744). New York: Basic Books.

Reisman, J., and Rabordy, S. (1993). *Principles of Psychotherapy with Children*, 2nd edition. New York: Maxwell Macmillan.

Riley, J. (1996a). Open secrets. *Newsday*, March 31, pp. A5, A31–32.

—— (1996b). When you can't keep a secret. *Newsday*, April 1, pp. A7, A24–26.

—— (1996c). Know and tell. *Newsday*, April 2, p. A6.

—— (1996d). Will bills cure ills? *Newsday*, April 3, pp. A8, A33.

Rind, D. M., et al. (1994). Effect of computer-based alerts on the treatment and outcomes of hospitalized patients. *Archives of Internal Medicine* 154:1511–1517.

Rosenthal, E. (1997). When healthier isn't cheaper. *The New York Times*, Week in review, Mar. 16, pp. 1, 4.

Rosenthal, L. (1987). *Resolving Resistance in Group Psychotherapy*. Northvale, NJ: Jason Aronson.

Rothman, D. H. (1996). *Networld!* Rocklin, CA: Prima Publishing.

Rubin, A. (1987). Case management. In *The Encyclopedia of Social Work, 18th edition*, ed. A. Minahan, pp. 212–222. Silver Spring, MD: National Association of Social Workers.

Saeman, H. (1994). Psychologists appear confident regarding future. *The National Psychologist*, March/April, pp. 1, 6–7.

—— (1996a). Psychologists cheer as top psychiatrist jeers managed care. *The National Psychologist*, May/June, p. 1.

—— (1996b). Psychologists frustrated with managed care, economic issues, but plan to 'hang tough,' survey reveals. *The National Psychologist*, January/February, pp. 1–2.

—— (1996c). 280 Long Island psychologists join 2,000 physicians in provider-owned HMO. *The National Psychologist*, March/April, p. 18.

—— (1996d). Chicago psychologist has built largest private EAP with 350 firms. *The National Psychologist*, April, pp. 6, 9, 11.

Safran, C. (1996). *Clinical Computing in Patient Care: Capturing the Clinical Encounter* (conference proceedings). Harvard Medical School, Department of Continuing Education, Boston.

Safran, C. et al. (1996). Effects of a knowledge-based patient record on adherence to practice guidelines. *M. D. Computing* 13(1):55–63.

Safran, C., Rind, D., Citroen, M., et al. (1995). Protection of confidentiality in the computer-based patient record. *Clinical Computing* 12(3):187–192.

Safran, J., and Segal, Z. (1996). *Interpersonal Process in Cognitive Therapy*. Northvale, NJ: Jason Aronson.

Sands, H. (1997). Untitled [Letter to the editor]. *NYS Psychologist,* January, p. 4.

Schaffer, S. (1994). Divorce mediation Part II. *NYSPA Notebook* 6(2):1.

—— (1995a). Consent agreements in forensic assessment. *NYSPA Notebook* 7(5):9, 30.

—— (1995b). Recent legal case news. *NYSPA Notebook*, 7(3), 9.

Schneider, A. J., and Laiken, D. S. (1980). *Listen to Me I'm Angry*. New York: William Morrow.

—— (1995a). *The Love Book*. New York: Bantam.

—— (1995b). *Stress Reduction/Double Induction.* (Audio tape.) Liberty, NY: CHILL.

Schore, A. (1994). *Affect Regulation and the Origin of the Self.* Mahwah, NJ: Erlbaum.

Schoub, B. (1994). *AIDS and HIV in Perspective: A Guide to Understanding the Virus and Its Consequences*. New York: Cambridge.

Schultz, E. (1994). Medical data gathered by firms can prove less confidential. *The Wall Street Journal*, May 18, pp. A1, A5.

Schwartz, J. (Director) (1996). *Health Care Tapes*. Association of Orthodox Jewish Scientists. 27 West 23rd Street, New York, NY 10010.

Seligman, M. (1993). *What You Can Change and What You Can't*. New York: Knopf.

—— (1995). The effectiveness of psychotherapy: The Consumer Reports Study. *American Psychologist* 50:965–974.

Serwer, A. (1996). The hidden growth stars. *Fortune*, Oct. 14, pp. 74–82.

Shafranske, E. (1996). *Religion and the Clinical Practice of Psychology*. Washington, DC: American Psychiatric Press.

Shapiro, E. (1994). *The boundaries are shifting: renegotiating the therapeutic frame.* Presentation at the International Scientific Symposium, "The Inner World in the Outer World," at the Austen Riggs Center, Stockbridge, MA, October 22–23.

—— (1996). *The inner world in the outer world.* Presentation before the Freudian Society, New York, NY, April.

Shapiro, F. (1995). *Eye Movement Desensitization and Reprocessing: Basic Principles, Protocols and Procedures*. New York: Guilford.

Shapiro, J. (1995). The downside of managed mental health care. *Clinical Social Work Journal* 23(4):441–451.

Shapiro, L. E. (1996). *12-Hour Therapy with Children.* King of Prussia, PA: Center for Applied Psychology.

Shectman, F. (1986). Time and the practice of psychotherapy. *Psychotherapy* 23:521–525.

Sherman, D. W. (1996). Taking the fear out of AIDS nursing. *Journal of the New York State Nurses Association* 27(1):4–8.

Shore, K. (1995a). *The immorality of managed competition and managed care.* Paper presented at the Preserving Psychotherapy Conference of the National Coalition of Mental Health Professionals and Consumers and Georgia Mental Health Coalition on Managed Care, Atlanta, GA, November 5.

—— (1995b). *Moving America beyond managed care and managed competition.* Paper presented at the Preserving Psychotherapy Conference of the National Coalition of Mental Health Professionals and Consumers and Georgia Mental Health Coalition on Managed Care, Atlanta, GA, November 5.

—— (1995c). Managed care: the subjugation of a profession. *Psychotherapy in Private Practice* 14(2):67–75.

Shugawat, L. (1996). Email listing [On-line news posting]. URL: *http://www.clinicalsw@e55.webcom.com*, June 4.

Shuit, D. P. (1994). Verdict heats up memory debate; Psychology: Experts on both sides of the issue say it will lead to more restrictions on therapists who work with patients' suppressed recollections, as well as more law. Los Angeles Times [WWW document]. URL: *http://www.elibrary.com/*, May 22.

—— (1996). Controversy grows over California Malpractice Cap; Courts: Doctors seek U.S. version of state's $250,000 limit for pain and suffering. Los Angeles Times. The Electric Library [On-line service]. URL: *http://www.elibrary.com/*, January 29.

Slade, W. V., Hichs, G. P., Reed, C. E., et al (1996). A computer-based medical history system. *New England Journal of Medicine* 274:194–198.

Sleek, S. (1996). New Jersey to toughen its regulations on HMOs. *APA Monitor*, April, p. 35.

Smith, R. N., Chen, C. C., Feng, F. F., and Gomez-Gauchia, H. (1993). A massively parallel memory-based story system of psychotherapy. *Computers and Biomedical Research* 26:415–423.

Smith-Bell, M., and Winslade, W. J. (1994). Privacy, confidentiality, and privilege in psychotherapeutic relationships. *American Journal of Orthopsychiatry* 64(2):180–193.

Snarr, B. B. (1995). Managed care: recent cases increase employers' liability risk [WWW document]. URL: *http://www.elibrary.com/*, November 1.

Solomon, J. (1996). Breaking the silence. *Newsweek*, May 20, pp. 21–22.

Special report finds Health Insurance Plan of Greater New York routinely fails to pay millions of dollars (1996). *The New York Times*, April, p. A1, 3.

Spielberger, C. D., and Sydeman, S. J. (1994). State-Trait Anxiety Inventory and State-Trait Anger Expression Inventory. In *The Use of Psychological Tests for Treatment Planning and Outcome Assessment*, ed. M. E. Maruish, pp. 292–321. Hillsdale, NJ: Erlbaum.

Spinhoven, P., Lobbc, R. M., and Rombouts, R. (1993). Feasibility of computerized psychological testing with psychiatric outpatients. *Journal of Clinical Psychology* 49(3): 440–447.

Spitz, H. (1996). *Group Psychotherapy and Managed Mental Health Care.* New York: Brunner/Mazel.

Spragins, E., Kahn, J., and Miller, A. (1996). America's Best HMOs. *Newsweek*, June 24, pp. 56–64.

Starfield, B., Powe, N. R., Weiner, J. R., et al. (1994). Costs vs. quality in different types of primary care settings. *Journal of the American Medical Association* 272(24):1903–1908.

Stearns, H. (1996). New legislation to protect genetic health privacy. *Oncology News International* 5:5,16.

Steenbarger, B. N. (1997). Alcoholism counseling: relevant research. *NYS Psychological Association Notebook IX*, January, p. 20.

Stein, A. (1996). Boulder therapists form group to operate outside managed care. *Boulder County Business Report*, January, pp. 21, 27.

Stevenson, M. R. (1996). Gambling addiction [Letter to the editor]. *APA Monitor*, February, p. 3.

Stone, A. (1995). Psychotherapy and managed care: the bigger picture. *Harvard Newsletter*, December, pp. 5–11.

Stone, A. A. (1995). Where will psychoanalysis survive? Keynote address to the American Academy of Psychoanalysis, December 9.

Strean, H. (1994). *Psychotherapy with the Orthodox Jew.* Northvale, NJ: Jason Aronson.

Survey: Psychologists appear confident regarding future (1994). *National Psychologist*, March/April, pp. 1, 6–7.

Tafrate, R. C. (1995). Evaluation of treatment strategies for adult anger disorders. In *Anger Disorders*, ed. H. Kassanove, pp. 109–128. Washington, DC: Taylor & Francis.

Tanaka-Matsumi, J. (1995). Cross-cultural perspectives on anger. In *Anger Disorders*, ed. H. Kassanove, pp. 81–89. Washington, DC: Taylor & Francis.

Tavris, C. (1989). *Anger: The Misunderstood Emotion.* (2nd ed.) New York: Touchstone.

Taylor, J. (1992). *Where People Fly and Water Runs Uphill.* New York: Warner Books.

Taylor, V., and Armsworth, J. (1996). Managed Care *News* Reports Fee Trends: Highlights of fee study results. NFSCSW [WWW document]. URL *http://www.webcom.com/nfscsw/*, January/February.

Texans for Lawsuit Reform (1996a). Poll summary [WWW document]. URL *http://www.tortreform.com.*

—— (1996b). Tort reform statistics [WWW document]. URL *http://www.tortreform.com.*

Texas Medical Association (1986). Managed care glossary [WWW document]. URL: *http://www.bcm.tmc.edu/ama-mss/glossary.html.*

Thomlinson, R. J. (1986). Behavior theory in social work practice. In *Social Work Treatment: Interlocking Theoretical Approaches*, ed. F. J. Turner, pp. 131–153. New York: Free Press.

Thompson, R., Jr., and Gustafson, K. (1996). *Adaptation to Chronic Child Disorders.* Washington, DC: American Psychological Association.

Tomsho, R. (1996). "Free Agent" doctors are selling practices, signing job contracts. *The Wall Street Journal*, March 12, pp. 1, A12.

Turkel, J. (1994). Disavowal and defensive alterations of cognitive style as a consequence of childhood trauma. In *Issues in Psychoanalytic Psychology* 16(2), ed. E. Kronish, pp. 191–209. New York: Washington Square Institute.

U.S. Healthcare chief will get $1 billion (1996). *The New York Times*, June 15, p. A14.

Vaill, P. B. (1996). *Learning as a Way of Being: Strategies for Survival in a World of Permanent White Water*. San Francisco: Jossey-Bass.

Van Biema, D. (1996). Of the soul. *Time*, June 24, pp. 64–68.

Vanderbas, G. R. (1995). Managing Chronic Illness. *APA Monitor*, August, p. 13.

The VBH Manual: Clinical Protocols and Procedures (1994). Falls Church, VA: Value Behavioral Health.

Walker, G. (1991). *In the Midst of Winter: Systemic Therapy with Families, Couples, and Individuals with AIDS Infections*. New York: Norton.

Wallis, C. (1996). Faith and healing. *Time*, June 24, pp. 58–62.

Watkins, S. (1989). Confidentiality and privileged communications: legal dilemma for family therapists. *Social Work* 34:133–136.

Weiner, B. A., and Wettstein, R. M. (1994). Confidentiality of patient-related information. *Archives of Ophthalmology* 112:1032–1036.

Weiner, R. H. (1995). The independent practice of psychology: an unfortunate oxymoron. *National Psychologist*, January/February, pp. 1, 6–7.

Weisberg, I. (1993). Brief time-limited psychotherapy. *International Journal of Communicative Psychoanalysis and Psychotherapy* 8(1):105–108.

Weise, E. (1996). What makes a hacker the world's most wanted? [WWW document]. URL: *http://www.sjmercury.com/info/subinfo.htm*, January 25.

Weiss, B. (1988). *Many Lives, Many Masters*. New York: Simon and Schuster.

Weissman, S. M. (1996). Damaged care for mental ills. *Legal Times*, March, pp. 25, 37–39.

Welch, B. (1996a). The death of managed care. *Coalition Report*. November 15, pp. 1, 7.

—— (1996b). Holding managed care accountable: the irony of malpractice law. Mental Health InfoSource [WWW document]. URL *http://www.mhsource.com*.

—— (1996c). One of managed care's earliest critics tells about law practice to defend m.c. victims. *National Psychologist*, March/April, p. 15.

Werner, H. D. (1986). Cognitive theory. In *Social Work Treatment: Interlocking Theoretical Approaches*, ed. F. J. Turner, pp. 91–129. New York: Free Press.

Whitman, G. (1996). From some states. *Coalition Report*, March/April, p. 9.

Williams, M. (1995). Tort reform: Is the system broken?: Debate begins to intensify over Ohio's efforts to limit lawsuits (First in a four-part series). Columbus Daily Reporter [WWW document]. URL *http://sddt.com/~columbus/Files2/tort.html*, December 26.

Wilson, E. O. (1975). *Sociobiology*. Cambridge, MA: Harvard University Press.

Wilson, H. (1995). *The Columbia Dictionary of Quotations: Microsoft Bookshelf '95* [Computer program]. Microsoft Corporation.

Wilson, K. (1993). It's getting easier to know you. Riding the Information Highway: *Newsday* Special Reprint, July, p. 27.

Winslow, R. (1996). Limiting drugs a doctor orders may cost more. *The Wall Street Journal*, March 20, pp. B1, B4.

Wired Magazine (1995). Are you in an Equifax database? [WWW document]. URL *http://www.fuzine.mt.cs.cmu.edu/mlm/online.html*.

Wolk, J. L., Sullivan, W. P., and Hartmann, D. J. (1994). The managerial nature of case management. *Social Work* 39:152–159.

Wolpe, J. (1990). *The Practice of Behavior Therapy*. 4th ed. New York: Pergamon.

Wulach, J. (1993). *Law and Mental Health Professionals: New York*. Washington, DC: American Psychological Association.

Wylie, M. S. (1994). Endangered species: The managed care revolution. *Family Therapy Networker*, March/April, pp. 20–34.

Yamaguchi, S., Kobayashi, S., Koide, H., and Tsunematsu, T. (1992). Longitudinal study of regional cerebral blood flow changes in depression after stroke. *Stroke* 23:1716–1722.

Yurkowski, W. (1996). How the latest health care legislation can affect your business. *Inside Business*, September, p. 25.

Zich, J. (1996). Medical malpractice reform good medicine? Health Care Liability Alliance [WWW document]. URL: *http://www.wp.com/hcla/hclanews.htm*, February 12.

APPENDICES

Forms

1. Consent Form
2. Sample Patient File
3. Payment and Session Monitor
4. Confidentiality Disclaimer
5. Outpatient Treatment Report
6. Insurance Abuse Report
7. HCFA Claim Form

Resources

1. Computer Software
2. HCFA Claim Forms
3. Internet
4. National 800 Hotlines
5. Suggested Reading
6. Sources for Assessment Materials
7. Professional Organizations
8. Specialties

FORMS

CONSENT FORM

TO WHOM IT MAY CONCERN:

I, (____________________________) hereby authorize
(Patient's Name)

(______________________________) to release my treatment records
(Therapist's Name)

and/or any information he or she deems necessary to the appropriate insurance or managed care company to facilitate continuity of care and reimbursement. This consent form will remain in effect until otherwise canceled by written notice sent to the therapist identified above.

____

Signature of Patient/Client Date:___________

SAMPLE PATIENT FILE

I. DEMOGRAPHICS	
Name:	☐ Male ☐ Female
Address:	Date of Birth:
City, State, Zip:	SS#:
Employer:	Insurance Co:
Address:	Mailing Address:
City, State, Zip:	
Telephone:	Contact:
Primary Care Physician:	Pin #:
Address:	
City, State, Zip:	
II. INSURANCE DATA	
Company Name:	
Address:	
City, State, Zip:	
Telephone:	Contact:
Telephone Shortcuts:	
Insurance/MC Requirements:	Policy #:
OTR due after session #:	Auth. #:
☐ Mail ☐ Fax ☐ Phone	
III. IMPAIRMENTS	
Presenting Problem:	
Precipitant/Trigger:	
Severity of Symptoms: ☐ Mild ☐ Moderate ☐ Severe	
IV. HISTORY	
Psychiatric History:	
Substance Abuse History:	
Relevant Medical History:	
V. SOCIAL	
Family Supports/Vulnerabilities:	
Other Social Supports/Vulnerabilities:	

VI. DIAGNOSIS—DSM-IV- MAS or ICD • 9 CODES				
AXIS I:	AXIS II:	AXIS III:	AXIS IV:	AXIS V:

VII. GOALS OF TREATMENT
1.
2.
3.
4.
VIII. TREATMENT PLAN
Session Frequency:
Medication:
Homework:
Support Groups:
Hypnosis:
Proposed Length of Treatment:
IX. INTERVENTIONS
1.
2.
3.
4.

X. DISCHARGE PLAN

XI. MENTAL STATUS EXAM & RISK ASSESSMENT

PATIENT PROGRESS NOTES

Name:		Modality: Ind. Psychotherapy
# Sessions Auth:	Date Effective:	OTR Due:
Session #:	Date:	Duration: 50 Min.
Problem:	Progress Rating:	
Comments:		

Provider:

PAYMENT AND SESSION MONITOR

Patient Name:	Insurance Co.:
Address:	Address:
City, State, Zip:	City, State, Zip:
D of B: Ist Visit:	Billing Address:
Mem. #:	
SS#:	Telephone:
Your Provider #:	Fax:
MCO Protocol:	Case Manager:
1.	PCP:
2.	Address:
3.	
	Psychiatrist:
1st Visit: CPT 90820 - 60 Min.	Address:
Subsequent Visits: 90844 - 50 Min.	

OTR Alert	#	Date of Visit	Auth No.	Auth Date #	End Date	Date OTR Filed	Co-Pay	Debit	Credit	Ins. Bal	Pt. Bal
	1										
	2										
	3										
	4										
	5										
	6										
	7										
	8										
	9										
	10										
	11										
	12										
	13										
	14										
	15										
	16										
	17										
	18										
	19										
	20										

CONFIDENTIALITY DISCLAIMER

CONFIDENTIAL

This fax transmission is private, privileged, and confidential, and is intended only for the professional use of the addressee. If you are not the addressee, or the agent responsible for delivering the fax unread to the addressee, please be advised that you have received this document in error, and that reading, copying, distributing, or disseminating any part of this document is strictly prohibited. If you have received this fax in error, please notify me immediately by calling (telephone number). Your courtesy in respecting the privacy of this communication is appreciated.

OUTPATIENT TREATMENT REPORT

GENERAL INFORMATION:	Date:
Provider:	MCO:
Address:	Address:
City, State, Zip:	City, State, Zip:
Lic/Cert #:	Case Mgr.:
	Phone: Fax:

PATIENT DATA:	
Patient's Name:	Date of Birth:
Address:	SS#:
City, State, Zip:	Initial Date of Service:
Member #:	Authorization #:
Telephone:	No of Sessions:
Insured's Name:	Date Effective:
Address:	Total Sessions to Date:
Employee SS#:	Release Signed: ☐ Date:
Group #:	

DIAGNOSIS:	
AXIS I: Primary:	Secondary:
AXIS II:	AXIS III:
AXIS IV: (Stressors):	
AXIS V: (GAF) Current: Average: Highest Past 12 Months:	

DESCRIPTION:
Document nature, severity, and duration of symptoms/behaviors.

CURRENT MENTAL STATUS:
Describe mood, judgment, dress, memory, intelligence, and risks of suicide or violence.

SUBSTANCE ABUSE:
☐ None ☐ Abuse ☐ Dependence ☐ Unstable remission
Identify substance and specify quantity/frequency:

BRIEF PSYCHOSOCIAL HISTORY:
Provide short history of central life role functions related to symptoms/behaviors.

TARGET IMPAIRMENTS:		
List all impairments/symptoms/problems. Rate Severity: 1 = Mild; 2 = Moderate; 3 = Severe. Specify Duration: 1 = < a Month; 2 = 1–6 Mos; 3 = 7–11 Mos; 4 = > a Yr.		
Impairments:	Severity:	Duration:
1.		
2.		
3.		
4.		
5.		

GOALS OF TREATMENT:
Describe the improved or adjusted behaviors that will result from treatment.
1.
2.
3.
4.
5.

INTERVENTIONS: (Methods of Achievement)
1.
2.
3.
4.
5.

TARGET SCHEDULE:	
Symptom:	Target Date(s):
1.	
2.	
3.	
4.	
5. PROPOSED TERMINATION DATE:	

PROGRESS SUMMARY:	DATE:
# Sessions used:	
# Sessions requested:	
Total # of sessions:	

PROPOSED TREATMENT MODALITY:
☐ Ind. ☐ Medication monitoring ☐ Group ☐ Family ☐ Collateral
☐ Community resources ☐ Self-Help

MEDICATION:	
☐ None ☐ Psychiatric ☐ Medical	
Specify dosage: Frequency:	
Prescribing physician:	Telephone:
☐ Psychiatrist ☐ Other MD	

Clinician's Signature:______________________________ Date: ____________

INSURANCE ABUSE REPORT

GENERAL INFORMATION	DATE:
*PROVIDER:	MCO:
ADDRESS:	ADDRESS:
CITY, STATE, ZIP:	CITY, STATE, ZIP:
PHONE:	PHONE:
LIC/CERT #:	*NAME OF REVIEWER:

(*You can leave these blank, but a better option is to include the names and mark the document CONFIDENTIAL.)

DESCRIPTION: (Describe patient in general terms, but do not identify. Briefly document nature of the abuse or problem.)

PLEASE DO NOT STAPLE IN THIS AREA

APPROVED OMB-0938-0008

PICA

HEALTH INSURANCE CLAIM FORM

PICA

1. MEDICARE (Medicare #) MEDICAID (Medicaid #) CHAMPUS (Sponsor's SSN) CHAMPVA (VA File #) GROUP HEALTH PLAN (SSN or ID) FECA BLK LUNG (SSN) OTHER (ID)

1a. INSURED'S I.D. NUMBER (FOR PROGRAM IN ITEM 1)

2. PATIENT'S NAME (Last Name, First Name, Middle Initial)

3. PATIENT'S BIRTH DATE MM DD YY SEX M F

4. INSURED'S NAME (Last Name, First Name, Middle Initial)

5. PATIENT'S ADDRESS (No., Street)

6. PATIENT RELATIONSHIP TO INSURED Self Spouse Child Other

7. INSURED'S ADDRESS (No., Street)

CITY STATE

8. PATIENT STATUS Single Married Other

CITY STATE

ZIP CODE TELEPHONE (Include Area Code) ( )

Employed Full-Time Student Part-Time Student

ZIP CODE TELEPHONE (INCLUDE AREA CODE) ( )

9. OTHER INSURED'S NAME (Last Name, First Name, Middle Initial)

10. IS PATIENT'S CONDITION RELATED TO:

11. INSURED'S POLICY GROUP OR FECA NUMBER

a. OTHER INSURED'S POLICY OR GROUP NUMBER

a. EMPLOYMENT? (CURRENT OR PREVIOUS) YES NO

a. INSURED'S DATE OF BIRTH MM DD YY SEX M F

b. OTHER INSURED'S DATE OF BIRTH MM DD YY SEX M F

b. AUTO ACCIDENT? PLACE (State) YES NO

b. EMPLOYER'S NAME OR SCHOOL NAME

c. EMPLOYER'S NAME OR SCHOOL NAME

c. OTHER ACCIDENT? YES NO

c. INSURANCE PLAN NAME OR PROGRAM NAME

d. INSURANCE PLAN NAME OR PROGRAM NAME

10d. RESERVED FOR LOCAL USE

d. IS THERE ANOTHER HEALTH BENEFIT PLAN? YES NO *If yes*, return to and complete item 9 a-d.

READ BACK OF FORM BEFORE COMPLETING & SIGNING THIS FORM.

12. PATIENT'S OR AUTHORIZED PERSON'S SIGNATURE I authorize the release of any medical or other information necessary to process this claim. I also request payment of government benefits either to myself or to the party who accepts assignment below.

SIGNED DATE

13. INSURED'S OR AUTHORIZED PERSON'S SIGNATURE I authorize payment of medical benefits to the undersigned physician or supplier for services described below.

SIGNED

14. DATE OF CURRENT: MM DD YY ILLNESS (First symptom) OR INJURY (Accident) OR PREGNANCY(LMP)

15. IF PATIENT HAS HAD SAME OR SIMILAR ILLNESS. GIVE FIRST DATE MM DD YY

16. DATES PATIENT UNABLE TO WORK IN CURRENT OCCUPATION FROM MM DD YY TO MM DD YY

17. NAME OF REFERRING PHYSICIAN OR OTHER SOURCE

17a. I.D. NUMBER OF REFERRING PHYSICIAN

18. HOSPITALIZATION DATES RELATED TO CURRENT SERVICES FROM MM DD YY TO MM DD YY

19. RESERVED FOR LOCAL USE

20. OUTSIDE LAB? YES NO $ CHARGES

21. DIAGNOSIS OR NATURE OF ILLNESS OR INJURY. (RELATE ITEMS 1,2,3 OR 4 TO ITEM 24E BY LINE)

1. ___ . __ 3. ___ . __

2. ___ . __ 4. ___ . __

22. MEDICAID RESUBMISSION CODE ORIGINAL REF. NO.

23. PRIOR AUTHORIZATION NUMBER

24. A						B	C	D		E	F	G	H	I	J	K
DATE(S) OF SERVICE From			To			Place of Service	Type of Service	PROCEDURES, SERVICES, OR SUPPLIES (Explain Unusual Circumstances)		DIAGNOSIS CODE	$ CHARGES	DAYS OR UNITS	EPSDT Family Plan	EMG	COB	RESERVED FOR LOCAL USE
MM	DD	YY	MM	DD	YY			CPT/HCPCS	MODIFIER							
1																
2																
3																
4																
5																
6																

25. FEDERAL TAX I.D. NUMBER SSN EIN

26. PATIENT'S ACCOUNT NO.

27. ACCEPT ASSIGNMENT? (For govt. claims, see back) YES NO

28. TOTAL CHARGE $

29. AMOUNT PAID $

30. BALANCE DUE $

31. SIGNATURE OF PHYSICIAN OR SUPPLIER INCLUDING DEGREES OR CREDENTIALS (I certify that the statements on the reverse apply to this bill and are made a part thereof.)

SIGNED DATE

32. NAME AND ADDRESS OF FACILITY WHERE SERVICES WERE RENDERED (If other than home or office)

33. PHYSICIAN'S, SUPPLIER'S BILLING NAME, ADDRESS, ZIP CODE & PHONE #

DR. MURIEL P. WARREN CSW
240 EAST 76TH STREET
NEW YORK, NY 10021
(212) 988-9602

PIN# **N18862** GRP#

(APPROVED BY AMA COUNCIL ON MEDICAL SERVICE 8/88)

PLEASE PRINT OR TYPE

FORM HCFA-1500 (12-90)
FORM OWCP-1500 FORM RRB-1500

BECAUSE THIS FORM IS USED BY VARIOUS GOVERNMENT AND PRIVATE HEALTH PROGRAMS, SEE SEPARATE INSTRUCTIONS ISSUED BY APPLICABLE PROGRAMS.

NOTICE: Any person who knowingly files a statement of claim containing any misrepresentation or any false, incomplete or misleading information may be guilty of a criminal act punishable under law and may be subject to civil penalties.

REFERS TO GOVERNMENT PROGRAMS ONLY

MEDICARE AND CHAMPUS PAYMENTS: A patient's signature requests that payment be made and authorizes release of any information necessary to process the claim and certifies that the information provided in Blocks 1 through 12 is true, accurate and complete. In the case of a Medicare claim, the patient's signature authorizes any entity to release to Medicare medical and nonmedical information, including employment status, and whether the person has employer group health insurance, liability, no-fault, worker's compensation or other insurance which is responsible to pay for the services for which the Medicare claim is made. See 42 CFR 411.24(a). If item 9 is completed, the patient's signature authorizes release of the information to the health plan or agency shown. In Medicare assigned or CHAMPUS participation cases, the physician agrees to accept the charge determination of the Medicare carrier or CHAMPUS fiscal intermediary as the full charge, and the patient is responsible only for the deductible, coinsurance and noncovered services. Coinsurance and the deductible are based upon the charge determination of the Medicare carrier or CHAMPUS fiscal intermediary if this is less than the charge submitted. CHAMPUS is not a health insurance program but makes payment for health benefits provided through certain affiliations with the Uniformed Services. Information on the patient's sponsor should be provided in those items captioned in "Insured": i.e., items 1a, 4, 6, 7, 9, and 11.

BLACK LUNG AND FECA CLAIMS

The provider agrees to accept the amount paid by the Government as payment in full. See Black Lung and FECA instructions regarding required procedure and diagnosis coding systems.

SIGNATURE OF PHYSICIAN OR SUPPLIER (MEDICARE, CHAMPUS, FECA AND BLACK LUNG)

I certify that the services shown on this form were medically indicated and necessary for the health of the patient and were personally furnished by me or were furnished incident to my professional service by my employee under my immediate personal supervision, except as otherwise expressly permitted by Medicare or CHAMPUS regulations.

For services to be considered as "incident" to a physician's professional service, 1) they must be rendered under the physician's immediate personal supervision by his/her employee, 2) they must be an integral, although incidental part of a covered physician's service, 3) they must be of kinds commonly furnished in physician's offices, and 4) the services of nonphysicians must be included on the physician's bills.

For CHAMPUS claims, I further certify that I (or any employee) who rendered services am not an active duty member of the Uniformed Services or a civilian employee of the United States Government or a contract employee of the United States Government, either civilian or military (refer to 5 USC 5536). For Black-Lung claims, I further certify that the services performed were for a Black Lung-related disorder.

No Part B Medicare benefits may be paid unless this form is received as required by existing law and regulations (42 CFR 424.32).

NOTICE: Any one who misrepresents or falsifies essential information to receive payment from Federal funds requested by this form may upon conviction be subject to fine and imprisonment under applicable Federal laws.

NOTICE TO PATIENT ABOUT THE COLLECTION AND USE OF MEDICARE, CHAMPUS, FECA, AND BLACK LUNG INFORMATION
(PRIVACY ACT STATEMENT)

We are authorized by HCFA, CHAMPUS and OWCP to ask you for information needed in the administration of the Medicare, CHAMPUS, FECA, and Black Lung programs. Authority to collect information is in section 205(a), 1862, 1872 and 1874 of the Social Security Act as amended, 42 CFR 411.24(a) and 424.5(a) (6), and 44 USC 3101;41 CFR 101 et seq and 10 USC 1079 and 1086; 5 USC 8101 et seq; and 30 USC 901 et seq; 38 USC 613; E.O. 9397.

The information we obtain to complete claims under these programs is used to identify you and to determine your eligibility. It is also used to decide if the services and supplies you received are covered by these programs and to insure that proper payment is made.

The information may also be given to other providers of services, carriers, intermediaries, medical review boards, health plans, and other organizations or Federal agencies, for the effective administration of Federal provisions that require other third parties payers to pay primary to Federal program, and as otherwise necessary to administer these programs. For example, it may be necessary to disclose information about the benefits you have used to a hospital or doctor. Additional disclosures are made through routine uses for information contained in systems of records.

FOR MEDICARE CLAIMS: See the notice modifying system No. 09-70-0501, titled, 'Carrier Medicare Claims Record,' published in the Federal Register, Vol. 55 No. 177, page 37549, Wed. Sept. 12, 1990, or as updated and republished.

FOR OWCP CLAIMS: Department of Labor, Privacy Act of 1974, "Republication of Notice of Systems of Records," Federal Register Vol. 55 No. 40, Wed Feb. 28, 1990, See ESA-5, ESA-6, ESA-12, ESA-13, ESA-30, or as updated and republished.

FOR CHAMPUS CLAIMS: PRINCIPLE PURPOSE(S): To evaluate eligibility for medical care provided by civilian sources and to issue payment upon establishment of eligibility and determination that the services/supplies received are authorized by law.

ROUTINE USE(S): Information from claims and related documents may be given to the Dept. of Veterans Affairs, the Dept. of Health and Human Services and/or the Dept. of Transportation consistent with their statutory administrative responsibilities under CHAMPUS/CHAMPVA; to the Dept. of Justice for representation of the Secretary of Defense in civil actions; to the Internal Revenue Service, private collection agencies, and consumer reporting agencies in connection with recoupment claims; and to Congressional Offices in response to inquiries made at the request of the person to whom a record pertains. Appropriate disclosures may be made to other federal, state, local, foreign government agencies, private business entities, and individual providers of care, on matters relating to entitlement, claims adjudication, fraud, program abuse, utilization review, quality assurance, peer review, program integrity, third-party liability, coordination of benefits, and civil and criminal litigation related to the operation of CHAMPUS.

DISCLOSURES: Voluntary; however, failure to provide information will result in delay in payment or may result in denial of claim. With the one exception discussed below, there are no penalties under these programs for refusing to supply information. However, failure to furnish information regarding the medical services rendered or the amount charged would prevent payment of claims under these programs. Failure to furnish any other information, such as name or claim number, would delay payment of the claim. Failure to provide medical information under FECA could be deemed an obstruction.

It is mandatory that you tell us if you know that another party is responsible for paying for your treatment. Section 1128B of the Social Security Act and 31 USC 3801-3812 provide penalties for withholding this information.

You should be aware that P.L. 100-503, the "Computer Matching and Privacy Protection Act of 1988", permits the government to verify information by way of computer matches.

MEDICAID PAYMENTS (PROVIDER CERTIFICATION)

I hereby agree to keep such records as are necessary to disclose fully the extent of services provided to individuals under the State's Title XIX plan and to furnish information regarding any payments claimed for providing such services as the State Agency or Dept. of Health and Humans Services may request.

I further agree to accept, as payment in full, the amount paid by the Medicaid program for those claims submitted for payment under that program, with the exception of authorized deductible, coinsurance, co-payment or similar cost-sharing charge.

SIGNATURE OF PHYSICIAN (OR SUPPLIER): I certify that the services listed above were medically indicated and necessary to the health of this patient and were personally furnished by me or my employee under my personal direction.

NOTICE: This is to certify that the foregoing information is true, accurate and complete. I understand that payment and satisfaction of this claim will be from Federal and State funds, and that any false claims, statements, or documents, or concealment of a material fact, may be prosecuted under applicable Federal or State laws.

Public reporting burden for this collection of information is estimated to average 15 minutes per response, including time for reviewing instructions, searching existing date sources, gathering and maintaining data needed, and completing and reviewing the collection of information. Send comments regarding this burden estimate or any other aspect of this collection of information, including suggestions for reducing the burden, to HCFA, Office of Financial Management, P.O. Box 26684, Baltimore, MD 21207; and to the Office of Management and Budget, Paperwork Reduction Project (OMB-0938-0008), Washington, D.C. 20503.

RESOURCES

Computer Software

All of the following software packages have problems. Some of them are backed by helpful and available technical support systems and some are not. Because most of them are expensive, it is wise to investigate any software in which you are interested very carefully before committing yourself to a package.

Applied Computing Services
2764 Allen Road West
Elk, WA 99009
800-553-4055

The Cure
45 Highland Road
Boxford, MA 01921
508-352-8909

Delphi/Psychotherapy Billing Software
PC Consulting Group; POB 69328
Portland, OR 97201
800-847-8446

Ea$y Billing
Maria Productions
524 Don Gaspar
Santa Fe, NM 87501
505-982-5321
easybilling@nets.com

Owen Consulting
192 Stanley Drive
Centereach, NY 11720
516-427-1874

$um Time Software
635 Franklin Avenue
New Orleans, LA 70117
800-767-5788

Sisyphus Software
771 Fifth Avenue
Salt Lake City, UT 84103-3511
800-487-1420

The Therapist
Beaver Creek Software
29508 N.E. Pheasant Ave.
Corvallis, OR 97333
503-752-5039
72613.367@compuserve.com

Therapist Helper
500 West Cummings Park; Suite 3150
Woburn, MA 01801-6514
800-343-5737

Therascribe
John Wiley & Sons Inc.
One Wiley Drive
Somerset, NJ 08875

HCFA Claim Forms

Listed below are some of the vendors from whom you may purchase HCFA-1500 claim forms:

American Medical Association
PO Box 10946
Chicago, IL 60610
Att: Order Dept.
1-800-621-8335

US Government Printing Office
Supt. of Documents
Washington, DC 20402
202-512-1800

Colwell Systems
PO Box 9024
Champaign, Il 61826-9024

Colwell and other supply companies provide forms for patient information, consent, and appointments, as well as several types of HCFA forms and mailing envelopes.

Internet

Mental Health/Managed Care:

American Academy of Child and Adolescent Psychiatry: http://www.aacap.org/web/aacap/
American Mental Health Alliance: http:www.mental-health-coop.com/
American Psychiatric Association: http://www.psych.org/
American Psychiatric Association: http://apsa.org/
American Psychoanalytic Association: http://apsa.org/
American Psychological Association PsychNet: http://www.apa.org
CyberPsych:
American Psychoanalytic Foundation
American Association of Suicidology
Society for the Exploration of Psychotherapy Integration
http://www.cyberpsych.org
Florida Mental Health Institute: http://www.fmhi.usf.edu/
Internet Mental Health Page: http://www.mentalhealth.com
Mental Health Inforsource: http://www.mhsource.com
Mental Health Net: http://www.cmhc.com
National Alliance for the Mentally Ill (NAMI) for consumers and family members: http://www.nami.org/
National Coalition for Mental Health Professionals and Consumers: http://www.execpc.com/~mastery/coalitionMain.html
National Committee for Quality Assurance (NCQA): http://www.ncqa.org/
National Federation of Societies for Clinical Social Workers: http://www.nfscsw.org/
National Institute of Mental Health: http://www.nimh.nih.gov/
Open Minds: The Behavioral Health Care Analyst: http://www.openminds.com
Pharmaceutical Information Network: http://pharminfo.com/
Prevention Online: http://www.health.org
PsychCentral: http://www.coil.com/~grohol/
Psychology Organizations on the Web: http://www.wesleyan.edu/psyc/psyc260/psych.htm
Psychotechnology Online: http://www.psychotechnology.com
Psychotherapy Finances: http://www.psyfin.com/
Psychscapes Worldwide: http://www.mental-health.com
SWAN–Social Workers Advocating Network Technologies: http://www.sc.edu/swan/national.html
Web Resources for Social Workers: http://www.colostate.edu/Depts/SocWork/webstuff.html

Privacy/Medical Records/Technology:

Center for Democracy and Technology: http://www.cdt.org/privacy/health/
Computer Professionals for Social Responsibility: http://www.cpsr.org/dox/home.html
Electronic Frontier Foundation (EFF): http://eff.org/
Electronic Policy Network (EPN): http://epn.org/
Electronic Privacy Information Center (EPIC): http://www.epic.org/
Medical Records Institute: http://www.medrecinst.com/
National Coalition for Patient Rights: http://www.tiac.net/users/gls/cprnu.html
Privacy International: http://www.privacy.org/pi/
Privacy Rights Clearinghouse: http://www.privacyrights.org/
Psychiatric Society for Informatics: http://www.psych.med.umich.edu/web/psi

Self-Help, Support Groups, and Specific Disorders

Alcoholics Anonymous: http://www.alcoholics-anonymous.org/
Alliance to Fight Eating Disorders: http://fsci.umn.edu/~AAABL/default.htp
American Self-Help Clearinghouse: http://www.cmhc.com/selfhelp/
Anxiety-Panic Page: http://www.algy.com/anxiety/
Borderline Personality Disorder: http://members.aol.com/BPDcentral/index.html
Depression Central: http://www.psycom.net/depression.central.html
Death, dying, and grief resources: http://www.cyberspy.com/%7Ewebster/death.html
International Society for Dissociative Disorders: http://www.issd.org/
Obsessive-compulsive disorder: http://www.fairlite.com/ocd/
Schizophrenia Home Page: http://www.schizophrenia.com
Sexual abuse: (newsgroup) http://alt.abuse.recovery, alt.sexual.abuse.recovery
Web of Addictions: http://www.well.com/user/woa/

Specialized Areas

(Addiction Resources) Web of Addictions: http://www.well.com/user/woa/
American Academy of Child and Adolescent Psychiatry: http://www.psych.med.umich.edu/web/aacap
Health Care Financing Administration (HCFA): http://www.hcfa.gov/
Idea Central Health Policy Page: http://www.epn.org/idea/health.html
National Institute of Mental Health Depression Awareness, Recognition and Treatment Program: http://www.nimh.nih.gov/publicat/eduprogs/dart.htm
Not-for-Profit Resources in Housing, Health, and Human Services: http://www.duke.edu/~ptavern/housing.html

National 800 Hotlines/ Information and Referral Numbers

Al-Anon Family Group Headquarters	1-800-356-9996
National Council on Alcoholism	1-800-NCA-CALL
National Institute on Drug Abuse	1-800-662-HELP
American Mental Health Fund	1-800-433-5959
National Aids Hotline:	1-800-342-2437
In Spanish	1-800-344-7432
National Aids Information Clearinghouse	1-800-458-5231
National Council on Child Abuse and Family Violence	1-800-222-2000
National Criminal Justice Referral System (Victims)	1-800-851-3420
National Foundation for Depressive Illness	1-800-248-4344
National Victims Resource Center	1-800-627-6872
National Sexual Addiction Hotline	1-800-321-2273
Parents Anonymous	1-800-421-0353

Suggested Reading

The Complete Psychotherapy Treatment Planner
Authors: Jongsman and Peterson
Publisher: John Wiley & Sons, Inc.
Year: 1995

Using DSM-IV
Authors: La Bruzza with Mendez-Villarrubia
Publisher: Jason Aronson
Year: 1994

The New Informants
Authors: Bollas and Sundelson
Publisher: Jason Aronson
Year: 1995

What Managed Care is Doing to Outpatient Mental Health: A Look Behind the Veil of Secrecy
Author: Miller
Publisher: Boulder Psychotherapists' Press, Inc.
Year: 1994

Sources for Assessment Materials

NCS Assessments
PO Box 1416
Minneapolis, MN 55440
Phone: 1-800-627-7271
Fax: 1-800-632-9011

Psychological Corporation
555 Academic Court
San Antonio, TX 78204-2498
Phone: 1-800-211-8378
Fax: 1-800-232-1223

EdITS Educational & Industrial Testing Service
PO Box 7234
San Diego, CA 92167
Phone: 1-619-222-1666
Fax: 1-619-226-1666

Longwood Division, Allyn and Bacon
PO Box 10695
Des Moines, IA 50336-0695
Phone: 1-800-278-3525

Childwork/Childsplay
PO Box 61586
King of Prussia, PA
Phone: 1-800-962-1141

Specializes in programs for play therapy and for self help.

Psychological and Educational Publications & Remedial Activities
1477 Rollins Road
Burlingame, CA 94010-2316
Phone: 1-800-523-5775
Fax: 1-800-447-0907

PAR Psychological Assessment Resources, Inc.
PO Box 998
Odessa, FL 33556
Phone: 1-800-331-8378
Fax: 1-800-727-9329

Professional Health Plan Publications
5856 College Avenue
Oakland, CA 94618

Provides assessment material specifically designed for MCOs.

ORTHO Interdisciplinary Approaches to Mental Health
Publication Sales Division
49 Sheridan Avenue
Albany, NY 12210

Cobb and Henry Publishers
1 Sutton Place
Hampton, VA 23666
Phone: 1-800-972-3273
Fax: 1-757-827-1060

Includes information about tests and measurements for Black populations.

Village Publishing
Custody Evaluation Products
73 Valley Drive
Furlong, PA 18925

MHS
908 Niagara Falls
North Tonawanda, NY 14020-2060
Phone: 1-800-456-3003
Fax: 1-416-424-1700

Professional Organizations

American Academy of Child and Adolescent Psychiatry
3615 Wisconsin Avenue NW
Washington DC 20016-3007
202-966-7300

American Mental Health Alliance (AMHA)
520 Commonwealth Avenue
Boston, MA 02215
617-536-7171

POB 1036
Cambridge, MA 02140
617-576-9900
http://www.mental-health-coop.coml

American Psychoanalytic Association
309 East 49th Street
New York, NY 10017
212-752-0450
http://www.apsa.org/

American Psychological Association
750 First Street NE
Washington DC 20002-4242
202-336-5500
http://www.apa.org

Boulder Psychotherapists' Guild, Inc.
350 Broadway, Suite 210
Boulder, CO 80303
303-444-1036
Fax: 303-494-3837

National Coalition for Patients' Rights
1644 Massachusetts Avenue
Lexington, MA 02173
617-433-0114
Fax: 617-861-0635

Computer-Based Patient Record Institute
1000 E. Woodfield Road, Suite 102
Schaumburg, IL 60173-4742
847-706-6746

Confidential Counseling Options (CCO)
Oakland County, Michigan
Telephone 810-988-6044
e-mail address: pef541@oeonline.com

Connecticut Psychotherapists' Guild
New Haven, CT
203-789-8208 (in New Haven)

800-731-8126 (outside New Haven)
Online address: http://members.aol.com/CPGuild

Medical Records Institute
567 Walnut Street, POB 289
Newton, MA 02160
617-964-3923

Mental Health Information Center
800-969-NMHA

National Coalition for Mental Health
Professionals and Consumers
POB 438
Commack, NY 11725-0438
Telephone/Fax: 516-424-5232

National Mental Health Association
1021 Prince Street
Alexandria, VA 22314-2971
703-684-7722

New England Coalition for Patient Rights
1644 Massachusetts Avenue
Lexington, MA 02173
617-433-0114

Privacy International
Washington Office
666 Pennsylvania Avenue SE, Suite 301
Washington, DC 20003

Privacy Rights Clearinghouse
University of San Diego School of Law
Center for Public Interest Law
5998 Alcala Park
San Diego, CA 92110-2492
619-260-4160

Private Practitioners Group (PPG)
3384 Long Beach Road (#229)
Oceanside, NY 11572
800-860-2688
Fax: in NY, 516-889-2688; others 800-860-2688

A Sample of Specialties

The following list contains examples of specialties among the hundreds of areas that might interest psychotherapists. The organizations and educational resources represent a few of the opportunities available for specialty education, training, and further information.

Specialty: Adoption

Type of work:	preadoption and postadoption counseling, working with attorneys, families, birth parents
Education:	child development, family studies National Adoption Assistance Training, Resource, and Information Network (NAATRIN): gopher://gopher-cec.mes.umn.edu:1300/00/resources/adoptINFO/
Organizations:	Association of American Nonprofit Adoption Agencies 111 Devon Cove Jacksonville, AR 72076 501-985-0172 Independent Adoption Center 800-877-6736
Journals:	Adoptive Families Magazine Issues in Adoption Advocacy
Internet:	Adoption Policy Resource Center: http://www.fpsol.com/adoption/advocates.html

Specialty: Custody Evaluation

Type of work:	Legal consultation, courts, private consultation
Education:	PACE Workshops (Professional Association of Custody Evaluators) 1-800-633-PACE
Organizations:	Professional Academy of Custody Evaluators http://www.custody-pace.org/
Journals:	The Custody Newsletter
Internet:	CCADE Web: http://forensic.nova.edu

Specialty: Disabilities

Type of work: working with physically, mentally, learning, and emotionally disabled children and adults

Organizations: American Association on Mental Retardation
444 North Capitol Street NW, Suite 846
Washington, DC 20001-1512
800-424-3688 or 202-287-1968

American Board of Disability Analysts (Education and Credentialing)
Park Plaza Medical Building
345 24th Avenue North, Suite 200
Nashville, TN 37203-1620
615-327-2994
Fax: 615-327-9235

Center for the Advancement of Rehabilitation and Disability Studies
55 Wheeler Street
Cambridge, MA 02138-1168
617-492-7100

National Alliance for the Mentally Ill
200 North Glebe Road, Suite 1015
Arlington, VA 22203-3754
703-524-7600

National Information Center for Children and Youth with Disabilities (NICHCY)
POB 1492
Washington, DC 20013-1492
800-695-0285

Internet: DisabilityNet: http://www.globalnet.co.uk/~
Institute on Disability & Human Development: http://www.uic.edu/depts/idhd/
MedWeb: http://www.gen.emory.edu/medweb.disabled.html

Specialty: Divorce Mediation

Type of work: conflict management, divorce process, working with attorneys
Education: workshops are held throughout the country through several sources, including:

Mediation Matters
Dr. Carl Schneider
3917 Dunnel Lane
Kensington, MD 20895
800-905-2221
301-933-8880

The Mediation Center, Inc.
440 East Broadway, Suite 340
Eugene, OR 97401
800-JDAGREE
541-345-1456

Organizations: Academy of Family Mediators
4 Militia Drive
Lexington, MA 02173
617-674-2662

Journals: Mediation Quarterly
Internet: Resources: http://www.igc.apc.org/tmc/

Specialty: Eating Disorders

Type of work: treating people with eating disorders individually, in groups, or with other family members
Education: Center for the Study of Anorexia and Bulimia
1 West 91st St.
New York, NY 10024
212-595-3449

Organizations: American Anorexia/Bulimia Association (AABA)
293 Central Park West
New York, NY 10024
212-501-8351

National Association of Anorexia Nervosa and Associated Disorders (ANAD)
Box 7
Highland Park, IL 60035
847-831-3438

National Association to Advance Fat Acceptance
POB 188620
Sacramento, CA 95818
916-558-6880

Journal: International Journal of Eating Disorders

Internet: Divorce Mediation Resources: http://www.conflictnet.org/tmc/div.html

Divorce Mediation Homepage: http://www.Fresno.edu/pacs/family.html

Specialty: Ecopsychology

Type of work: combining wellness, ecology, and psychology; an especially important field for MCOs and other business and government agencies

Education: Institute of Global Education
[A United Nations Non-Governmental Organization]
Department of Integrated Ecology
POB 1605
Friday Harbor, WA 98250
360-378-6313

Organizations: Project Nature Connect
POB 1605
Friday Harbor, WA 98250
360-378-6313

Internet: Project Nature Connect: http://www.pacificrim.net/~nature/welcome.html

Specialty: Eye Movement Desensitization and Reprocessing (EMDR)

Type of work: Interactional, standardized approach to therapy to accelerate treatment of self-esteem disorders, particularly those related to trauma

Organizations: EMDR Institute
POB 51010
Pacific Grove, CA 93950-6010
408-372-3900

Internet: http://www.emdr.com/

Specialty: Forensics

Type of work: work with criminal justice system, psychological testing, disability evaluation, evaluation and treatment of post-traumatic stress disorder, expert testimony, consultation to attorneys in areas such as custody decisions, conflict resolution, jury selection, behavioral styles, presentation skills, expert witness, mediator in custody disputes

Education: John Jay College of Criminal Justice
899 Tenth Avenue
New York, NY
212-237-8878

National University
4025 Camino del Rio South
San Diego, CA 92108-4107
619-563-7436

University of Alabama at Birmingham
University Station
Birmingham, AL 35294
205-934-2069

Organizations: American Board of Professional Psychology
2100 East Broadway, Suite 313
Columbia, MO 65201-6082
314-875-1267

Journals:	American Journal of Forensic Psychology
Internet:	Psychiatry and the Law: http://ua1vm.edu/~jhooper/tableofc.html

Specialty: Hypnosis

Type of work:	hypnotherapy
Education:	American Institute of Hypnotherapy 16842 VonKarman Avenue, Suite 475 Irvine, CA 92714 800-872-9996
	Milton H. Erickson Foundation 3606 North 24th Street Phoenix, AZ 85016 602-956-6196
Organizations:	National Board of Hypnosis Education and Certification 197 Glenwood Road Delond, FL 32720 904-738-0408
Internet:	Resources: http://www.concentric.net/~pbunnell/hypnosis.shtml
	http://www.hypnosis.com

Specialty: Industrial/Organizational

Type of work:	government, consulting firms, academic, research, public and private industry: personnel selection, criterion development, training, performance appraisal, motivation, job satisfaction, group processes, decision-making, productivity, organizational change
Education:	Purdue University Department of Psychological Sciences 1364 Psychological Sciences Building W. Lafayette, IN 47907-1364 317-494-6063

	Texas A&M Department of Psychology College Station, TX 77843 409-845-7146
Organizations:	Society for Industrial and Organizational Psychology (SIOP) P.O. Box 87 Bowling Green, OH 43402-0087
Journals:	The Industrial Psychologist (TIP)
Internet:	TIP: http://cmit.unomaha.edu/TIP/TIP.html
Resources:	http://www.ccnet.com/~bluenote/welcome.html

Specialty: Neuro-Linguistic Programming (NLP)

Type of work:	behavioral technology to creating healthy relationships
Education:	Neuro-Linguistic Programming 24 East 12th Street New York, NY 10003 212-647-0860 (in NY) 201-509-9599 (in NJ) 800-4-ACT-NLP Fax: 201-509-2326
Organizations:	Society of Neuro-Linguistic Programming 44 Montgomery Street, 5th Floor San Francisco, CA 94104 415-955-0541
Journals:	NLP World
Internet:	Resources: http://www.actwin.com/nlp/ Society of NLP: http://www. Purenlp.com/society.htm

Specialty: Sport Psychology

Type of work:	aggression control, attentional focus, burnout, competition, confidence, goal-setting, imagery, and increasing teamwork abilities

Education:	Directory of Graduate Programs in Applied Sport Psychology Fitness Information Technology, Inc. POB 4425 University Avenue Morgantown, WV 26504 304-599-3482 800-477-4348
Organizations:	Association for the Advancement of Applied Sport Psychology Dept. Of Physical Education University of North Carolina Chapel Hill, NC 27599-8700
Journals:	Journal of Sports and Exercise Psychology The Sport Psychologist Quest
Internet:	Sport Psychology http://serves.bmod.athalbascav.ca/html/aupr/spmt.htm Mind Tools http://www.gasov.edu/psychweb/mtsite/page11.html

Specialty: Trauma

Type of work:	post-traumatic stress disorder, emotional trauma, traumatic stress for individual, group, or large-scale disasters
Education:	Clinical Laboratory and Education Division National Center for PTSD VA Palo Alto Health Care System 3801 Miranda Avenue Palo Alto, CA 94304 415-493-5000
Organizations:	National Center for Post Traumatic Stress Disorders VA Medical Center White River Junction, VT 802-296-5132

	International Society for Traumatic Stress Studies (ISTSS) 60 Revere Drive, Suite 500 Northbrook, IL 60062 847-480-9028
Journals:	Traumatology (electronic journal) Journal of Traumatic Stress PTSD Research Quarterly
Internet:	Resources: http://gladstone.uoregon.edu/~dvb/trauma. htm http://www.long-beach.va.gov/ptsd/stress.html

GLOSSARY

MANAGED CARE GLOSSARY

Read this Glossary and conquer the managed care miasma! by *Les DelPizzo* exclusively for Mental Health Net

Last updated: January 19, 1996

This Glossary is a compilation from some very expert sources, heavily amended and reformatted to permit quick and easy referral. This can be used both to get key staff "up to speed" and for training purposes.

I used an italicized font to signal directions, market preference, and editorial comment about concepts. I would welcome any comments or additions to this glossary and shall treat it as a "work in progress" rather than the "end of the road." I have begun to add many items from the field of information technology, since this technology shall, in many cases, be the engine of change.

A

accountable health plan (AHP)

A regional (geographic) joint venture between practitioners and institutions (insurance companies, HMOs, or hospitals) that would assume responsibility and risk for delivering medical care to a specific population or group. Physicians and other providers would either own, work for, or contract with these health plans. *Note that this concept includes both payers and providers in a linked system. These plans generally have some incentive to develop preventive programs and to emphasize wellness. Is publicly accountable for the impact of its services on the health status of a population. This was a major concept in Clinton health reform package, but is being picked up in the marketplace. Florida, for instance, uses this term in explicitly in recent state law.* Often referred to as *community care network*, *organized system of care*, and *IDS* (*in-*

tegrated delivery system) or *IHDS* (*integrated health delivery system*). Also known as *community accountable healthcare networks* (*CAHNs*) or *health purchasing alliances*.

actuary

A person who determines insurance policy rates, reserves, and dividends, as well as conducts various other statistical studies. *You don't develop capitated rates, or agree to a capitated contract without one of these working for you in some capacity.* (See *capitation* below.)

admissions per 1,000

An indicator calculated by taking the total number of inpatient and/or outpatient admissions from a specific group (e.g., employer group, HMO population at risk), for a specific period of time (usually one year), dividing it by the average number of covered members in that group during the same period, and multiplying the result by 1,000. This indicator can be calculated for behavioral health or any disease in the aggregate and by modality of treatment (e.g., inpatient, residential, and partial hospitalization, etc.). *Such measures are commonly used by managed care entities to evaluate utilization management performance.*

adverse selection

Attracting members as enrollees into a health plan who are sicker than the general population (specifically, members who are sicker than was anticipated when the budget for medical costs was developed). Such members tend to use services at higher rates than other member populations. *Can quickly put you out of business in a capitated environment, unless you can re-negotiate rates or figure out why such a plan enrollment pattern is occurring and are able to do something about it. Traditionally, this has been the problem of the plan sponsor or its insurance company, as opposed to providers within the plan. With the advent of AHPs below, and a number of other risk-sharing strategies, however, the provider may be significantly impacted by this phenomenon.*

administration services only (ASO)

A relationship between an insurance company or other management entity and a self-funded plan or group of providers in which the insurance company or management entity performs administrative services only, such as billing, practice management, or marketing, and does not assume any risk.

alternate delivery systems

Health services provided in other than an inpatient, acute-care hospital. Examples within general health services include skilled and intermediary nursing facilities, hospice programs, and home health care. *Alternate delivery systems are designed to provide needed services in a more cost-effective manner. Most of the services provided by community mental health centers fall into this category.*

application integrators

Software that transparently provides application-to-application functionality, primarily through data conversion and transmission, while eliminating the need for custom programming. Also referred to as *application integration gateway*, *application interface gateway*, *integration engine*, or *intelligent gateway*. *This type of software is key to developing networks of information systems, making client-specific information available in real time to all members of an IHDS.*

asynchronous transfer mode (ATM)

A type of cell switching LAN/WAN technology that transfers information in a compressed mode at speeds of gigabits (billions of bits) per second. Is most useful for transmission of high-resolution images and real-time video images, as well as voice, data, video, and other types of information. Viewed as the future network of choice because of its many advanced capabilities. An operational definition of "broad bandwidth." *Could be the means to link the full continuum of care in a real time, "Hi, how are you?" mode. Would permit specialists to treat patients hundreds of miles away; would permit "on call" accessibility to scarce specialists, including behavioral health specialists.*

audit of provider treatment or charges

A qualitative or quantitative review of services rendered or proposed by a health provider. The review can be carried out in a number of ways: a comparison of patient records and claim form information, a patient questionnaire, a review of hospital and practitioner records, or a pre- or post-treatment clinical examination of a patient. Some audits may involve fee verification. *Something we had better get used to being subject to, since this is usually first type or "first generation" managed care approach.*

C

capitation

A method for payment to providers, common or targeted in most managed care arenas. Unlike the older fee-for-service arrangement, in which the provider is paid per procedure, capitation involves a prepaid amount per month to the provider per covered member (PMPM). The provider is then responsible for providing all contracted services (such as behavioral health) required by members of that group during that month for the fixed fee, regardless of the amount of charges incurred. In such an arrangement, the provider is now *at risk*, picking up risk that the payer or employer used to have exclusively in fee-for-service or indemnity arrangements. Management services, too, may be capitated. In such contracts, the contracting party is required to provide all management services (precertification, utilization review, case management, discharge planning, etc.) required for the fixed fee, while the costs of treatment services are paid separately. *This last model relating to management services is the way much managed behavioral healthcare is handled presently. A managed care organization (MCO) will contract with an HMO or a major insurer to manage a behavioral health "carve out." (See below.) The MCO provides these management services for a fixed charge per member per month (PMPM) and subcontracts with providers, usually at a discounted fee-for-service, to serve the covered members.*

carve-outs

A payer strategy in which a payer separates ("carves-out") a portion of the benefit, such as behavioral health, and hires a managed behavioral health program (MBHP) or managed care organization (MCO) to provide these benefits. *This permits the payer to create a behavioral health benefits package, get to market quicker with such a package, and have greater control of their costs. Many HMOs and insurance companies adopt this strategy because they do not have in-house expertise related to behavioral health or the service "carved out."*

case rate

Flat fee paid for a client's treatment based on his diagnosis and/or presenting problem. For this fee the provider covers all of the services the client requires for a specific period of time. Also *bundled rate*, or *flat fee-per-case. Very often used as an intervening step prior to Capitation. In this model, the provider is accepting some significant risk, but does have considerable flexibility in how it meets the client's needs. Keys to success in this mode: (1) properly pricing case rate, if provider has control over it, and (2) securing a large volume of eligible clients.*

character-based terminal

A type of data terminal that displays only alphanumeric or text characters and character-based graphics. Lacks the ability to display bit-mapped graphics that are required by GUI programs and operating systems such as Windows and X-Windows, which runs on Unix-based systems. *A primitive type of hardware, one best avoided, if costs permit. Real time access of client data and conferencing will require more sophisticated (and expensive) hardware.*

community health information network (CHIN)

An integrated collection of computer and telecommunication capabilities that permit multiple providers, payers, employers, and related healthcare entities within a geographic area to share and communicate client, clinical, and payment information. Also known as *community health management information system.*

clinic without walls (CWW)

Similar to an independent practice association (see IPA below), this type of physician or provider grouping represents a legal and formal entity. Under such arrangements, the legal entity provides administrative and support services to each physician/provider and the provider continues to practice in his/her own facility. The provided services can include marketing, billing and collection, staffing, management, and the like. *This arrangement permits providers to present a single "face" to the managed care marketplace with a minimum of day-to-day disruption. Key to its success, however, is its ability to really impose or create common billing and support services. This type of arrangement is often a transitional stage to more integrated arrangements.*

clinical data depository

That component of a computer-based patient record (CPR) which accepts, files, and stores clinical data over time from a variety of supplemental treatment and intervention systems for such purposes as practice guidelines, outcomes management, and clinical research. May also be called a *data warehouse.*

clinical decision support

The capability of a data system to provide key data to physicians and other clinicians in response to "flags" or triggers, which are functions of embedded, provider-created rules. *A system that would alert case managers that a client's eligibility for a certain service is about to be exhausted would be one example of this type of capacity. Also a key functional requirements to support clinical or critical pathways* (see below).

clinical or critical pathways

A "map" of preferred treatment/intervention activities. Outlines the types of information needed to make decisions, the timelines for applying that information, and what action needs to be taken by whom. Provides a way to monitor care "in real time." These pathways are developed by clinicians for specific diseases or events. *Proactive providers are working now to develop these pathways for the majority of their interventions and developing the software capacity to distribute and store this information.*

closed panel

A type of benefit plan in which plan members are permitted to receive services only through a specific limited number of providers. Usually not applicable to emergency care. *The provider's nightmare: the panel closes and they are on the outside looking in. The consumer's nightmare: their favorite or long-time physician or provider is not in the panel under their healthcare plan.*

collections per 1,000

An indicator calculated by taking the total collections for services received by a specific group (e.g., employer group, or group for which payer or provider are at risk) for a specific period of time, dividing it by the average number of covered members or lives in that group during that period, and multiplying the result by 1,000. This indicator may be calculated for behavioral health care in aggregate, and/or by treatment modality of treatment (e.g., inpatient, residential, partial hospitalization, and outpatient). A measure used to evaluate utilization management performance. *Proactive providers should be developing the capacity to measure their performance along such dimensions.*

community rating

The practice of some prepayment plans whereby rates are calculated using a broad range of populations in a community or region. Result is that net rate of premiums for plan subscribers are reasonably uniform and not dependent on individual claim experience or the experience of any group. This is the rating methodology required of federally qualified HMOs and of HMOs under the laws of many states, and occasionally indemnity plans under certain circumstances. Under such a rating system, the HMO is permitted to factor in differences for age, sex, mix (average contract size), and industry factors; not all factors are necessarily allowed under state laws. *By averaging costs of treatment over large populations, this method is probably fairest. Can raise rates for plans serving low-use beneficiaries such as young, healthy people. Can lower rates for plans with adverse selection, those whose members may be older and more dependent upon receiving health care.* (See *experience rating* below for alternative way of arriving at rates.)

computer-based patient record (CPR)

A term for the process of replacing the traditional paper-based chart through automated electronic means; generally includes the collection of patient-specific information from various supplemental treatment systems (i.e., a day program and a personal care provider); its display in graphical format; and its storage for individual and aggregate purposes. Also called *electronic medical record, on-line medical record, paperless patient chart.*

concurrent review

A routine review by an internal or external utilization reviewer, during the course of a patient's treatment, to determine if continued treatment is *medically necessary* (see below). *This usually occurs for inpatient, residential, and partial hospitalization treatment, though it is becoming more frequent for outpatient as well.*

continued stay review

A review conducted by an internal or external auditor to determine if the current place of service is still the most appropriate to provide the level of care required by the client.

cost shifting

The practice by some providers of redistributing the (negative) difference between normal charges and amounts received from certain payers by increasing charges made to other payers. *Should really be called "charge shifting." Is fairly endemic in a fee-for-service environment; becomes nearly impossible as the environment moves to managed care. Best means to eliminate this practice: universal coverage of all consumers.*

D

database management system (DBMS)

An information processing concept introduced in the late 1970s that separated data from the computer applications that created or processed that data, thus making data more accessible and minimizing the amount of programmer time needed to maintain computer programs.

Important concept because most CHINs or large-scale computer-based record systems will depend upon this crucial separation between data and systems that generate or process it.

days (or visits) per 1,000

An indicator calculated by taking the total number of days (for inpatient, residential, or partial hospitalization) or visits (for outpatient) received by a specific group for a specific period of time (usually one year). This number is then divided by the average number of covered members or lives in that group during the same period and multiplied by 1,000. A measure used to evaluate utilization management performance.

diagnosis-related groups (DRGs)

Payment system that reimburses health-care providers a fixed amount for all care in connection with a standard diagnostic category. Instituted by Medicare for the payment for hospital services and now used by many insurance companies. *A form of case rate payment system.*

direct contracting

Providing health services to members of a health plan by a group of providers contracting directly with an employer, thereby butting out the middleman or third-party insurance carrier. *This can be provider heaven, since middleman–MCO–is cut out and provider gets some portion of the money usually made by it. Key is to price services correctly, since provider is usually at full risk in this situation. Takes a strong IDS or AHP to pull this off.*

discounted fee-for-service

An agreed upon rate for service between the provider and payer that is usually less than the provider's full fee. This may be a fixed amount per service or a percentage discount. *Providers generally accept such contracts because they represent a means to increase their volume or reduce their chances of losing volume.*

disease management

A type of product or service now being offered by many large pharmaceutical companies to get them into broader healthcare services. Bundles use of prescription drugs with physician and allied professionals, linked to large databases created by the pharmaceutical companies, to treat people with specific diseases. The claim is that this type of service provides higher quality of care at more reasonable price than alternative, presumably more fragmented, care. *The development of such products by hugely-capitalized companies should be all the indicator necessary to convince a provider of how the healthcare market is changing. Competition is coming from every direction—other providers of all types, payers, employers (who are developing their own in-house service systems), the drug companies.*

drug utilization review (DUR)

Either concurrent and retrospective management of an insured population's drug utilization. The goal of such management is to reduce the cost of drug therapies. Methods used include substitution of generic drugs for name brands, using a formulary to limit the universe of drugs that can be prescribed, use of co-payments for prescriptions, and encouraging the use of drugs that will trigger rebates or discounts.

E

electronic data interchange (EDI)

The electronic exchange of business information in a standardized, structured, machine-processable format; electronically communicating business-to-business information, including client-related data.

electronic fund transfers (EFT)

The transfer of money between businesses and individuals by use of computer-generated debit and credit entries rather than checks or cash. *How progressive behavioral health entities should bill for Medicaid and how they should get paid by them and by Federal agencies with whom they have grants.*

enrolled group

Persons with the same employer or with membership in an organization in common, who are enrolled collectively in a health plan. Often there are stipulations regarding the minimum size of the group and the minimum percentage of the group that must enroll before the coverage is available. Same as *contract group*.

enrollee

Any person eligible, as either a subscriber or a dependent, in an employee benefit plan. (Synonyms: beneficiary, eligible individual, member, participant)

exclusive provider organization (EPO)

A type of provider organization similar to an HMO. Such entities often use PCPs as gatekeepers, often capitate providers, have a limited provider panel, and use an authorization system. These entities are "exclusive" because the member must remain within the network to receive benefits. The main difference from an HMO is that EPOs are generally regulated under insurance regulations rather than HMO regulations. Many states refuse to permit the development of EPOs, claiming that they are really HMOs.

ERISA–Employee Retirement Income Security Act of 1974

Also called the Pension Reform Act, this act regulates the majority of private pension and welfare group benefit plans in the U.S. It sets forth requirements governing, among many areas, participation, crediting of service, vesting, communication and disclosure, funding, and fiduciary conduct. *Key legislative battleground now, because ERISA exempts most large self-funded plans from state regulation and, hence, from any reform activities undertaken at state level–which is now the arena for much health-care reform.*

experience

A term used to describe the relationship of premium to claims for a plan, coverage, or benefits for a stated time period. Usually expressed as a percent or ratio (see also *medical loss ratio* (*MLR*).

experience rating

Determining the premium rate for a group risk, wholly or partially, on the basis of that group's experience or previous use of health benefit compared to premiums paid. The opposite of *community rating* above.

F

fee-for-service

A traditional means of billing by health providers for each service performed, with payment in specific amounts for specific services rendered (as opposed to retainer, salary, or other contract arrangements). Both third party payers and direct pay patients are billed in this manner. *Though much beloved by most providers, this is a dying practice.*

fee schedule

A listing of fees or allowances for specified medical or health procedures, which usually represents the maximum amounts the program or plan will pay for specified procedures. (Synonym: *table of allowances*)

flat fee-per-case

Flat fee paid for a client's treatment based on his diagnosis and/or presenting problem. For this fee the provider covers all of the services the client requires for a specific period of time. See *case rate*, above. *Often characterizes "second generation" managed care systems. After the MCOs squeeze out costs by discounting fees, they often come to this method. If provider is still standing after discount blitz, this approach can be good for provider and clients, since it permits a lot of flexibility for provider in meeting client needs.*

formatting and protocol standards

Data exchange standards which are needed between CPR systems, as well as the CPR and other provider systems, to ensure uniformity in how data is collected, stored, and presented. *Proactive providers are current in their knowledge of these standards and are working to make sure that their data systems conform to these standards, where possible.*

G

gatekeeper

An individual, usually a clinician, who controls the access to healthcare services for members of a specific group. In many HMO settings, this gatekeeper is the primary care physician (PCP) or his/her staff. In other health care delivery systems (and in HMOs in which behavioral health services are contracted out), the gatekeeper is often a case manager of the (behavioral) health organization.

graphical user interface (GUI)

A software or operating system interface that displays "real" pictures on the screen. These pictures may represent other things—icons. GUIs permit the use of screen elements such as windows, scrollbars, buttons, pointers, and such. *Think of Windows, which you undoubtedly have on your desktop.*

gross charges per 1,000

An indicator calculated by taking the gross charges incurred by a specific group for a specific period of time, dividing it by the average number of covered members or lives in that group during the same period, and multiplying the result by 1,000. This is calculated for behavioral health care in the aggregate and by modality of treatment (e.g., inpatient, residential, partial hospitalization, and outpatient). A measure used to evaluate utilization management performance.

gross costs per 1,000

An indicator calculated by taking the gross costs incurred for services received by a specific group for a specific period of time, dividing it by the average number of covered members or lives in that group during the same period, and multiplying the result by 1,000. This is calculated for behavioral health care in the aggregate and by modality of treatment (e.g., inpatient, residential, partial hospitalization, and outpatient). A measure used to evaluate utilization management performance. *This is the key concept for the provider. What matters is our cost and, in managed care, we must control this indicator and make sure it is below our collections per 1,000.*

group model

A type of HMO. In this model, an HMO contracts with a medical group for the provision of healthcare services. The relationship between the HMO and the medical group is generally very close, although there are wide variations in the relative independence of the group from the HMO. A form of *closed panel* health plan.

H

HCFA 1500

The Health Care Finance Administration's standard form for submitting physician service claims to third party (insurance) companies.

***health insurance purchasing cooperative* (*HIPC*)**

A government or quasi-government entity established to purchase bulk health insurance for businesses and individuals. Not too different from a wholesaler in the retail business. Its intent is to purchase health insurance for the cooperative's members at prices and terms more favorable than would generally be available to the participants. *Was a key concept in Clinton health plan and died with that legislation. The market is developing somewhat similar entities, however, some even with governmental participation* (see *health plan purchasing cooperatives* below).

***health level seven* (*HL7*)**

An existing *formatting and protocol standard*, it is an interface specification that operates at the application level for transmitting health-related data. This standard has largely been used for transmission of data among departments within institutions for orders, clinical observations, test results, etc. Specific parts of HL7 have applicable CHIN use where such data needs to be transmitted between institutions and systems.

***health maintenance organization* (*HMO*)**

The definition of an HMO has evolved constantly. Originally, an HMO was defined as a prepaid organization that provided health care to voluntary enrolled members in return for a preset amount of money on a PMPM (per member per month) basis. With the increase of self-insured business and of other arrangements that might not involve prepayment, that definition is no longer accurate. Presently, the definition needs to encompass two key elements: a health plan that places at least some of the providers at risk for medical expenses, and a health plan that utilizes PCPs (primary care physicians) as gatekeepers (although there are some HMOs that do not). Obtaining care without a primary care physician's referral, or obtaining care from a non-network member, usually results in no payment for services by the payer organization.

***health plan purchasing cooperative* (*HPPC*)**

Critical piece of Clinton plan. Now being developed in market with demise of proposed legislation. Permits creation of purchasing agent for large groups of employers in a region. This "purchasing agent" would shop for best price and best outcomes. Would provide small employers some market muscle and might encourage them to provide health coverage. *Because small business was one of most vociferous opponents of federal health plan, it remains to be seen how active it shall be in using this mechanism.*

I

***incurred but not reimbursed* (*IBNR*)**

Refers to claims that reflect services already delivered, but, for whatever reason, have not yet been reimbursed. These are bills "in the pipeline." *This is a crucial concept for proactive providers who are beginning to explore arrangements that put them in the role of adjudicating claims—as the result, perhaps, of operating in a sub-capitated system (see below). Failure to account for these potential claims could lead to some very bad decisions. Good administrative operations have fairly sophisticated mathematical models to estimate this amount at any given time.*

indemnity health insurance

A traditional health insurance plan with little or no benefit management, a fee-for-service reimbursement model, and few restrictions on provider selection. *Think of a dinosaur.*

independent physician association; individual practice association; independent provider association (IPA)

This set of initials is one of the most fluid now in circulation. Originally, it meant a type of health maintenance organization allowing physicians to work out of their own offices instead of a central facility. These HMOs typically are formed and operated by physicians and marketed to employers. Under this arrangement, physicians still see their individual patients, as well as patients from the HMO. *Today, this set of initials also includes entities that contract with groups of providers, including corporate providers such as behavioral health centers. Each provider agrees to see patients/clients from plans who contract with the HMO of which the IPA is a part and to serve these clients for agreed-upon fees. Such IPAs often are not associated with a single HMO, but serve a number of them under contract. This is especially the case in specialty services such as behavioral health. This model is another example of entities that are in the "wholesale" as opposed to the retail business, since IPAs tend to contract with payers who market their own plans to employers.*

integrated (health) delivery system (IDS/I(H)DS)

This is the "Holy Grail" right now of healthcare providers. Linkage of all regional services—vertical and horizontal—into one legal entity able to negotiate with the marketplace. In its most integrated form, even includes insurance or financing function, so that there is no division between provider and payer (see *accountable health plan*. Also called *integrated medical system*).

integrated services digital network (ISDN)

Communication protocols developed by telephone companies to permit telephone networks to carry data, voice, video, and other source material digitally. Has large bandwidth, permitting fast and accurate transmission of large amounts of data. *Usually a fairly large one-time cost to get each workstation ISDN-able and fairly large costs to use on an ongoing basis. Yet, potential to transmit so much data reliably makes this mode very attractive for entities developing CHINs or networks. As cost comes down, this may be the preferred way to develop communication networks for providers.*

interface

A point of means of interaction between two systems. Your keyboard is an interface, as is your monitor screen. Common interactions between systems in the healthcare environment include patient/client demographic, claims/accounts receivable, and clinical orders. These large volume interactions require system-to-system interfaces. *Such interactions can occur in "real time" or in batch mode. In real time or interactive mode, interaction directly impacts database—you and data base are in "Hi, how are ya?" mode; in batch mode, interactions are "batched" for later processing. In a managed care system, real time interaction is almost always required. A case manager must know what resources a client has expended, to make resource allocation decisions about a client.*

L

legacy systems

Computer applications—both hardware and software—that have been inherited through previous acquisition and installation. Most often, these systems run business applications that are not integrated with each other. Newer systems which stress open design and distributed processing capacity are gradually replacing such systems.

local access transport area (LATA)

A defined region in which a telephone and long distance carrier operates. *Important concept for those CHINs that depend upon phone lines. When creating communications networks, you try to avoid crossing boundaries of these, if possible, since costs escalate dramatically when there is a need to communicate over more than one LATA.*

local exchange carrier (LEC)

The telephone company that provides and supports the local connection to the public switched telephone network. In many areas of the U.S., the LEC is one of the seven regional bell operating companies (RBOCs) or "Baby Bells." *These LECs become crucial partners for any organization or group of organizations seeking to develop a CHIN or, more conservatively, simply seeking to integrate their information system across many sites.*

M

managed behavioral health program (MBHP)

An organization that assumes the responsibility for managing the behavioral health benefit for an employer or payer organization under a *carve out* arrangement. The management may range from utilization management services to the actual provision of the services through its own organization or provider network. Reimbursement may be on a fee-for-service, shared risk, or full-risk basis. *Also called a managed care organization or MCO, though this is a specialty MCO.*

managed health care

A system that uses financial incentives and management controls to direct patients to providers who are responsible for giving appropriate care in cost-effective treatment settings. Such systems are created to control the cost of health care. *Note that there is no direct reference to quality in this definition.*

master patient/member index

An index or file with a unique identifier for each patient or member that serves as a key to a patient's or member's health record.

medically necessary

Services or supplies which meet the following tests:

- they are appropriate and necessary for the symptoms, diagnosis, or treatment of the medical condition;

they are provided for the diagnosis or direct care and treatment of the medical condition;

they meet the standards of good medical practice within the medical community in the service area;

they are not primarily for the convenience of the plan member or a plan provider; and

they are the most appropriate level or supply of service which can safely be provided.

This standard is becoming the most important one for providers to focus upon. Note that many of the rehabilitation services common to behavioral healthcare, especially to severely disabled populations, may not meet such a test, or do so only by stretching their meaning.

***medical loss ratio* (*MLR*)**

The amount of revenues from health insurance premiums that is spent to pay for the medical services covered by the plan. Usually referred to by a ratio, such as 0.96–which means that 96% of premiums were spent on purchasing medical services. *The goal is to keep this ratio below 1.00–preferably in the 0.80 range, since the MCO's or insurance company's profit comes from premiums. Currently, successful HMOs do have MLRs in the 0.70–0.80 range.*

MSO

One of the following:

medical staff organization An organized group of physicians, usually from one hospital, formed into an entity able to contract with others for the provision of services, or

management (or medical) services organization An entity formed by, for example, a hospital, a group of physicians, or an independent entity, to provide business-related services such as marketing and data collection to a grouping of providers like an IPA, PHO or CWW. *This second definition is becoming almost exclusive usage.*

***multiple employer trust* (*MET*)**

A legal trust established by a plan sponsor that brings together a number of small, unrelated employers for the purpose of providing group medical coverage on an insured or self-funded basis. *Not quite a health plan purchasing cooperative, but along the same lines. More market-oriented and usually smaller in scale.*

N

network model

A health plan that contracts with multiple physician groups or other providers to deliver health care to members. Generally limited to large single or multi-specialty groups. Distinguished from group model plans that contract with a single medical group, from IPAs that contract through an intermediary, and from direct contract plans that contract with individual physicians in the community. *Many current behavioral health-care networking efforts are attempts to create service systems along this line, or to integrate behavioral health-care practices into such entities.*

O

object oriented database

Database organized around an object model, as opposed to relational or flat databases. "Objects" are anything: video clips, files, reports, and so on. This model seeks to group many different types and sources of data as objects and to create a common way to deal with them. Allows modular development of software and better reflects the way people really think. *This is the latest generation of software.* (See *relational data model* below.)

out-of-area benefits

Benefits supplied by a plan to its subscribers or enrollees when they need services outside the geographic limits of the HMO. These benefits usually include emergency care benefits, plus low fee-for-service payments for nonemergency care.

P

PCP capitation

A reimbursement system for health-care providers of primary-care services who receive a pre-payment every month. The payment amount is based on age, sex and plan of every member assigned to that physician for that month. Specialty capitation plans also exist, but are little used. *PCPs contract with specialists to get their service. When pay to specialist is also capitated, this is a sub-capitation system. This model is the specialists' nightmare; makes their income completely dependent upon the PCP. In this context, behavioral health providers are usually viewed as specialists. Suggests a need to be very close to primary care physicians, and another reason to seek integration with them.*

per member per month (*PMPM*)

Specifically applies to a revenue to or cost by a provider for each enrolled member each month.

per member per year (*PMPY*)

Same as above, as applies to year.

per thousand members per year (*PTMPY*)

A common way of reporting utilization. The most common example is hospital utilization, expressed as *days PTMPY. For outpatient-oriented providers, this indicator would reflect VISITS PTMPY.*

physician-hospital organization (*PHO*)

An arrangement among physicians and hospital(s) wherein a single entity, the PHO, agrees to provide services to insurers' subscribers for a single price. Formerly called a MeSH or medical staff-hospital organization. Often superseded by a medical foundation, which carries out similar role, but which is more integrated in its governance and operation. *One of the most common and active structural developments in health care. Just about every hospital is seeking to develop one of these with its medical staff–or a portion of it–so that together they can provide a single "face" to the managed care market.*

point-of-care technology

Those technologies that enable physicians and other clinicians to electronically record findings, enter orders, and review information from the location at which care is provided. *A good example of "real time" interaction. Input from clinician directly changes database. At the heart of "tele-medicine."*

point-of-service (POS)

A type of benefit plan in which the insured person can choose to use a nonparticipating provider at a reduced coverage level and with more out-of-pocket cost. Such POS plans combine both HMO-like systems with indemnity systems. Often known as open-ended HMOs or PPOs, these plans permit insured to choose providers outside the plan, yet are designed to encourage the use of network providers. *One of the most popular plans with consumers and employers. Represents area of greatest HMO growth.*

precertification

The prior authorization required by some payers before health benefit payments will be authorized.

predetermination

An administrative procedure whereby a health provider submits a treatment plan to a third party before treatment is initiated. The third party usually reviews the treatment plan, monitoring one or more of the following: patient's eligibility, covered service, amounts payable, application of appropriate deductibles, copayment factors, and maximums. Under some programs, for instance, predetermination by the third party is required when covered charges are expected to exceed a certain amount. Similar processes: *pre-authorization, precertification, pre-estimate of cost, pretreatment estimate, prior authorization.*

preferred provider organization (PPO)

A variation of traditional fee-for-service care arrangements. A group of physicians, dentists, and/or hospitals and other practitioners contracts with a payer to provide employees with services at competitive rates. The employee is not penalized or prevented from using his or her regular physician, even if that physician does not participate in the PPO; in such cases, however, the participant usually pays a higher fee or co-payment. PPOs usually provide incentives for provider participation, such as a competitive rate structure or the implication of increased volume. In addition, PPOs generally use primary care physicians to assure that hospitalization occurs only when absolutely necessary, with extensive concurrent utilization review.

prepaid group practice plan

A plan under which contractually specified health services are rendered by participating physicians to an enrolled group of persons, with a fixed periodic payment in advance made by or on behalf of each person or family.

primary care provider (PCP)

A primary care provider such as a family practitioner, general internist, pediatrician, and sometimes an ob/gyn. Generally, a PCP supervises, coordinates, and provides medical care to members of a plan. The PCP may initiate all referrals for specialty care. *Within behavioral health, case managers are often the PCP; role often done by outpatient therapist. Alternatively, it is possible to conceive of a system in which behavioral health services are integrated into the PCP practice directly.*

profile

Aggregated data in formats that display patterns of health-care services over a defined period of time.

profile analysis

Review and analysis of profiles to identify and assess patterns of health-care services.

provider organization

A practice, clinic, mental health center, hospital, or other organization that is employed by managed health programs to provide treatment services.

R

relational data model

A database management scheme that permits reports to be pulled from many different files, provided there is a common—or related—element linking all the files. *This is currently the most powerful way of developing databases. Slowly being supplanted by object-oriented databases noted earlier.*

resource-based relative value scale (RBRVS)

A Medicare weighting system to assign units of value to each CPT code (procedure) performed by physicians and other providers. The number of units or value for each procedure includes a portion for physician skill, expenses associated with the procedure, and geographic area. *Loved by "process" docs such as PCPs, since adoption of this scale by Medicare increased their pay; despised by "transaction" docs such as specialists and surgeons, since they lost money per transaction.*

retrospective review process

A review that is conducted after services are provided to a patient. The review focuses on determining the appropriateness, necessity, quality, and reasonableness of health care services provided. *Becoming seen as least desirable method; supplanted by CONCURRENT reviews.*

risk sharing

A method by which medical insurance premiums are shared by plan sponsors and participants. In contrast to traditional indemnity plans in which insurance premiums belonged solely to insurance company that assumed all risk of using these premiums. *Key to this approach is that the premiums are ONLY payment providers receive; provides powerful incentive to be parsimonious with care.*

S

self-funded health plans

Plans that provide for the reimbursement of medical expenses incurred by an employee, his/her spouse, or his/her dependents by the employer or a group of employers, as opposed to an insurance company. In such arrangements, the employer assumes all the risk, unless it can share some of it with a managed care entity or a group of providers. Many variations of this approach are possible. It is possible to insure some benefits and self-insure others; to self-insure or self-fund all benefits up to a certain aggregate claim level; or to set certain individual claim limits for self-funding and insure above that level (see *self-insurance* below).

self-insurance

A program for providing group insurance with benefits financed entirely through the internal means of the policyholder, as opposed to purchasing coverage from commercial carriers. *These plans and those directly above are exempt from ERISA and from most regulation. Thus, they are much used by large employers.*

sub-capitation

An arrangement that exists when an organization being paid under a capitated system contracts with other providers on a capitated basis, sharing a portion of the original capitated premium. *Can be done under carve-out, with the providers being paid on a PMPM basis.*

T

telnet

The TCP/IP (Internet) standard high-level protocol for establishing terminal connections to a host computer over a network. Allows users to access a remote host (computer) as if their terminal were directly connected to it. *A must for "real time" networks.*

third-party administrator (TPA)

Usually an out-of-house professional firm providing administrative services, such as paying claims, collecting premiums, and carrying out other administrative support services, for employee benefit plans (synonyms: *administrative agent, carrier, insurer, underwriter*).

treatment episode

The period of treatment between admission and discharge from a modality (e.g., inpatient, residential, partial hospitalization, and outpatient). *Many healthcare statistics and profiles use this unit as a base for comparisons.*

U

uniform bill 1992 (UB-92)

Bill form used to submit hospital insurance claims for payment by third parties. Similar to HCFA 1500, but reserved for the inpatient component of health services.

utilization

Can be expressed in a variety of ways:

The extent to which a given group uses specified services in a specified period, expressed as the number of services used per year per 1,000 or per 1,000 persons eligible for the services. Utilization rates may be expressed in other types of ratios, such as per eligible persons covered.

The extent to which the members of a covered group use specified services over a specific period, in the aggregate. Usually expressed as the number of services used per year. Utilization rates are established to help in comprehensive health planning, budget review, and cost containment.

V

value added networks (VANs)

Integrated networks that combine transmission and applications on a single network, offering enhanced services that change the data in some desirable way upon entry and/or exit. Permit data communications between similar or dissimilar equipment. These services—packet assembly/disassembly, protocol/speed/code conversions—permit communication across different hardware and software. Thus, the value-added. *When you hear about the Information Highway, these VANs are a critical component of it. The biggest companies in America and abroad are working to develop these value-added capacities, so that communications can occur relatively transparently across all types of hardware and software. CHINs and the development of any integrated information systems will be greatly enhanced as these giants develop and deliver these services.*

W

withhold pool

The amount withheld from a PCP's capitation payment or a specialist's payment amount to cover expenditures greater than budgeted or expected in serving a specified enrollee group. *This is one of the most common ways to incentivize specialists–read "behavioral health providers"–under managed care. If utilization is less than withhold pool, or if pool relatively unused, specialists get some portion of that pool back as payment.*

INDEX